THE APPLICATIONS OF BIOINFORMATICS IN CANCER DETECTION

ANNALS OF THE NEW YORK ACADEMY OF SCIENCES
Volume 1020

THE APPLICATIONS OF BIOINFORMATICS IN CANCER DETECTION

Edited by Asad Umar, Izet Kapetanovic, and Javed Khan

The New York Academy of Sciences
New York, New York
2004

Library of Congress Cataloging-in-Publication Data

Applications of Bioinformatics in Cancer Detection Workshop (2002: National Institutes of Health).
   The applications of bioinformatics in cancer detection / edited by Asad Umar, Izet Kapetanovic, and Javed Khan.
      p.; cm. — (Annals of the New York Academy of Sciences; v. 1020)
      Includes bibliographical references and index.
      ISBN 1-57331-510-9 (cloth: alk. paper) — ISBN 1-57331-511-7 (pbk.: alk. paper)
   1. Cancer—Diagnosis—Data processing—Congresses. 2. Medical informatics—Congresses. 3. DNA microarrays—Diagnostic use—Congresses.
      [DNLM: 1. Computational Biology—methods—Congresses. 2. Neoplasms—diagnosis—Congresses. QZ 241 A6515 2004] I. Umar, Asad. II. Kapetanovic, Izet. III. Khan, Javed, M.D. IV. Title. V. Series.
Q11.N5 vol. 1020
   [RC270]
   500 s—dc22
   [616.99/40

                                         2004006687

GYAT / PCP
Printed in the United States of America
ISBN 1-57331-510-9 (cloth)
ISBN 1-57331-511-7 (paper)
ISSN 0077-8923

ANNALS OF THE NEW YORK ACADEMY OF SCIENCES

Volume 1020
May 2004

THE APPLICATIONS OF BIOINFORMATICS IN CANCER DETECTION

Editors
ASAD UMAR, IZET KAPETANOVIC, AND JAVED KHAN

This volume is the result of the **Applications of Bioinformatics in Cancer Detection Workshop**, sponsored by the Division of Cancer Prevention, National Cancer Institute, National Institutes of Health, and held August 6–7, 2002, in Bethesda, Maryland.

CONTENTS

Preface

PETER GREENWALD

Division of Cancer Prevention, National Cancer Institute, National Institutes of Health, Bethesda, Maryland, USA

The workshop and the proceedings of the Applications of Bioinformatics in Cancer Detection present a framework and recommendations provided by the leading researchers in computational and cancer biology to develop, design, and implement bioinformatics approaches to the science of cancer prevention.

We should note two very interesting trends in biomedical research. First is the trend toward technology-driven rather than hypothesis-driven advances. Second is a greater appreciation of the need for integrative science. Molecular biology has been largely influenced by the reductionism—the attempt to explain all biological processes by the same explanations (as by physical laws) that chemists and physicists use to interpret inanimate matter. Now, with the large amounts of data, we see the need for syntheses, understanding, and translational approaches; hence, the need for aggressive development of the field of bioinformatics.

As new and more efficient technologies for cancer detection, screening, surveillance, and diagnosis are being developed at a rapid rate, our dependence on bioinformatics tools is becoming more apparent. Application of these new technologies, especially for early detection of cancer, is likely to have a profound effect on public health, but several barriers have to be overcome to achieve this goal.

Importance of early cancer detection is exemplified by the fact that, if all colorectal cancer cases were detected when localized, the overall 5-year survival rates could improve from around 60% to 90%. As a matter of fact, the National Cancer Institute Colorectal Cancer Progress Review Group predicted that wider use (defined as doubling the current colorectal screening rate to 60%) could save >20,000 lives annually. Early detection is also a key to management of breast, ovarian, prostate, and other cancers. The 5-year survival rate for breast and prostate cancer patients with localized, early-stage disease is 85% to 95% and remains high at 10 years.

With the advent of multiplex, high-throughput technologies and sophisticated bioinformatics tools discussed here, researchers are beginning to use techniques made possible by the rapidly advancing fields of genomics and proteomics.

One example of the rapidly proliferating use of new tools is the science of proteomics—studies of the global patterns of protein expression in individual cells, tissues, or body fluids. Cancer cells may produce unique proteins, or proteins in

Address for correspondence: Peter Greenwald, M.D., Dr.Ph., Director, Division of Cancer Prevention, National Cancer Institute, National Institutes of Health, 6130 Executive Boulevard, Room 2040, MSC 2580, Bethesda, MD 20892-7309. Voice: 301-496-6616; fax: 301-496-9931.
pg37g@nih.gov

Ann. N.Y. Acad. Sci. 1020: ix–x (2004). © 2004 New York Academy of Sciences.
doi: 10.1196/annals.1310.001

different quantities, compared to normal cells. As evident from several recent clinically relevant publications, it seems that more and more of these studies are yielding novel data with far-reaching implications, and clinicians and health care researchers are starting to recognize proteomics as a new tool in the early diagnosis of cancer and in the prediction of clinical outcomes. For the time being, though, the sophistication of the techniques used in protein analysis, as well as the automation and computational processes necessary to handle large amounts of complex, multi-variate data, will probably restrict these diagnostic tests to well-equipped and experienced laboratories. However, as seen historically with all technologies, the accessibility of these tools will become more generally available as the number of users increases and the field matures.

Proceedings: The Applications of Bioinformatics in Cancer Detection Workshop

IZET M. KAPETANOVIC,[a] ASAD UMAR,[b] AND JAVED KHAN[c]

[a]Chemopreventive Agent Development Research Group, [b]Gastrointestinal and Other Cancer Research Group, Division of Cancer Prevention, and [c]Oncogenomics Section, Pediatric Oncology Branch, National Cancer Institute, Bethesda, Maryland, USA

ABSTRACT: The Division of Cancer Prevention of the National Cancer Institute sponsored and organized the Applications of Bioinformatics in Cancer Detection Workshop on August 6–7, 2002. The goal of the workshop was to evaluate the state of the science of bioinformatics and determine how it may be used to assist early cancer detection, risk identification, risk assessment, and risk reduction. This paper summarizes the proceedings of this conference and points out future directions for research.

KEYWORDS: bioinformatics; data mining; cancer; early detection; risk assessment; genomics; proteomics; drug discovery

INTRODUCTION

The Division of Cancer Prevention (DCP) of the National Cancer Institute (NCI) sponsored and organized the Applications of Bioinformatics in Cancer Detection (ABCD) Workshop on August 6–7, 2002. Speakers included representatives from government, academia, and industry in the area of bioinformatics as applied or applicable to cancer prevention. The goal of the workshop was to evaluate the state of the science of bioinformatics and determine how it may be used to assist early cancer detection, risk identification, risk assessment, and risk reduction. In the context of the workshop, a broad definition of bioinformatics was employed, that is, application of computer processes to solve biological problems; or, as defined on the NCI Web site, "bioinformatics is the development and application of computational tools and approaches for expanding the use of biological, medical, behavioral, or health data, including those required to acquire, store, organize, archive, analyze, or visualize such data" (http://otir.cancer.gov/tech/bioinformatics.html/).

Recent technological advances in biology and biomedical areas are resulting in a large accumulation of complex and multivariate data, and the problem is how to optimize and make most efficient use of this deluge of information. A systematic approach to data collection, storage, analysis, and representation is needed. Advances in theoretical and computational tools are providing opportunities for thorough data

Address for correspondence: Izet M. Kapetanovic, Chemopreventive Agent Development Research Group, Division of Cancer Prevention, National Cancer Institute, Bethesda, MD 20892-7322. Voice: 301-435-5011; fax: 301-402-0553.
 kapetani@mail.nih.gov

Ann. N.Y. Acad. Sci. 1020: 1–9 (2004). © 2004 New York Academy of Sciences.
doi: 10.1196/annals.1310.002

mining in these vast collections of information. Data mining is a process of extracting "useful" information from a large collection of data. The goal is to enable and facilitate the process of going from data collection to knowledge acquisition. However, this path from data collection to knowledge acquisition is difficult and uncertain due to the intricacies of biological systems, the multivariate nature of data, and an overabundance of complex, nonlinear relationships. In the area of cancer prevention, we would like to be able to identify signs and risks early on and prior to onset of clinical disease and thereby be able to intervene appropriately and in a timely fashion.

There are two general approaches to data mining: theory-driven and data-driven. Theory-driven approaches are more established, but require assumptions about the underlying relationships and more extensive statistical, mathematical, and computer knowledge. The newer data-driven methods, on the other hand, do not require a priori knowledge about the relevant theory or all possible nonlinear relationships, and they do not make assumptions about statistical distributions. The latter are more suited to finding hidden features in data where none are visible by conventional statistical methods or by human decision alone. They have learning and adaptive capability and the ability to handle imprecise and multivariate and multidimensional information. For example, data-driven methods have an ability to achieve nonintuitive, complex nonlinear separation between patient classes and they can help identify a disease pattern even if all individual biomarkers are within an established reference range or, conversely, identify a nondisease pattern when all individual biomarkers are outside of the known reference range. In another words, the relationship of these biomarkers to each other may be more important than their individual absolute levels. These computational techniques are also referred to as machine learning or artificial intelligence. They hold a promise to be able to process and analyze huge amounts of noisy data coming simultaneously from many different inputs. Recognizing the ever-growing role of computational methodologies in medicine, the FDA has issued guidance for this purpose: "Guidance for the Content of Premarket Submissions for Software Contained in Medical Devices" (http://www.fda.gov/cdrh/ode/57.html/).

Examples of bioinformatics tools and techniques include principal component analysis, hierarchical clustering, artificial neural networks, fuzzy logic, neuro-fuzzy logic, genetic and evolutionary algorithms, and support vector machines. A recent book[1] describes and discusses various data mining techniques. Their ability to reduce dimensionality and generalize through nonlinear approximation and interpolation is the common thread among them. In that, they can generate outputs from previously unseen inputs (unsupervised learning) or from previously learned inputs (supervised learning). These computational methodologies are also classified as "soft computing" (http://www.soft-computing.de/)[2] because they utilize tolerance for imprecision and uncertainty to produce new information via approximation. In essence, these techniques are general approximators of any multivariate nonlinear function. It is increasingly recognized that bioinformatics tools hold promise in early detection, risk identification, risk assessment, and risk reduction, thereby facilitating effective approaches for the chemopreventive intervention. Specific areas amenable to bioinformatics include the following:

- Pattern clustering
- Classification
- Gene and protein array analysis

- Image and signal processing
- Decision support
- Database mining.

A brief overview of commonly used bioinformatics tools and their applications was included in the workshop booklet and is discussed in some detail in the following chapter. In addition, newer, more innovative bioinformatics methods are discussed. Furthermore, specific bioinformatics techniques are discussed in detail, and present examples of their use in cancer early detection, risk assessment, and prognosis are provided.

Several general themes relating to the use of bioinformatics in medical research and clinical application were also addressed during the workshop. Issues that warrant consideration and further attention were identified. It was rightfully acknowledged that bioinformatics holds a significant potential to enable, facilitate, and expedite progress in early detection and risk identification, assessment, and reduction of cancer.

EXAMPLES AND PROOF OF PRINCIPLE

Dr. Michael Bittner (National Human Genome Research Institute, NIH, Bethesda, MD) opened the workshop with a basic observation about cellular memory and inertia that was later also echoed by Dr. Arul Chinnaiyan (University of Michigan, Ann Arbor, MI). The idea presented was that cells, in general, display great inertia and normal cells exhibit very stable gene expression. Different tissues show different expression of unique genes and a different pattern of expression of more common genes. Perturbations of normal tissues tend to result in relatively minor changes in gene expression that are reversible on return of tissue to its normal state. This leads to a premise that phenotype differences should be detectable based on concerted changes in expression of genes beyond a certain threshold level. Cells tend to follow a chosen path until dysregulated, which then may lead to cancer. The goal here would be to identify highly discriminatory genes between different phenotypes, such as normal and diseased, diseased responsive to treatment and diseased unresponsive to treatment, susceptible to disease and not susceptible to disease, etc. For example, Dr. Bittner presented data showing WNT5A gene expression to be discriminatory and an important marker in human melanoma progression.[3] It was correlated with greater motility and invasiveness and appeared to have a strong correlation with the survival phenotype. A number of different bioinformatics approaches and applications were described during the workshop for distinguishing different cancer-related phenotypes.

In order to identify genes that best discriminate between normal and disease (cancerous) phenotypes, Dr. Joseph Ibrahim (University of North Carolina, Chapel Hill, NC) applied **Bayesian** method utilizing **Markov chain Monte Carlo** techniques for DNA microarray analysis. This method has the advantage of being able to handle small sample size and allow incorporation of other already available information such as historical data or expert opinion. Another Bayesian approach, **Bayesian Decomposition**, was employed by Dr. Michael Ochs (Fox Chase Cancer Center, Philadelphia, PA) to identify participating pathways based on changes in gene expression.[4] This approach works backwards, using observed changes in mRNA to discover changes in signaling that cause them. The ability of Bayesian Decomposition to assign genes to multiple coexpression groups (multiple coregulation) and encode biological information into the system makes it very suitable for this task and overcomes the limitations of other systems. This approach holds promise in helping to identify errors in signaling pathways that can act as cancer triggering mechanisms and to evaluate how these signaling pathway errors are affected by intervention.

Dr. Margaret Shipp (Dana Farber Cancer Institute, Boston, MA) and Dr. Chinnaiyan demonstrated use of combined genomic, proteomic, and clinical data in their respective studies of cancer-related phenotypes. With the aid of supervised learning (weighted voting with cross-validation testing and support vector machine algorithms), Dr. Shipp was able to identify signatures of outcome in large B cell lymphoma and rational targets of intervention.[5] This study was able to correlate PKC-beta mRNA and protein expression with enzymatic activity and led to the design of a clinical trial with a selective PKC-beta inhibitor to decrease proliferation and increase apoptosis. Dr. Chinnaiyan combined the use of high-density DNA microarrays to identify candidate genes, tissue microarrays to validate the gene expression at the protein level, and clinical information to enable making an association in prostatic cancer.[6] Unsupervised average linkage hierarchical clustering of genes into benign and malignant clusters was employed, with further clustering of the malignant cluster. Using the above general approach, hepsin (a transmembrane serine protease) was shown to be upregulated in prostatic cancer, with the highest hepsin expression found in the precursor lesion, prostatic intraepithelial neoplasia (PIN).

The development, optimization, and use of a robust **artificial neural network** classifier to handle four different diagnostic categories (lymphoma, Ewing's sarcoma, rhabdomyosarcoma, neuroblastoma) of small round blue-cell tumors were described by Dr. Javed Khan (National Cancer Institute, NIH, Bethesda, MD). The classifier was optimized for sensitivity and specificity and used to identify the most important and relevant genes in this classification.[7]

Proteomic fingerprinting provides information that is complementary to genomic fingerprinting or phenotyping. Proteins impart cellular functionality as they carry out most of the work of the cells and also represent the majority of drug targets. Based on an assumption that there are hidden diagnostic signatures in serum, Dr. Emanuel Petricoin III (CBER, FDA, Bethesda, MD) applied bioinformatics tools to demonstrate that serum proteomic patterns reflect tissue pathologic states, as in the case of ovarian[8] or prostatic cancer. There are plans to also extend this approach to other organs. **Pattern recognition** and classification required less than 1 μL of raw unfractionated serum. This approach utilized a supervised genetic algorithm to iteratively seek combination of mass-to-charge (m/z) values that can be used to classify samples and unsupervised **Kohonen SOMs** (self-organized maps) as a fitness test. The system was designed to learn and adapt with new data. The results of the study led to a PMA (premarket approval) application to FDA requesting clearance to market a class III medical device. In addition to identifying proteomic patterns, it is also useful to identify proteins themselves. Dr. Vineet Bafna (Celera, Rockville, MD) described **SCOPE**, a probabilistic model for scoring tandem mass spectra against a peptide database.[9] This approach can be employed to identify and characterize proteins differentially expressed in diseased vs. normal tissues and thereby discover diagnostic markers and targets for intervention.

Dr. Robert Murphy (Carnegie Mellon University, Pittsburgh, PA) proposed a different approach based on differences in subcellular distribution of some proteins between normal and cancerous tissues: "location proteomics".[10] Supervised learning was used to generate a "class" of patterns for subcellular structures of interest from images of localization of different proteins, extract subcellular localization features (SLF, numerical values describing the distribution of the protein within the cells) independent of cell position and rotation, and enable classification methods to learn to distinguish classes based on the features. Projected use of this approach is to monitor dynamic properties of proteins, relate them to changes with disease state and therapeutic intervention, and apply them to screening, detection, and intervention.

In addition to genomic and proteomic areas, bioinformatics also plays a critical role in imaging. Dr. Matthew Freedman (Georgetown University, Washington, D.C.) described **CAD** (computer-aided detection) and **CADX** (computer-aided diagnosis) approaches to improve small lung cancer detection and evaluation of response to anti-estrogen therapeutic intervention for mammary tumors. Dr. Carlos Andrés Peña-Reyes (Swiss Federal Institute of Technology, Lausanne, Switzerland) described the **COBRA system** (computer-assisted case interpretation) for modeling the human decision process, not human reasoning, in breast cancer risk assessment based on mammograms.[11] It uses **fuzzy Co-Co** (cooperative coevolutionary) methodology, that is, two evolutionary algorithms, one searching for labels and the other for rules. This divide-and-conquer approach is believed to provide a better search power at a lesser computational cost. It holds promise in improvements in sensitivity and specificity.

In order to streamline, optimize, and expedite drug discovery and development process, *in silico* methods based on integration of biology, chemistry, medicine, and information technology were proposed. AnVil received two Small Business Innovation Research (SBIR) awards from NIH to develop computational tools for discovery of cancer drugs. Dr. John McCarthy (AnVil, Inc., Burlington, MA) described his company's approach combining data mining, high-dimensional analysis and visualization, statistics, and domain expertise to convey information, extract knowledge, and identify structures, patterns, anomalies, trends, and relationships. Using their proprietary technology, they generated diagnostic predictor and treatment outcome predictor for AML and ALL leukemia based on genomic profile and proposed a 76-gene chip for these applications in personalized medicine. They also employed a similar approach for a lung cancer DNA chip and chemical structure–based predictive toxicology. Dr. Ganesh Vaidyanathan (DuPont de Nemours & Co., Wilmington, DE) described **InfoEvolve**™, a set of empirical modeling tools for transitioning from data to knowledge and based on **information theory** and **genetic algorithm**. Its advantages are that it can build models with both low bias (low errors during training) and low variance (low errors during validation) without requiring a compromise between the two. It can be used to discover important inputs, build predictive models along the line of information-weighed **Bayesian modeling**, and identify strategies for discovering and designing compounds with desired biological activities. This modeling approach was shown useful in drug discovery in that it allowed sampling of fewer compounds in order to get a certain fraction of active ones.

It is recognized that cancer is a complex and multifactorial collection of diseases and that individual variables (biomarkers and indicators of cancer phenotype) are not adequately predictive or discriminatory. Dr. Judith Dayhoff (Complexity Research Solutions, Inc., Silver Spring, MD) described integrated use of **multivariate analysis**, **artificial neural networks**, and complementary statistical tools in aiding early cancer detection and risk assessment.[12] This approach employs composite medical index or panel of biomarkers (clinical, genomic, proteomic, biochemical, imaging, etc.) rather than individual variables. It is patient-specific in that individual patient's information is entered into a neural network and index reflecting that patient's status or risk is obtained. Several medical examples, including oncology, were presented. She also pointed out that the amount of data is not as important as data being sufficiently represented along the boundaries of the discrimination problem. Adding small amount of random noise to provide more data points around the boundaries for training neural networks is often helpful.

SOFTWARE TOOLS

A need for open source software tools in public domain was recognized, and Sandrine Dudoit (University of California at Berkeley, Berkeley, CA) and John Quackenbush (The Institute for Genomic Research [TIGR], Rockville, MD) described two sets of resources for genomic microarray analysis at Bioconductor (http://www.bioconductor.org/) and TIGR (http://www.tigr.org/software/), respectively.

The **Bioconductor project**[13] makes available an open source and open development software to assist biologists and statisticians in the area of bioinformatics. Its primary emphasis is on inference using cDNA microarrays. It consists of several modules that facilitate the analysis and comprehension of genomic data and allow efficient representation and manipulation of large and complex data sets of multiple types. Bioconductor packages include tools for preprocessing cDNA microarray data (similar package is also available for the Affymetrix platform): **marrayClasses** (classes and methods for cDNA microarray data), **marrayInput** (data input for cDNA microarrays), **marrayNorm** (location and scale normalization for cDNA microarray data), and **marrayPlots** (diagnostic plots for cDNA microarray data); as well as tools for differential gene expression: **multtest** (multiple hypothesis testing) and **ROC** (receiver operating characteristic approach). In addition to making software tools readily available, it also provides a platform for rapid design and deployment of quality software.

Another set of tools is available at TIGR Web site (http://www.tigr.org/software/). There, one can find a variety of standard operating procedures and software tools that are freely available to the scientific community, including **Resourcerer** (database for annotating and linking microarray resources within and across species), **MIDAS** (Microarray Data Analysis System for microarray data quality filtering and normalization that allows raw experimental data to be processed through various data normalizations, filters, and transformations via a user-designed analysis pipeline), **MADAM** (Microarray Data Manager, to load and retrieve microarray data to and from a database), **MultiExperiment Viewer** (MEV, Java application designed to allow the analysis of microarray data to identify patterns of gene expression and differentially expressed genes, and providing large number of different data mining tools), and **Array Viewer** (software tool designed to facilitate the presentation and analysis of microarray expression data, leading to the identification of genes that are differentially expressed).

Other more specific tools are also available, such as **dChip** (DNA chip analyzer; http://www.dchip.org/), which was described by Dr. Cheng Li (Harvard University,

Boston, MA). The dChip is a tool for normalization and estimation of expression levels in multiple oligonucleotide experiments based on a multiplicative model.[14] It employs a probe-sensitivity index to capture the response characteristic of a specific probe pair from multiple chips and calculates model-based indices and thereby detects outlier probe sets. It also provides hierarchical clustering and **principal components analysis** (PCA).

STANDARDIZATION

In order to facilitate management, sharing, and mining of huge amounts of complex microarray data being generated, establishing of standards is of paramount importance. **Microarray Gene Expression Data (MGED) Society** (http://www.mged.org/) is an international organization aiming to establish and implement standards for microarray data annotation and exchange, including facilitating the creation of related databases and public repositories and development of data analysis tools. It aims to make huge amounts of genomic and proteomic data broadly accessible. **MIAME** (Minimum Information about a Microarray Experiment) is a defined standard or a set of guidelines outlining the *minimum* information required to unambiguously interpret microarray data and allow access and subsequent independent verification (http://www.mged.org/workgroups/miame/miame.html).[15]

Several prominent journals, including *The Nature* and *The Lancet*, have recently endorsed MIAME as a standard requirement for authors submitting microarray data for publication. In addition, *The Nature* will also require submission of microarray data to a public database (http://www.ebi.ac.uk/arrayexpress/ and http://ncbi.nlm.nih.gov/geo/).

There are also standardization efforts for protocols in microarray data analysis, such as the one by **CAMDA** (Critical Assessment of Microarray Data Analysis; http://www.camda.duke.edu/).

MICROARRAY CROSS-PLATFORM META-ANALYSIS

Presently, genomic studies are most prevalent and common. In spite of this, these studies are limited to small data sets (limited number of samples) and data sets on different platforms (oligo, cDNA, ink-jet, etc.). In addition, technologies involved in genomic sample processing and analysis are changing and evolving and there are continual improvements of experimental protocols for samples and microarrays. Therefore, there is a need for building models across platforms and with combined data sets. This would provide a more general approach and more reproducible and comprehensive models and decrease system-specific biases and idiosyncrasies. In addition, it would provide opportunity to validate models using data from other laboratories and larger data sets. Dr. Chinnaiyan stressed a need to cross-validate or interstudy-validate multiple data sets *in silico* and demonstrated use of meta-analysis of microarray data to identify dysregulation pathways.[16] α-Methylacyl coenzyme A racemase (AMACR), involved in β-oxidation of fatty acids, was identified as a possible tissue biomarker for prostate cancer (sensitivity of about 97% and specificity of about 100% in diagnosing prostate cancer needle biopsies) following meta-analysis of 4 independent gene expression data sets.[6] Dr. Pablo Tamayo (Whitehead Institute, MIT, Cambridge, MA) described use of a **Large Bayes Inference with Relative Features** approach. It involves rescaling data from individual data sets, merging and normalization, relative feature extraction, discretization and selection, creation of a database of labeled frequent item sets (combinations of frequently observed features' values or common occurrences in the data), and building a Bayes classifier using a product approximation. The advantages of a Bayes classifier are that it works with a small number of data points, with missing values and features, and with large data dimensionality, and combines supervised and unsupervised methods. Application and benefits of this approach were demonstrated across platforms (leukemia and lymphoma subclasses) and combined data sets (4-class adenocarcinoma data set).

FUTURE DIRECTIONS

Question and discussion sessions were lively and stimulated a lot of thought. Comments and recommendations tended to be general in nature—not specific, but applicable to cancer prevention. The following "needs" were identified:

- Bioinformatics analysis should be incorporated into the experimental design from the beginning, not as an afterthought.
- More holistic approach should be employed incorporating genomic, proteomic, biochemical, pathological, and clinical data. Model development should be based on both clinical and molecular information. Different variables should be considered in relation to each other rather than independently.
- Standard operating procedures (SOPs) should be developed for collection, handling, storage, annotation (in computable form), and analysis of specimens. They should have portability and be independent of a specific laboratory.
- There is a need for more prospective studies.
- Larger well-annotated data sets should be established to get around the limitations associated with having the number of variables greater than the number of samples by several orders of magnitude. Annotation of data sets should be into functional categories that are relevant to cancer. Large data sets could be attained by combining data sets, using cooperative group studies with a large number of subjects, and using experimental animal studies to validate bioinformatics tools and as a proof of principle.
- Public repositories/warehouses should be established for samples (biorepositories), data, bioinformatics tools, and standardized data sets. These could then be used for validation and data mining.
- Further developments are needed in computational tools for data analysis across protocols, platforms, multiple data sets, and independent laboratories.
- Selection and implementation of "gold standard(s)" for validation are needed. RT-PCR was proposed as the most accepted standard in genomics, but its implementation has drawbacks. Another approach was to establish "reference laboratories" for validations.

- Publications should include adequate information to evaluate, reproduce, and *in silico* validate computational methods and results.
- Cross-training opportunities should be made available and encouraged, if not required, between biology/medicine and computation/bioinformatics.
- Funding should be made available for training, study sections for technology-driven (as opposed to hypothesis-driven) proposals, and SBIR projects.
- It would be worthwhile to establish and maintain a list of commercially and publicly available computational tools along with a brief description and general rating in terms of overall quality, capabilities, and usefulness.
- Greater effort is needed in development and validation of text mining algorithms.

REFERENCES

1. HASTIE, T., R. TIBSHIRANI & J. FRIEDMAN. 2001. The Elements of Statistical Learning: Data Mining, Inference, and Prediction. Springer-Verlag. New York/Berlin.
2. KECMAN, V. 2001. Learning and Soft Computing. MIT Press. Cambridge, MA.
3. WEERARATNA, A.T., Y. JIANG, G. HOSTETTER *et al.* 2002. Wnt5a signaling directly affects cell motility and invasion of metastatic melanoma. Cancer Cell **1**: 279–288.
4. MOLOSHOK, T.D., R.R. KLEVECZ, J.D. GRANT *et al.* 2002. Application of Bayesian decomposition for analyzing microarray data. Bioinformatics **18**: 566–575.
5. SHIPP, M.A., K.N. ROSS, P.B. TAMAYO *et al.* 2002. Diffuse large B-cell lymphoma outcome prediction by gene-expression profiling and supervised machine learning. Nat. Med. **8**: 68–74.
6. RUBIN, M.A., M. ZHOU, S.M. DHANASEKARAN *et al.* 2002. α-Methylacyl coenzyme A racemase as a tissue biomarker for prostate cancer. JAMA **287**: 1662–1670.
7. KHAN, J., J.S. WEI, M. RINGNER *et al.* 2001. Classification and diagnostic prediction of cancers using gene expression profiling and artificial neural networks. Nat. Med. **7**: 673–679.
8. PETRICOIN, E.F., A.M. ARDEKANI, B.A. HITT *et al.* 2002. Use of proteomic patterns in serum to identify ovarian cancer. Lancet **359**: 572–577.
9. BAFNA, V. & N. EDWARDS. 2001. SCOPE: a probabilistic model for scoring tandem mass spectra against a peptide database. Bioinformatics **17**(suppl. 1): S13–S21.
10. BOLAND, M.V. & R.F. MURPHY. 2001. A neural network classifier capable of recognizing the patterns of all major subcellular structures in fluorescence microscope images of HeLa cells. Bioinformatics **17**: 1213–1223.
11. PEÑA-REYES, C.A. & M. SIPPER. 2000. Evolutionary computation in medicine: an overview. Artif. Intell. Med. **19**: 1–23.
12. DAYHOFF, J.E. & J.M. DELEO. 2001. Artificial neural networks: opening the black box. Cancer **91**: 1615–1635.
13. DUDOIT, S. & Y.H. YANG. 2003. Bioconductor R packages for exploratory analysis and normalization of cDNA microarray data. *In* The Analysis of Gene Expression Data: Methods and Software. Springer Pub. New York.
14. LI, C. & W.H. WONG. 2001. Model-based analysis of oligonucleotide arrays: expression index computation and outlier detection. Proc. Natl. Acad. Sci. USA **98**: 31–36.
15. BRAZMA, A., P. HINGAMP, J. QUACKENBUSH *et al.* 2001. Minimum information about a microarray experiment (MIAME)—toward standards for microarray data. Nat. Genet. **29**: 365–371.
16. RHODES, D.R., T.R. BARRETTE, M.A. RUBIN *et al.* 2002. Meta-analysis of microarrays: interstudy validation of gene expression profiles reveals pathway dysregulation in prostate cancer. Cancer Res. **62**: 4427–4433.

Overview of Commonly Used Bioinformatics Methods and Their Applications

IZET M. KAPETANOVIC,[a] SIMON ROSENFELD,[b] AND GRANT IZMIRLIAN[b]

[a]Chemopreventive Agent Development Research Group and [b]Biometry Research Group, Division of Cancer Prevention, National Cancer Institute, Bethesda, Maryland, USA

ABSTRACT: Bioinformatics, in its broad sense, involves application of computer processes to solve biological problems. A wide range of computational tools are needed to effectively and efficiently process large amounts of data being generated as a result of recent technological innovations in biology and medicine. A number of computational tools have been developed or adapted to deal with the experimental riches of complex and multivariate data and transition from data collection to information or knowledge. These include a wide variety of clustering and classification algorithms, including *self-organized maps* (SOM), *artificial neural networks* (ANN), *support vector machines* (SVM), *fuzzy logic*, and even hyphenated techniques as *neuro-fuzzy networks*. These bioinformatics tools are being evaluated and applied in various medical areas including early detection, risk assessment, classification, and prognosis of cancer. The goal of these efforts is to develop and identify bioinformatics methods with optimal sensitivity, specificity, and predictive capabilities.

KEYWORDS: bioinformatics; data mining; cancer; early detection; risk assessment; hierarchical clustering; neural networks; support vector machines; fuzzy logic; genomics; proteomics; drug discovery

INTRODUCTION

Technological advances in biological and biomedical areas, especially in genomics and proteomics, are resulting in huge amounts of high-dimensional data with the number of "features" or "predictors" exceeding sample size by orders of magnitude. This new statistical paradigm, termed a "curse of dimensionality", has required the medical researchers to turn to the fields of **artificial intelligence** and **machine learning** in their quest for adequate analysis tools. Analogously as the recognition of the field of medical statistics as a specialized area of applied statistics resulted in the development of numerous new statistical methodologies, the fields of artificial intelligence and machine learning are currently being retooled and refined to suit the practical needs of bioinformatics. Integration of modern computational tools in bioinformatics and innovative high-throughput biotechnologies carry with them a great

Address for correspondence: Izet M. Kapetanovic, Chemopreventive Agent Development Research Group, Division of Cancer Prevention, National Cancer Institute, Bethesda, MD 20892-7322. Voice: 301-435-5011; fax: 301-402-0553.
kapetani@mail.nih.gov

Ann. N.Y. Acad. Sci. 1020: 10–21 (2004). © 2004 New York Academy of Sciences.
doi: 10.1196/annals.1310.003

impact potential in health care. The **-omic** (comprehensive analysis of components within a biological grouping, i.e., proteomics for proteins) revolution is stimulating development of new and reinvention of older computational methods. This review describes some of the commonly used and evolving bioinformatics methods and data mining tools and includes examples of their application to early cancer detection or diagnosis, risk identification, risk assessment, and risk reduction. It is not intended to be exhaustive, but only to present a brief overview. Individual topics are discussed in a more comprehensive manner in separate chapters in this volume. Another chapter reviews newer computational methods in cancer-related bioinformatics.

BIOINFORMATICS METHODS

Clustering

An excellent survey of the material on clustering techniques in microarray data analysis is Tibshirani *et al.*[1] (http://www-stat.stanford.edu/~tibs/research.html/). Clustering methods are used to arrange cell lines and genes in some natural order, with similar cell lines (and/or genes) placed close together. There are two major approaches to clustering: bottom-up and top-down. **Hierarchical clustering** is a bottom-up clustering method that starts with each cell line (gene) in its own cluster. It works by agglomerating the closest pair of clusters at each stage, successively combining clusters until all of the data are in one cluster. A number of methods are in common use for measuring the similarity of the expression profiles, such as **Euclidean distance**, **Pearson correlation**, **Manhattan distance**, and others.[2] The relationships between each sample (or gene) is represented by a hierarchical tree, the **dendrogram**, which can be cut at any level to yield a specified number of clusters. Top-down clustering starts with a preset specified number of clusters and initial positions for the cluster centers. The **K-means** is used to reposition the cluster centers through the following steps: (1) observations are assigned to the closest cluster center to form a partition of the data; (2) the observations in each cluster are averaged, producing new values for the center vector of that cluster. Steps 1 and 2 are iterated, and the process converges to the minimum of total within cluster variance. Tree-structured vector quantization carries out K-means clustering in a top-down, binary manner. It is commonly used in image and signal compression. The **principal components analysis** (PCA), when applied to the genes, finds the linear combinations of gene expressions having the highest variance. Similarly, when applied to cell lines, it finds the highest variance linear combination of the cell lines. The correlation of each gene with the leading principal component provides a way of sorting (clustering) the genes as well as cell lines. The self-organizing map (SOM) is similar to K-means clustering, with the constraint that the cluster centers are restricted to remain in a one- or two-dimensional manifold. An iterative procedure is used to readjust the positions of the centers. There is a similarity between SOMs, multi-dimensional scaling, and principal components. In a comparative study, it was reported that K-means clustering produces tighter clusters than hierarchical clustering, but the latter tends to produce a greater number of smaller clusters, potentially a valuable feature for discovery.[1]

Unlike K-means clustering, hierarchical clustering produces an ordering of the objects, which can be informative for data display. Because SOMs are constructed from a two-dimensional representation of the data, it is a good idea to check the resulting predicted classes against an algorithm that functions directly in the original dimension of the data set, such as K-means.

The above methods are the one-way clustering techniques; however, the use of two-way clustering, that is, simultaneous clustering both the genes and cell lines, has also been investigated.[1] A simple approach to this problem is to apply a one-way clustering method separately to the genes and to the cell lines. Block clustering, in contrast, uses both gene and cell line information to simultaneously cluster both. The two-way clustering procedures seek a global organization of genes and cell lines. This study reported that these types of procedures are able to discover gross global structure, but may not be effective for discovering finer detail. In response to this finding, a new method called **gene shaving** was proposed. The gene shaving technique can search for sets of genes that optimally separate the cell lines.[3] The algorithm begins by finding a nested sequence of candidate clusters, with all gene clusters in the initial position and one gene cluster in the final position.

Artificial Neural Networks

Artificial neural networks (ANN), modeled after normal brain processes and neurophysiological learning, are powerful computational tools for multifactorial classification and multivariate nonlinear regression. Technological advances and availability of computational power brought by the era of personal computers made ANN a popular method for routine analysis in a wide spectrum of scientific and engineering applications, including automatic target recognition, stock market analysis, expert systems, pattern recognition, medical imaging, and DNA microarray analysis. However, ANN methodologies often represent more art than science. Many decisions related to the choice of ANN structure and parameters are often completely subjective. Theoretical recommendations for the size of training data set are lacking, and an optimum size is almost never available in practice. Special attention also has to be paid to avoid overtraining that would result in memorization instead of gener-alization of the data. Therefore, there is a considerable uncertainty in the optimal design of the ANN architecture. The final ANN solution may be influenced by a number of factors (e.g., starting weights, number of cases, and their order during the training phase, number of training cycles, etc.).

Bootstrap sampling (random sampling with replacement) to produce a large number of individual neural networks was one proposed approach addressing this problem.[4] Parametric or nonparametric statistical analysis of the resultant distribu-tion of neural networks would yield predictive intervals. ANN is a strongly nonlinear approximation and, therefore, the topology of the objective function in the space of the ANN parameters is usually very complex. In particular, the objective function may contain many local minima, and gradient methods of optimization, such as Newton-Raphson, steepest descent, etc., can easily lead the minimization procedure to one of these local minima, resulting in very suboptimal weights. To avoid this problem, a number of sophisticated optimization algorithms have been developed, such as **genetic algorithm**, **simulated annealing**, and various versions of **stochastic optimization**.

Genetic algorithms are based on the concept of natural selection, survival of the fittest. Using principles of inheritance, mutation and/or cross-over, genetic algorithms generate a series of random potential solutions (population) and use objective fitness function to evaluate each member of the population. The probability of a particular gene being copied in the next generation (reproduction) is determined by its fitness (i.e., its contribution to the objective function). The reiterative process continues with the fitter members until the fittest member of the population is identified as the optimized solution. It has been shown theoretically and computationally that such a process provides a random walk in the space of the ANN parameters toward minimum of the objective function. A fundamental advantage of the genetic algorithm is that in principle it is able to find the global minimum. Genetic algorithms are highly intensive computationally and require millions of readjustments ("generations") of the objective function to reach a convergence.

Simulated annealing is another method of finding a global minimum. The set of arguments of the objective function (the ANN weights, for example) are likened to a thermodynamic system. Objective function is considered as its energy, and the search for the minimum is analogous to the search of thermodynamically stable state with the lowest energy possible. It was shown that simulated annealing has a high probability to converge to a global minimum. Similar to genetic algorithm, simulated annealing is highly computationally intensive.

There are many versions of stochastic optimization. Their common theme is a random walk in the phase space toward the minimum of objective function. The arguments of objective function are perturbed randomly. The new set of parameters are accepted if the objective function is decreasing. The whole process is often likened to the random walk of a drunken person in his/her attempt to find the way home. A surprising feature of this kind of algorithm is that average time required to reach the goal is often smaller than that resulting from exact analysis and prediction of each step. The advantages of stochastic algorithms are especially noticeable for the random walk in high-dimensional space. Generally speaking, this family of algorithms does not guarantee convergence to the global minimum. However, a great advantage of stochastic optimization methods is that, unlike the gradient methods, they generally do not require computation of the objective function gradients. Taking into account high dimension of the parameter space and high computational cost of the gradient evaluation, this feature is highly important and makes the convergence process comparatively fast.

Despite all the obstacles and difficulties in design and training of ANNs, there are numerous examples of highly successful applications of ANNs. Recently, a marked increase in application of ANNs in biomedical areas, especially in cancer research, has been observed. It is currently widely recognized that cancer risk evaluation based on a single or few biomarkers may not be possible. ANN is inherently suited in this regard because of its ability to perform simultaneous analysis of large amounts of diverse information. **ROC** (receiver operating characteristics curve) methodology, which is frequently used as a measure of classification performance, has been adapted to evaluation of the ANN performance.[4,5] The y-axis and x-axis on the ROC curves represent sensitivity and specificity, respectively, and the area under the curve is an indication of how well the independent variable separating two dichotomous classes performs.

Support Vector Machine

An important recent innovation in the statistical learning theory is the support vector machine (SVM).[6] SVM represents a particular instance of a large class of learning algorithms known as kernel machines and is a powerful supervised algorithm for classification. This algorithm projects data into higher dimensional space where two classes are linearly separable. It finds a hyperplane in the space of the data points that separates two classes of data and maximizes the width of a separating band between the data points and the hyperplane. The support vectors are defined as the ones nearest to this margin, and only the support vectors define the model and need to be stored. There are many fundamental advantages of the SVM algorithms compared with other methods. First, unlike ANN, SVM produces a unique solution because it is basically a linear problem and does not have such a pitfall as multiple local minima. Second, SVM is inherently able to deal with very large amounts of dissimilar information. Third, the discriminant function is characterized by only a comparatively small subset of the entire training data set, thus making the computations noticeably faster. SVM is a highly promising tool in genomics and proteomics.

Boosting

Abundance of exploratory tools, each possessing their pros and cons, creates a difficult problem of selecting the best of them. It seems to be a good idea to try to combine their strengths for creating an even more powerful tool. To a certain extent, this idea has been implemented in a new family of classification algorithms known under the general term "boosting". **Boosting** was proposed in a series of groundbreaking works.[7] Boosting is a general method for combining many weak classifiers to produce a stronger classifier. Boosting sequentially applies a classification algorithm to reweighed versions of the training data and then takes a weighted majority vote of the sequence of classifiers thus produced. For many classification algorithms, this simple strategy results in a dramatic improvement in performance. This seemingly mysterious phenomenon can be understood in terms of well-known statistical approaches, such as additive models and maximum likelihood.[8]

Bagging

Another technique that has evolved as a mechanism for improving existing classification algorithms is "**Bagging**", an acronym for (B)ootstrap (Agg)regation.[9] Given a particular classifier and a data set, bagging proceeds by drawing B bootstrap samples from the data set (random sample with replacement of equal size). Each bootstrap sample trains a classifier. Since sampling with replacement tends to pick from those already sampled about a third of the time, a bootstrap sample of size n contains roughly $2n/3$ unique samples. Consequently, $n/3$ of the original sample is left out. The validation step is carried out by predicting class membership, for each of the n elements of the original sample, using the (roughly) $B/3$ classifiers that element did not train. Final class membership is predicted using the most popular vote. The point of bagging a classifier is to pick a middle way between overfitting (low variance, but high bias) and oversmoothing (low bias, but high variance). A very promising new tool that incorporates bagging in a very clever way is **random**

forests.[10–12] This tool performs bagging on classification (or regression) trees with the added novel idea of random feature set selection each time a node is split during the training process. This has the effect of decorrelating the ensemble of classification/regression trees and helps to strengthen the divide between training and validation. An especially nice additional property of random forest is that it performs so well with practically no real tuning parameters. The random forest algorithm has recently been successfully applied in the analysis of proteomics data.[13]

Fuzzy Logic

The real world, including that of medicine, is imprecise, vague, and ambiguous, that is, fuzzy. Lotfi Zadeh, the founder of fuzzy logic, proposed that one could exploit tolerance for imprecision and partial truths to achieve tractability, robustness, interpretability, and decreased computational cost. Fuzzy logic deals with ambiguity and vagueness, as opposed to probability that involves uncertainty and likelihood. A distinction between fuzzy and binary or crisp logic is that the former involves concepts of more or less or degree of membership (partial set membership) or continuity as opposed to yes or no or absence or presence or discreteness. Fuzzy logic uses the linguistic variable (i.e., computing with words instead of numbers). It provides a mathematical tool for representing and manipulating information in a way that resembles human communication and reasoning processes. It embeds existing structured human knowledge into workable mathematics. A typical fuzzy inference system includes fuzzification (classifying numeric data into fuzzy sets), knowledge/rule base (employing linguistic reasoning with "if … then" rules mapping the input into output variables), inference engine (applying the rule base to the fuzzy set to obtain a fuzzy outcome), and defuzzification process (converting the fuzzy outcome to a crisp one).

Nowadays, fuzzy logic devices are present in many everyday consumer products (e.g., automobile brakes, camera and camcorder autofocus, meteorology instrumentation, intravenous infusion pumps, kitchen devices, etc.). Theory and applications of fuzzy logic in medicine have been reviewed in several recent publications.[14–18] Some of the fuzzy techniques that have been employed for biomedical data analysis include fuzzy clustering, fuzzy classification, and hybrid systems, such as combinations of fuzzy logic and neural networks (neuro-fuzzy networks), genetic algorithm, evolutionary algorithm, or discrete wavelet transforms. For example, the advantage of some hybrid methods like neuro-fuzzy systems is that they combine the advantages of fuzzy systems that deal with explicit knowledge (understood and explainable) and neural networks that deal with implicit knowledge (acquired by learning).

APPLICATIONS

Genomics in Early Cancer Detection and Classification

The innovative technologies of gene expression analysis are providing promising tools for the identification of cancer cell signatures and cancer molecular targets, thereby facilitating early detection of cancer and intervention. Computational methods used for microarray data analysis have been reviewed.[19] Perou *et al.*[20] used hierarchical clustering for human breast tumor classification and identification of molecular portraits. Alizadeh et al.[21] studied gene expression in the three most prevalent adult lymphoid malignancies. Two previously unrecognized types of diffuse large B-cell lymphoma, with distinct clinical behaviors, were identified based on gene expression data and were shown to have markedly different median survival, even within a low-risk profile, according to the currently accepted diagnostic criteria. Two-way hierarchical clustering on cell lines and on genes was used to identify the two tumor sub-classes, as well as to group genes with similar expression patterns across the three different samples. However, these results were obtained after thresholding, which is a step fraught with problems over validity. Using a gene shaving technique, it was possible to duplicate two subtypes with differing median survival in an unsupervised manner, without thresholding.[3] Hierarchical clustering has several drawbacks (non-uniqueness, inversion problems, grouping based on local decision, lack of an opportunity to reevaluate the clustering, etc.) and other approaches have also been employed. Unsupervised methods, such as the Kohonen SOMs, have been used for gene clustering in promyelocytic leukemia.[22]

Use of supervised methods for microarray data analysis has also been recently reviewed.[23] Supervised ANNs have been used to classify estrogen receptor status in human breast tissue following PCA to reduce the dimensionality[24] and correctly classify the small, round blue-cell tumor subtypes and identify possible gene targets for therapy.[25] Others have successfully applied ANN to distinguish among subtypes of neoplastic colorectal lesions and showed that ANN outperformed hierarchical clustering in classification power and was able to distinguish between 27 different subtypes of neoplastic colorectal lesions.[26] SVMs have also been successfully applied in microarray gene expression analysis,[27] tumor classification,[28,29] cancer diagnosis,[30] and prognosis.[31] A group at Stanford developed supervised learning software for genomic expression data mining and made it available from their Web site (http://www-stat.stanford.edu/~tibs/SAM/index.html/).[32] It is in the form of an Excel add-in and is applicable to cDNA, oligo, SNP, and protein array data. It correlates expression data to clinical parameters. A fuzzy logic approach to identify connected networks of genes describing how the genes interrelate has also been proposed.[33]

Proteomic Profiling, Bioimaging, and Pattern Recognition

Proteomics is the analysis of the proteome, which is a term applied to the proteins expressed by the genome of a species. Importance of the problem was recently emphasized by founding the Human Proteome Organization (HUPO) (http://www.hupo.org/) with the aim of elucidating the human proteome. In general, there is a poor correlation between mRNA and protein levels.[34] In addition, genomics does not provide information regarding posttranslational events (such as phosphorylation, acetylation, lipidation, glycosylation, or ubiquitination). Proteome imparts cellular functionality as proteins carry out most of the work of the cell. The majority of drug targets are proteins. Proteomic fingerprinting provides complementary information to genomic fingerprinting. Proteins can serve as markers and targets of chemoprevention. Newer technological advances have enabled growth and interest in proteomics. Some of the tools presently available or under development include **surface-enhanced**

laser desorption/ionization time-of-flight (SELDI-TOF) and **matrix-assisted laser desorption/ionization time-of-flight** (MALDI-TOF), mass spectrometric (MS) techniques, **surface plasmon resonance** (SPR) technology, **laser capture microdissection** (LCM), and a number of protein, antibody, and tissue microarrays.

There are a number of difficulties inherent in proteomic research. For example, estimated number of proteins in the proteome exceeds that of genes in the genome by more than an order of magnitude. There is no PCR equivalent to amplify protein signal. Proteins are in a continual dynamic flux depending on cellular status and activity. Proteomic research will lead to new developments in identification and detection of biomarkers, recognition of new drug targets, individualized patient therapy, and enhancements in rational drug design. These new technologies have facilitated disease detection and diagnosis based on protein fingerprinting, relying on multiple instead of single protein biomarkers. It is not simply a matter of presence or absence of number of proteins, but rather their relative amounts to each other. This realization led to a considerable improvement in predictability. Bioinformatics tools are critical in the analysis of the huge amount of data being generated by the newer parallel analytical techniques.

Appropriate combinations of analytical and bioinformatics tools have been used to define an optimum discriminatory proteomic pattern in women without sign of disease, early-stage ovarian cancer, late-stage ovarian cancer, and benign diseases.[35] In this study, genetic algorithm and unsupervised SOM were used to analyze SELDI-TOF data from serum proteins applied to a hydrophobic interaction protein chip. In order to identify 5 proteins with different relative abundances between two training sets, on the order of 10^{20} combinations would be required and would be overwhelming even with today's computer technology. However, the problem can be greatly simplified by use of a genetic algorithm. Petricoin *et al.*[35] report that this approach yielded 100% sensitivity, 95% specificity, and 94% predictability.

Another study presented promising preliminary results in using neural network with a back-propagation algorithm for the tumor classification and biomarker identification of human astrocytoma based on tissue protein data.[36] Qu *et al.*[37] applied a modified AdaBoost algorithm proposed by Freund and Schapire.[7] Using this algorithm, 97% sensitivity and specificity have been achieved in discrimination between healthy men and those with prostate cancer and benign prostate hyperplasia based on serum protein data. The same group also obtained satisfactory results (positive predictive value of 91% for general population) for early detection of prostate cancer based on serum protein fingerprinting with a decision tree classification algorithm.[38]

ANN is also a powerful tool for **image analysis** and **pattern recognition**. It is the technique behind the FDA-approved computer-assisted diagnosis instrumentation ImageChecker® that is used to analyze digital mammograms and draws the physician's attention to suspicious features that may be indicative of cancer (http://www.r2tech.com/prd/prd001.html/).

ANNs have been used to classify patterns of subcellular structures in fluorescence microscope images of HeLa cells.[39] Images of subcellular structures were parameterized using an elaborate system of 37 geometric and texture features. The 37 vectors of these features were used as input vectors for the back-propagation ANN. The ANN was able to successfully recognize all 10 subcellular structures used in the training process. This method allows monitoring of dynamic protein properties and relates them to changes with disease states and therapeutic intervention.

Usefulness of fuzzy logic was demonstrated in **computer-aided cancer detection** in the areas of bioimaging, classification, and pattern recognition. A fuzzy logic approach was used in detection of lobulated and microlobulated masses in digital mammography,[40] and fuzzy-neural and feature extraction techniques were employed for detecting and diagnosing microcalcifications on digital mammograms.[40] A breast cancer diagnosis system (BCDS) combined a fuzzy microcalcification detection algorithm with a feature extraction method and a back-propagation neural network (BPNN) for classification of benign or malignant microcalcifications with 89% classification rates.[41]

Multifactorial Analysis of Early Detection, Risk Identification, Risk Assessment, and Risk Reduction of Cancer

Cancer is a complex, multifactorial collection of diseases. The goal of chemoprevention is to identify risks, assess risks, detect early, and intervene to reduce risk of cancer prior to the appearance of clinical signs and pathological abnormalities. Individual variables (biomarkers and indicators of cancer) are not adequately predictive or discriminatory. However, simultaneous consideration of multiple factors (**composite medical index** or **panel of markers**) should provide a more useful indication into the initiation, progression, and reversal of carcinogenesis. A further complication is that the predictability of an outcome is not based on presence or absence of several biomarkers or their linear summation, but on a complex, nonlinear relationship between them. The challenge is to identify suitable composite medical indices that would provide acceptable sensitivity, specificity, and predictability.

Different multivariate analytical tools have been employed to identify a composite variable for early detection, risk identification, risk assessment, and risk reduction of cancer. ANNs have been frequently used in cancer detection, cancer classification, and prognosis.[4,25,26,36,42,43] Inputs into ANNs can include data from any or all of the following: clinical findings, clinical chemistry, gene microarrays, protein microarrays, biomarkers, genetic factors, environmental factors, etc. The output variable represents a **composite variable** or a predicted outcome (in terms of a cancer risk or prognosis) for the individual patient.[4]

Other computational methodologies that have been shown to be useful in the area of diagnosis, classification, and prediction based on multifactorial analysis include SVMs,[30,31] genetic algorithms and SOMs,[35] and fuzzy logic.[44]

The fuzzy logic approach in conjunction with a panel of biomarkers demonstrated accuracy, sensitivity, and specificity in the diagnosis and classification of lung cancer.[44] For example, this study was able to distinguish malignant versus benign cases with a sensitivity of 88% and a specificity of 86%. It was also able to discriminate between non-small-cell carcinoma (NSCLC) versus small-cell carcinoma (SCLC) with sensitivity and specificity of 91% and 91% and squamous versus adenocarcinoma with sensitivity and specificity of 77% and 79%, respectively. This approach was especially effective in early stages of cancer and in patients with all marker levels in the gray area. Another study[45] employed genetic algorithm to automatically produce a fuzzy BCDS in relation to the Wisconsin Breast Cancer Diagnosis (WBCD) database. This **fuzzy-genetic** approach provided a high classification performance and interpretability. Subsequently, these same authors[46] introduced a combination of a fuzzy system and a **cooperative coevolutionary** approach in the area of breast cancer diagnosis. Evolutionary methods are search or optimization techniques and are especially useful in search of large and complex spaces. Cooperative coevolutionary approach involves two coevolving cooperative species (database membership function and a rule base). Two genetic algorithms (subset of evolutionary algorithms) were used to control the evolution of two populations. The advantages of this approach were that it provided higher classification performance with a lower computational cost than other systems.

In all cases, these multifactorial computational methodologies have enabled or significantly improved detection, classification, or prognosis of cancer over evaluations based on a single variable.

Drug Discovery

Pharmaceutical companies recognize the value of the huge amounts of data being generated by new **-omics** and high-throughput technologies, and are trying to leverage these data into drug discoveries with the help of evolving bioinformatics tools. In an effort to streamline, expedite, and optimize drug discovery and development, pharmaceutical companies are actively incorporating bioinformatics into their practices. As a result, new fields such as **chemogenomics**, **chemical genomics**, and **chemical genetics** have emerged. Although definitions for these fields vary and overlap, these areas encompass new approaches to drug discovery and therapeutic target identification/validation.[47–49] The idea behind them is that drugs can be used to identify new therapeutic targets, and targets can be used to identify new drugs in the context of genomics/proteomics. In a sense, chemical genomics integrates chemical structure space and biological structure space and provides an *in silico* approach to drug discovery and optimization. There are a number of new companies with a primary focus on chemical genomics that have emerged recently and are developing their versions of the chemical genomic mousetraps. In addition, another related **-omic** discipline has emerged: pharmacogenomics.[50] **Pharmacogenomics** is a discipline examining an individual's response to drugs based on an individual's genetic makeup. It promises to enable optimized, personalized therapy for each patient. Advances in biological, analytical, and computational technologies have allowed for emergence of innovative **computer-aided drug design** (CADD). Genetic algorithms are frequently used in CADD.[51,52] New data mining techniques and visualization tools can be used to characterize effects of chemopreventive intervention and thereby facilitate drug discovery. The expectation is that they will be useful in identifying appropriate targets, suitable biomarkers, and more fitting drug agents.

REFERENCES

1. TIBSHIRANI, R., T. HASTIE, M. EISEN *et al.* 1999. Clustering methods for the analysis of DNA microarray data. Technical report. Stanford University. Stanford, CA.
2. JAGOTA, A. 2001. Microarray data analysis and vizualization. Department of Computer Engineering, University of California, Santa Cruz. Santa Cruz, CA.
3. HASTIE, T., R. TIBSHIRANI, M.B. EISEN *et al.* 2000. "Gene shaving" as a method for identifying distinct sets of genes with similar expression patterns. Genome Biol. **1**(2): 0003.1–0003.21 (http://genomebiology.com/2000/1/2/research/0003/).
4. DAYHOFF, J.E. & J.M. DELEO. 2001. Artificial neural networks: opening the black box. Cancer **91**: 1615–1635.

5. DeLeo, J.M. & J.E. Dayhoff. 2001. Medical applications of neural networks: measures of certainty and statistical tradeoffs. *In* International Joint Conference on Neural Networks (IJCNN '01), pp. 3009–3014. IEEE Press. New York.
6. Vapnik, V.N. 1998. Statistical Learning Theory. Wiley. New York.
7. Freund, Y. & R.E. Schapire. 1996. Experiments with a new boosting algorithm. *In* Machine Learning. Proceedings of the Thirteenth International Conference, pp. 148–156. Morgan Kaufmann. San Francisco.
8. Friedman, J., T. Hastie & R. Tibshirani. 1996. Additive statistical regression: a statistical view of boosting. Ann. Stat. **28:** 337–407.
9. Hastie, T., R. Tibshirani & J. Friedman. 2001. The Elements of Statistical Learning, Springer Pub. New York.
10. Breiman, L. 2001. Random forests. Mach. Learn. **45**(1): 5–32.
11. Breiman, L. 2002. A Manual on Setting Up, Using, and Understanding Random Forests V3.1 (http://oz.berkeley.edu/users/breiman/using_random_forests_v3.1.pdf/).
12. Liaw, A. & M. Weiner. 2003. The Random Forest Package in R (http://cran-us-r.project.org/).
13. Xiao, Z., B. Luke, G. Izmirlian *et al.* 2003. Submitted.
14. Vitez, T.S., R. Wada & A. Macario. 1996. Fuzzy logic: theory and medical applications. J. Cardiothorac. Vasc. Anesth. **10:** 800–808.
15. Steimann, F. 1997. Fuzzy set theory in medicine. Artif. Intell. Med. **11:** 1–7.
16. Kuncheva, L.I. & F. Steimann. 1999. Fuzzy diagnosis. Artif. Intell. Med. **16:** 121–128.
17. Abbod, M.F., D.G. von Keyserlingk, D.A. Linkens *et al.* 2001. Survey of utilization of fuzzy technology in medicine and healthcare. Fuzzy Sets Syst. **120:** 331–349.
18. Mahfouf, M., M.F. Abbod & D.A. Linkens. 2001. A survey of fuzzy logic monitoring and control utilisation in medicine. Artif. Intell. Med. **21:** 27–42.
19. Quackenbush, J. 2001. Computational analysis of microarray data. Nat. Rev. **2:** 418–427.
20. Perou, C.M., T. Sorlie, M.B. Eisen *et al.* 2000. Molecular portraits of human breast tumours. Nature **406:** 747–752.
21. Alizadeh, A.A., M.B. Eisen, R.E. Davis *et al.* 2000. Distinct types of large B-cell lymphoma identified by gene expression profiling. Nature **403:** 503–511.
22. Tamayo, P., D. Slonim, J. Mesirov *et al.* 1999. Interpreting patterns of gene expression with self-organizing maps: methods and application to hematopoietic differentiation. Proc. Natl. Acad. Sci. USA **96:** 2907–2912.
23. Ringner, M., C. Peterson & J. Khan. 2002. Analyzing array data using supervised methods. Pharmacogenomics **3:** 403–415.
24. Gruvberger, S., M. Ringner, Y. Chen *et al.* 2001. Estrogen receptor in breast cancer is associated with remarkably distinct gene expression patterns. Cancer Res. **61:** 5979–5984.
25. Khan, J., J.S. Wei, M. Ringner *et al.* 2001. Classification and diagnostic prediction of cancers using gene expression profiling and artificial neural networks. Nat. Med. **7:** 673–679.
26. Selaru, F.M., Y. Xu, J. Yin *et al.* 2002. Artificial neural networks distinguish among subtypes of neoplastic colorectal lesions. Gastroenterology **122:** 606–613.
27. Brown, M.P.S., W.N. Grundy, D. Lin *et al.* 2000. Knowledge-based analysis of microarray gene expression data by using support vector machines. Proc. Natl. Acad. Sci. USA **97:** 262–267.
28. Furey, T.S., N. Cristianini, N. Duffy *et al.* 2000. Support vector machine classification and validation of cancer tissue samples using microarray expression data. Bioinformatics **16:** 906–914.
29. Yeang, C-H., S. Ramaswamy, P. Tamayo *et al.* 2001. Molecular classification of multiple tumor types. Bioinformatics **17**(suppl. 1): S316–S322.
30. Ramaswamy, S., P. Tamayo, R. Rifkin *et al.* 2001. Multiclass cancer diagnosis using tumor gene expression signatures. Proc. Natl. Acad. Sci. USA **98:** 15149–15154.
31. Shipp, M.A., K.N. Ross, P. Tamayo *et al.* 2002. Diffuse large B-cell lymphoma outcome prediction by gene-expression profiling and supervised machine learning. Nat. Med. **8:** 68–74.
32. Tusher, V.G., R. Tibshirani & G. Chu. 2001. Significance analysis of microarrays applied to the ionizing radiation response. Proc. Natl. Acad. Sci. USA **98:** 5116–5121.

33. WOOLF, P.J. & Y. WANG. 2000. A fuzzy logic approach to analyzing gene expression data. Physiol. Genomics **3:** 9–15.
34. PRATT, J.M., J. PETTY, I. RIBA-GARCIA *et al.* 2002. Dynamics of protein turnover, a missing dimension in proteomics. Mol. Cell. Proteomics **1:** 579–591.
35. PETRICOIN, E.F., A.M. ARDEKANI, B.A. HITT *et al.* 2002. Use of proteomic patterns in serum to identify ovarian cancer. Lancet **359:** 572–577.
36. BALL, G., S. MIAN, F. HOLDING *et al.* 2002. An integrated approach utilizing artificial neural networks and SELDI mass spectrometry for the classification of human tumours and rapid identification of potential biomarkers. Bioinformatics **18:** 395–404.
37. QU, Y., B-L. ADAM, Y. YASUI *et al.* 2002. Boosted decision tree analysis of surface-enhanced laser desorption/ionization mass spectral serum profiles discriminates prostate cancer from noncancer patients. Clin. Chem. **48:** 1835–1843.
38. ADAM, B-L., Y. QU, J.W. DAVIS *et al.* 2002. Serum protein fingerprinting coupled with a pattern-matching algorithm distinguishes prostate cancer from benign prostate hyperplasia and healthy men. Cancer Res. **62:** 3609–3614.
39. BOLAND, M.V. & R.F. MURPHY. 2001. A neural network classifier capable of recognizing the patterns of all major subcellular structures in fluorescence microscope images of HeLa cells. Bioinformatics **17:** 1213–1223.
40. KOVALERCHUK, B., E. TRIANTAPHYLLOU, J.F. RUIZ *et al.* 1997. Fuzzy logic in computer-aided breast cancer diagnosis: analysis of lobulation. Artif. Intell. Med. **11:** 75–85.
41. VERMA, B. & J. ZAKOS. 2001. A computer-aided diagnosis system for digital mammograms based on fuzzy-neural and feature extraction techniques. IEEE Trans. Inf. Technol. Biomed. **5:** 46–54.
42. ERREJON, A., E.D. CRAWFORD, J. DAYHOFF *et al.* 2001. Use of artificial neural networks in prostate cancer. Mol. Urol. **5:** 153–158.
43. XU, Y., F.M. SELARU, J. YIN *et al.* 2002. Artificial neural networks and gene filtering distinguish between global gene expression profiles of Barrett's esophagus and esophageal cancer. Cancer Res. **62:** 3493–3497.
44. KELLER, T., N. BITTERLICH, S. HILFENHAUS *et al.* 1998. Tumor markers in the diagnosis of bronchial carcinoma: new options using fuzzy logic–based tumour marker profiles. J. Cancer Res. Clin. Oncol. **124:** 565–574.
45. PEÑA-REYES, C.A. & M. SIPPER. 1999. A fuzzy-genetic approach to breast cancer diagnosis. Artif. Intell. Med. **17:** 131–155.
46. PEÑA-REYES, C.A. & M. SIPPER. 2000. Evolutionary computation in medicine: an overview. Artif. Intell. Med. **19:** 1–23.
47. LENZ, G.R., H.M. NASH & S. JINDAL. 2000. Chemical ligands, genomics, and drug discovery. Drug Discovery Today **5:** 145–156.
48. DEAN, P.M. & E.D. ZANDERS. 2002. The use of chemical design tools to transform proteomics data into drug candidates. Biotechniques Suppl. **32:** S28–S33.
49. ZHENG, X.F. & T.F. CHAN. 2002. Chemical genomics: a systematic approach in biological research and drug discovery. Curr. Issues Mol. Biol. **4:** 33–43.
50. MCLEOD, H.L. & W.E. EVANS. 2001. Pharmacogenomics: unlocking the human genome for better drug therapy. Annu. Rev. Pharmacol. Toxicol. **41:** 101–121.
51. PEGG, S.C., J.J. HARESCO & I.D. KUNTZ. 2001. A genetic algorithm for structure-based *de novo* design. J. Comput. Aided Mol. Design **15:** 911–933.
52. TERFLOTH, L. & J. GASTEIGER. 2001. Neural networks and genetic algorithms in drug design. Drug Discovery Today **6**(suppl.): S102–S108.

New Developments in Cancer-Related Computational Statistics

SIMON ROSENFELD

Biometry Research Group, Division of Cancer Prevention, National Cancer Institute, National Institutes of Health, Department of Health and Human Services, Rockville, Maryland 20892, USA

ABSTRACT: A brief overview is presented of recently developed and currently emerging statistical and computational techniques that have been proved to be highly helpful in handling the avalanche of the new type of data generated by modern high-throughput technologies in experimental biology. The review, in no way comprehensive, focuses attention on Bayesian Networks, Hidden Markov Chain, and methods of chaotic dynamics for time-course genomic data; innovative methods in optimization and clustering; and multiple testing in the context of identification of differentially expressed genes.

KEYWORDS: Bayesian networks; expression profiles; microarray; multiple testing; hidden Markov chain; support vector machines; optimization

INTRODUCTION

In the recently formulated *challenge goal to eliminate suffering and death due to cancer by 2015*, NCI Director Dr. von Eschenbach emphasized the importance of the "seamless 3D approach" to cancer research, that is, efficient combination of discovery, development, and delivery. Each of these areas is now unthinkable without a broad involvement of powerful computational methodologies for data analysis and decision making. In recent years, bioinformatics has become an arena of active experimentation with innovative statistical tools utilizing immense computational power of modern computers. In this paper, we review several recently developed and currently emerging mathematical and statistical methodologies that have been shown to be highly promising in cancer-related bioinformatics.

BAYESIAN NETWORKS

Bayesian network (BN) is a model for representing uncertainty in knowledge. Uncertainty arises in a variety of situations such as uncertainty in the experts them-

Address for correspondence: Simon Rosenfeld, Biometry Research Group, Division of Cancer Prevention, National Cancer Institute, National Institutes of Health, Department of Health and Human Services, EPN 3136, 6130 Executive Boulevard, Rockville, MD 20892. Voice: 301-496-7748; fax: 301-402-0816.
sr212a@nih.gov

Ann. N.Y. Acad. Sci. 1020: 22–31 (2004). © 2004 New York Academy of Sciences.
doi: 10.1196/annals.1310.004

selves concerning their own knowledge, uncertainty inherent in the domain being modeled, uncertainty in the knowledge of an engineer trying to translate the knowledge, and just plain uncertainty as to the accuracy and actual availability of knowledge. BN uses probability theory to manage uncertainty by explicitly representing the conditional dependencies between the different knowledge components. This provides an intuitive graphical visualization of the knowledge including the interactions among the various sources of uncertainty.

In probabilistic reasoning, random variables (RV) are used to represent events and/or objects in the world. By making various instantiations to these RVs, we can model the current state of the world. Thus, this will involve computing joint probabilities of the given RVs. Unfortunately, the task is nearly impossible without additional information concerning relationships between the RVs. In order to simplify the problem, we consider the following chain rule decomposing the joint distribution of a complex event into the probabilities of simpler ones:

$$P(A_1,A_2,A_3,A_4,A_5) = P(A_1 | A_2,A_3,A_4,A_5)P(A_2 | A_3,A_4,A_5)P(A_3 | A_4,A_5)P(A_4 | A_5)P(A_5)$$

where $P(A_1,A_2,A_3,...)$ is the joint probability of the events $A_1,A_2,A_3,...$, and $P(A_1 | A_2,A_3,...)$ is a conditional probability of the event A_1 given that the events $A_2,A_3,...$, have actually taken place.

BN[1] takes this process further by making the important observation that certain RV pairs may become uncorrelated once information concerning some other RVs is known. More precisely, we may have the following independence condition:

$$P(A | C_1,...,C_n, U) = P(A | C_1,...,C_n)$$

for some collection of RVs named U. Intuitively, we can interpret this as saying that A is determined by $C_1,...,C_n$ regardless of U. Combined with the chain rule, these conditional independencies allow us to replace the terms in the chain rule with the smaller conditionals. There are two types of computations performed with BN: *belief updating* and *belief revision*. Belief updating is concerned with the computation of probabilities over RVs, while belief revision is concerned with finding the maximally probable global assignment. Belief revision can be used for modeling explanatory and diagnostic tasks.

BNs are well suited for handling heterogeneous information and may serve as a natural framework for translation of laboratory findings to bedside decision making. A promising implementation of BN was recently reported by Roberts *et al.*[2,3] Screening mammography is an effective method for detecting early breast cancer in asymptomatic women, even though as many as 75% of certain mammograms fall into indeterminate grades of radiological suspicion, prompting a follow-up breast biopsy. However, one would like to avoid recommending unnecessary biopsy not only because of risk of physical and psychological trauma, but also because biopsies may confound later mammographic findings by producing radiographic abnormalities. The BN model[2,3] implemented in the software package *MammoNet* represents a decision support tool to aid in evaluation of mammographic findings. The RVs are divided into three logical classes: demographic features, mammographic indications, and physical findings. Demographic features include such parameters as age, age of menarche, age of first live birth, and number of first-degree relatives with breast cancer. Mammographic indications include characteristics of calcifications, developing density, and architectural distortions. Physical findings consist of symptoms such as pain and nipple discharge. The next step in the model building is establishing causal relations between variables. Some of these relations are comparatively easy to formulate (e.g., breast cancer causes calcification, breast cancer causes pain, etc.). Others, such as relations between developing masses and calcification, are more difficult to formulate due to a lack of reliable information in the literature. In such cases, the probabilistic relations between variables are formulated using expert opinions. BN, in a nutshell, represents a set of probabilistic statements quantifying a priori information about the variables. Given an input query and a set of evidence formulas, the BN generator creates the structurally simplest network to compute the posterior probability of the outcome. The performance of the package *MammoNet* has been evaluated using the receiver operating characteristic (ROC) curves and it was found[2] that the BN outperforms the artificial neural network models and expert mammographers in similar tasks.

Further development of BN technique has been undertaken by Antal *et al.*[4] The two-step methodology consists of dual representation of the belief (Bayesian) networks and black-box regression models. At the first step, the belief network is used to elicit and represent the domain knowledge. At the next step, the belief network is transformed into an informative prior distribution for black-box models. At the last step, these prior distributions are used as a basis for the black-box methods such as logistic regression or artificial neural networks. The methodology has been applied to the medical classification task of discriminating between benign and malignant ovarian tumors. There are four categorical inputs (locularity, menopausal status, papillation, and bilaterality) and six continuous inputs (color score, resistance index, age, level of CA125, parity, and amount of ascites). The expert knowledge formalized in these parameters, after a proper assimilation within the BN, is used for the prediction of the only output parameter, the probability of pathology. The authors[4] report 12% misclassification rate and the ROC area under the curve as high as 0.905, which signify a tangible success on the current stage of methodology development.

TEMPORAL DYNAMICS OF EXPRESSION PROFILES

A general purpose in many time-course experiments is to characterize temporal patterns of gene expression. In principle, temporal profiling offers the possibility of observing the cellular mechanisms in action. Most of the traditional clustering approaches are based on the assumption that each gene-specific set of observations consists of independent identically distributed random values. This assumption does not hold in the time-course experiments, where each expression profile is probabilistically dependent on the previously observed profiles. Analysis of this type of observation is a traditional area of the multivariate time series analysis. However, similar to other problems in functional genomics, being under the "curse of dimensionality", there is a substantial difference with the classical multivariate time series analysis: the number of observed states of the time series is orders of magnitude smaller than the dimensions of the vectors characterizing these states. Independent dimensionality reduction in each of these vectors does not solve the problem because, generally speaking, different groups of genes may play a dominant role at different stages of temporal evolution. In order to overcome this fundamental obstacle, several distinct approaches are currently being developed.

The approach, combining clustering with explicit inclusion of temporal dynamics through autoregressive model fitting, has been suggested by Ramoni et al.[5] In this approach, the agglomerative clustering is applied to the entire time series in a step-up manner, producing the cluster-specific sets of average autoregressive coefficients. Once the procedure terminates, the autoregressive coefficients are reevaluated through the multivariate procedure within each cluster. The procedure has been applied to study the transcriptional response of human fibroblasts to serum. The study used the sequence of 13 two-dye cDNA arrays with 517 genes responding to treatment over the course of 24 hours. It has been shown that application of this methodology was able to successfully identify four different temporal behaviors, unlike the standard methods that merge all 517 genes into one cluster. Note that, contrary to the K-means or self-organizing maps (SOM) clustering procedures, no a priori assumptions about the number of clusters and/or their location in the parameter space are required.

Any parametric model-based approach invites routine criticism that the applicability of a model to the data at hand is usually unknown and difficult to verify, given a small number of samples usually available. For example, in the above-cited approach, the assumption that the time series are stationary, that is, that their statistical characteristics do not depend on time, plays an important role in estimating the autoregression coefficients. In particular, this assumption implies that applying a stationary random disturbance to the entire genome does not cause any permanent damage nor long-lasting changes, which may not be true for a living cell. On the other hand, this assumption is difficult to verify if only a short time series is available. This is why, in the absence of direct knowledge of underlying dynamics, the nonparametric approaches are perceived to be more attractive.

An attempt to overcome the above-mentioned limitations has been undertaken by Yuan et al.:[6] instead of a time series technique, a more general technique of hidden Markov model (HMM) has been utilized. In this model, a time-course behavior is governed by two independent probabilistic mechanisms: the conditional distributions at each time and the process describing the evolution of states over time. It is further assumed that the expression pattern (termed here as "state") for each gene can be described by a Markov chain, with a matrix of conditional probabilities (a.k.a. "transitional matrix") to be estimated from data. Generally speaking, this matrix has the size of the number of genes squared, thus making the computational burden insurmountable in any practical applications. In order to reduce dimensionality, one of the traditional approaches, such as those based on t test, is used to limit consideration to a comparatively small, but still fairly ample pool of the most significant genes. The authors[6] applied their methodology in three case studies and in each of them managed to find the significant genes that were not detected by other methods, but whose significance was subsequently validated by the Northern blot hybridization. The main lesson learned from this work is the fact that, despite an immense complexity of computations, the method proved to be feasible, thus promising valuable applications in functional genomics.

Both of the above reviewed approaches do not possess a natural facility to take into account a priori biological knowledge about the genomic mechanisms under consideration. A valuable framework for incorporating the previously accumulated structured knowledge into any current microarray data analysis is provided by databases produced by the Gene Ontology Consortium (http://www.geneontology.org/). Assimilating the newly generated data within the pool of previously established information creates vast new possibilities for data analysis and applications. An example of such a fruitful synergy is described in reference 7, where the relationships between gene expressions as functions of time and their involvement in a given biological process are analyzed. The biological knowledge expressed by Gene Ontology is used to generate a rule model associating the knowledge with minimal characteristic features of temporal gene expression profiles. This model allows learning and classification of multiple biological roles for each gene and can predict participation of genes in a biological process, even despite their contradictory behavior. This kind of methodology may prove to be pivotal for future developments by permitting a more focused experimental approach to elucidate the biological roles of genes.

The problem of visualization of temporal behavior in high-dimensional systems has been extensively studied in statistical mechanics and dynamics of chaotic systems.[8,9] Some of the ideas developed in these areas may be successfully transplanted into microarray data analysis. A common method for visualizing high-dimensional data is principal component analysis, where, instead of considering a complex behavior of 10,000 parameters simultaneously, we confine our attention to the first two or three principal components. A different approach has been suggested by Rifkin and Kim,[10] where visualization of temporal evolution in gene expressions is performed using the methods of chaotic dynamics. Suppose that there is a sequence of expression profiles $x_g(t)$, where g is the index of a gene and t is time. We select a set of fixed vectors v_m, $m = 1, \ldots, M$, in the state space of expression profiles and consider the scalar products $S_m(t) = v_m \cdot x(t)$. For each of these linear combinations, we form a 3D space consisting of $S_m(t)$, $S_m(t+1)$, and $S_m(t+2)$ and observe the 3D curves (trajectories) reflecting evolution of the expression profiles with time. At first glance, this kind of transformation seems too simplistic to produce any valuable result. However, as shown by the authors,[10] the possible patterns of behavior depicted by these trajectories are surprisingly diverse and may serve as the basis for classification, discrimination, and pattern recognition. An advantage of such an approach is that it maps the high-dimensional space into a set of simple low-dimensional patterns that are easy to parameterize and visualize. The authors have demonstrated their approach in action by applying it to the analysis of periodic processes in the *Saccharomyces cerevisiae* cell cycle. There is no doubt that this kind of approach may serve as a useful tool in any time-course data analysis.

COMPUTATIONAL ISSUES

Historically, cluster analysis was among the first methods applied to microarray data and still retains the reputation of a highly valuable tool. The cluster analysis has a long history of development with innumerable variations of its key components, and it seems surprising that it is still possible to augment it with anything substantially new. Support vector clustering (SVC) represents a new important development in cluster analysis. It takes advantage of support vector machines (SVM) and combines analytic flexibility with computational power. SVM implements the following idea: it maps the input vectors x into a suitably predefined high-dimensional feature space Z and, in this space, an optimal discriminating hyperplane is constructed.[11,12] Such a mapping into a high-dimensional space may consist, for example, in considering, together with the input vectors x, all the bilinear combinations of their components. At first sight, this mapping does not seem to make the problem simpler because now, instead of working in the input space with dimension ~10,000, we are dealing with the feature space with dimension ~50,000,000. The trick, however, is that, instead of the complex problem of nonlinear discrimination in the input space, we now face a much simpler problem of linear discriminant analysis that requires only the minimization of a simple quadratic function in the high-dimensional feature space. This paradoxical strategy proves to be highly computationally efficient. The advantage of SVM when applied to the microarray-based cancer research was expressively demonstrated by Brown et al.[13] and Ben-Hur et al.[14] The SVC methodology[14] takes a further step in this direction by performing cluster analysis in the high-dimensional feature space. The key idea underlying the clustering procedure is based on the observation that, given a pair of data points belonging to different clusters, any path connecting them must exit from the corresponding envelope spheres in the feature space. A unique advantage of SVC is that it can generate cluster boundaries of arbitrary shape, whereas other algorithms are most often limited to hyperellipsoids. In particular, SVC has the capacity to detect the clusters located within other clusters, which is completely impossible for the standard clustering procedures. The SVC methodology opens new vast possibilities in many areas of computational bioinformatics.

Optimization pervades all the areas of computational mathematics and statistics. Whatever methodology is being applied, whether it is neural network training or maximum likelihood estimation or cluster analysis, it usually ends up with minimization of a certain function in the space of parameters it depends on. Practical feasibility of many innovative procedures is directly dependent on the ability to solve the optimization problems. In bioinformatics, a necessity to work in a very high dimensional space imposes tough requirements on speed, memory, and accuracy of computations. Even slight progress in these areas produces a noticeable effect in the computational world. Development of the simultaneous perturbation stochastic approximation (SPSA) algorithm for stochastic optimization became a groundbreaking event in computational mathematics.[15,16] Generally speaking, there are many versions of stochastic optimization, and the idea that they all have in common is a random walk in the parameter space toward the minimum of the objective function. All the arguments of the objective function are perturbed randomly. The new set of parameters is accepted if the objective function is progressively decreasing. A great advantage of the stochastic optimization methods is that generally they do not require, contrary to the gradient methods, computation of the objective function gradients. Taking into account a high dimension of the parameter space and high computational cost of the gradient evaluation, this feature is very important and makes the convergence process comparatively fast, thus making the stochastic optimization the method of choice in many applications. The SPSA algorithm makes a fundamental step further in the same direction: instead of independent random perturbation of all the variables, at each step of minimization only one perturbation with carefully chosen parameters is used, regardless of the dimension of the parameter space. As a result, this algorithm converges $p/2$ times faster than the standard (gradient) optimization algorithms (p is the dimension of the parameter space). For example, in a typical case of artificial neural network (ANN) training with 200 parameters to be evaluated, it would mean 100 times acceleration. Another advantage of SPSA is that it is reasonably tolerable to noise in data. SPSA showed phenomenal effectiveness in high-dimensional problems and is especially useful for the training of ANN. There are numerous applications of SPSA in many areas including many medical applications.[17] However, so far, SPSA does not seem to have attracted much attention of the experts in bioinformatics and computational biology. It is our view that SPSA would make a tremendous impact on the effectiveness of solving computational problems in these areas of research.

MULTIPLE TESTING

As was nicely expressed by Page et al.,[18] a rapidly developing area of statistical bioinformatics requires both "playful creativity" and "scientific hard-mindedness". The above-reviewed techniques represent striking examples of fertile mathematical imagination, or "playful creativity". Even when supported by rigorous mathematical results, these techniques usually contain so many free tune-up parameters left to the investigator's discretion that a final result of the analysis may rarely be called completely objective or rigorously established. Mathematical statistics has always been leaning toward the "scientific hard-mindedness" in its attempt to formulate a problem in precisely defined terms and to follow mathematically faultless procedures. The problem of multiple testing is one such area where rigorous mathematical statistics, motivated by needs of functional genomics, is currently making rapid progress.

A central problem in microarray data analysis is the identification of differentially expressed genes. A conventional approach to solving this kind of problem in a univariate case would consist in formulating the null hypothesis of absence of differential expression followed by an attempt to reject this hypothesis using an appropriate test. A commonly accepted quantitative measure for characterizing the outcome of testing is the P value equal to the probability of committing the type I error, that is, rejecting the null hypothesis when in fact it is true. In the microarray context, it would mean declaring the gene differentially expressed when in fact it is not. If, for example, a P value is 0.01, then it would mean, roughly speaking, that in 99 cases our statement would be true if an experiment was repeated 100 times. This level of reliability seems sufficiently high for any practical purpose. However, this is not the case in the microarray experiments. Each microarray represents a set of 10,000 of such univariate experiments performed simultaneously; thus, if in each of them the probability to commit the type I error is only 0.01, then up to 100 genes would be declared differentially expressed, even when there is no difference between samples.

The problem of finding an appropriate generalization of the hypotheses testing procedures in the multidimensional case is addressed in the multiple testing theory.[19–23] There are a number of obstacles to finding such a generalization. First, the distributions of expression intensities, generally speaking, are not known a priori; therefore, the gene-specific P values cannot be computed based on any known distributions. In order to overcome this difficulty, the permutation distribution is used for computing the P values. Unfortunately, the idea of permutation is applicable only when a comparatively large number of replicates is available, say above 8, which is not always the case in practical situations. Second, the gene-specific test statistics, generally speaking, are not independent due to a tendency of genes to act in a concerted manner within the biological pathways. Ignoring this circumstance leads to decreasing the test power. There are two big groups of methods for controlling error rates in microarray experiments: the family-wide error rate (FWER) and the false-discovery error rate (FDR). FWER attempts to control the array-wide probability of type I error. Different approaches to FWER, such as Bonferroni, Hochberg, Holm, Sidak, minP, and maxT, reflect their different abilities to handle such features as correlation between the gene-specific test statistics, absence of parametric knowledge about their distributions, and computational efficiency.[20] FDR reflects a different philosophical view on the error control. Rather than controlling the family-wide probability of type I error, FDR estimates the proportion of falsely discovered genes among those that are declared significant. Transition from FWER to FDR reflects a fundamental paradigm shift that is rarely, to our best knowledge, discussed in the literature. FDR control assumes that it is admissible to commit a certain (presumably small) number of erroneous statements about the gene significance because any promising finding must be validated in an independent experimental setting. Figuratively speaking, in this framework of thinking, a statistician declines to take full responsibility for the data analysis, but provides a biologist with the best possible recommendations for a follow-up study. Quantification of FDR is better suited to the realities of the world of experimental biology. The simplest approach to FDR has been implemented in the method by Benjamini and Hochberg (BH/FDR) controlling the expected proportion of falsely discovered genes among those genes declared significant,[24] and was further refined for handling dependency between the test statistics by Benjamini and Yekutieli.[25] The drawback of the latter two approaches is that they do not control the actual proportion in any given microarray experiment, but only the expectation. Meanwhile, the variability of the sample FDRs may be intolerably high. It is our personal experience that the performance of the BH/FDR becomes very poor when the number of replicates is small and/or the levels of over-expression are not expected to be high. An attempt to overcome the drawbacks of BH/FDR is undertaken by Korn et al.,[19] where the procedure has been developed to control the actual, rather than expected, number of the falsely discovered genes. This procedure is highly computationally intensive and its actual usability in practical analysis is currently under investigation. It should be noted that existing methods of controlling FWER and FDR do not explicitly define an exact meaning of the notion of differential expression, leaving this definition to the biologist's responsibility. This means that it is tacitly recognized that the microarray experiment by itself is not expected to produce a final result of investigation into gene activity, but requires a priori knowledge for establishing feasible thresholds and a posteriori validation of findings. A comprehensive discussion of the current state of the art in multiple testing and its usability in practical analysis of expression arrays is presented in the report by Ge et al.[21] It is clear that, despite substantial progress and an avalanche of notable publications, a satisfactory solution to this important problem is still ahead.

CONCLUSIONS

Modern desktop or laptop computers are comparable in power with the most powerful supercomputers of the late 1980s. An easy widespread access to computational tools promotes a rapid proliferation of sophisticated mathematical techniques into the routine practice in every area of human knowledge. A brief review of methods presented here is just a glimpse of recent innovations in computational statistics directly related to bioinformatics and, more specifically, to cancer research. At first sight these methodologies may seem difficult to comprehend, especially for the researchers lacking rigorous mathematical and/or statistical training. However, it might be a timely reminder that only a decade ago the concept of cluster analysis was also often considered as highly abstract, but now is generally accepted as a fairly straightforward, if not simplistic, tool. It seems reasonable to expect that many of the emerging mathematical techniques currently undergoing experimental testing will become routine instruments of bioinformatics in the near future.

REFERENCES

1. PEARL, J. 1988. Probabilistic Reasoning in Intelligent Systems: Networks of Plausible Inference. Morgan Kaufmann. San Mateo, CA.
2. ROBERTS, L., C. KAHN & P. HADDAWAY. 1995. Development of a Bayesian Network for Diagnosis of Breast Cancer. IJCAI-95 Workshop on Building Probabilistic Networks. AI Palais de Congres. Montreal, Quebec, Canada.
3. KAHN, C., L. ROBERTS, K. SHAFFER & P. HADDAWAY. 1997. Construction of a Bayesian network for mammographic diagnosis of breast cancer. Comput. Biol. Med. 27(1): 19–29.
4. ANTAL, P., G. FANNES, D. TIMMERMAN et al. 2003. Bayesian applications of belief networks and multilayer perceptions for ovarian tumor classification with rejection. Artif. Intell. Med. 29(1–2): 39–60.
5. RAMONI, M., P. SEBASTIANI & I. KOHANE. 2002. Cluster analysis of gene expression dynamics. Proc. Natl. Acad. Sci. USA 99(14): 9121–9126.
6. YUAN, M., C. KENDZIORSKI, F. PARK et al. 2003. Hidden Markov models for microarray time course data in multiple biological conditions. Technical Report no. 178. Department of Biostatistics and Medical Informatics, University of Wisconsin.
7. LAGREID, A., T. HVIDSTEN, H. MIDELFART et al. 2003. Predicting gene ontology biological process from temporal gene expression patterns. Genome Res. 13: 965–979.
8. ABARBANEL, H. 1993. The analysis of observed chaotic systems. Rev. Mod. Phys. 65: 1331–1392.
9. TAKENS, F. 1984. Detection of strange attractors in turbulence. Lect. Notes Math. 898: 366.
10. RIFKIN, S. & J. KIM. 2002. Geometry of gene expression dynamics. Bioinformatics 18(9): 1176–1183.
11. VAPNIK, V. 1999. The Nature of Statistical Learning Theory. Springer Pub. New York.
12. FUREY, T., N. CRISTIANI, N. DUFFY et al. 2000. Support vector machine classification and validation of cancer tissue samples using microarray expression data. Bioinformatics 16(10): 906–914.
13. BROWN, M., W. GRUNDY, D. LIN et al. 2000. Knowledge-based analysis of microarray gene expression data by using support vector machines. Proc. Natl. Acad. Sci. USA 97(1): 262–267.
14. BEN-HUR, A., D. HORN, H. SIEGELMAN & V. VAPNIK. 2001. Support vector clustering. J. Mach. Learn. Res. 2: 125–137.
15. SPALL, J. 1998. Implementation of the simultaneous perturbation algorithm for stochastic optimization. IEEE Trans. Aerosp. Electronic Syst. 34: 817–823.
16. SPALL, J. 2000. Adaptive stochastic approximation by the simultaneous perturbation method. IEEE Trans. Autom. Control 45(10): 1839–1853.
17. GERENCSER, L., G. KOZMAN & Z. VAGO. 1998. SPSA for non-smooth optimization with application in ECG analysis. Proceedings of the 37th IEEE Conference on Decision and Control, Tampa, FL.
18. PAGE, G., J. EDWARDS, S. BARNES et al. 2003. A design and statistical perspective on microarray gene expression studies in nutrition: the need for playful creativity and scientific hard-mindedness. Nutrition 19: 997–1000.

19. KORN, E., J. TROENDLE, L. McSHANE & R. SIMON. 2001. Controlling the number of false discoveries: application to high-dimensional genomic data. NCI Technical Report no. 003.
20. DUDOIT, S., J. SHAFFER & J. BOLDRICK. 2003. Multiple hypothesis testing in microarray experiments. Stat. Sci. **18**(1): 71–103.
21. GE, Y., S. DUDOIT & T. SPEED. 2003. Resampling-based multiple testing for microarray data analysis. Test **12**(1): 1–77.
22. STOREY, J. 2002. A direct approach to false discovery rate. J. R. Stat. Soc. **B64**(3): 479–498.
23. STOREY, J. & R. TIBSHIRANI. 2003. Statistical significance for genome-wide studies. Proc. Natl. Acad. Sci. USA **100**(16): 9440–9445.
24. BENJAMINI, Y. & Y. HOCHBERG. 1995. Controlling the false discovery rate: a practical and powerful approach to multiple testing. J. R. Stat. Soc. **B57**: 289–300.
25. BENJAMINI, Y. & D. YEKUTIELI. 2001. The control of the false discovery rate in multiple testing under dependency. Ann. Stat. **29**(4): 1165–1188.

Bioinformatics Strategies for Translating Genome-Wide Expression Analyses into Clinically Useful Cancer Markers

DANIEL R. RHODES[a] AND ARUL M. CHINNAIYAN[a,b,c]

[a]Department of Pathology, [b]Department of Urology, and [c]Comprehensive Cancer Center, University of Michigan Medical School, Ann Arbor, Michigan 48109, USA

ABSTRACT: The DNA microarray has revolutionized cancer research. Now, scientists can obtain a genome-wide perspective of cancer gene expression. One potential application of this technology is the discovery of novel cancer bio-markers for more accurate diagnosis and prognosis, and potentially for the earlier detection of disease or the monitoring of treatment effectiveness. Because microarray experiments generate a tremendous amount of data and because the number of laboratories generating microarray data is rapidly growing, new bioinformatics strategies that promote the maximum utilization of such data are necessary. Here, we describe a method to validate multiple microarray data sets, a Web-based cancer microarray database for biomarker discovery, and methods for integrating gene ontology annotations with microarray data to improve candidate biomarker selection.

KEYWORDS: cancer; biomarkers; bioinformatics; meta-analysis; microarray

INTRODUCTION

Advances in DNA microarray technologies have led to an explosion of cancer gene expression profiling studies revealing a number of potential cancer markers: both tissue markers that may aid in more accurate diagnosis and prognosis, and potential serum markers that may aid in the early detection of cancer and in monitoring the effectiveness of therapy. The task of translating genome-wide expression data into clinically useful biomarkers poses many challenges, one being the selection of the most promising potential markers for future studies and another being the careful validation of markers on a large cohort of clinical samples. Because this validation process can be labor- and resource-intensive, the task of selecting candidate markers becomes very important. Furthermore, because a relatively small number of labora-tories are applying DNA microarray technology and generating genome-wide expres-sion data, the task of making gene expression data and analysis methods available to the cancer research community is equally important. With the rising flood of cancer

Address for correspondence: Arul M. Chinnaiyan, M.D., Ph.D., Assistant Professor of Pathology and Urology, Director of the Pathology Microarray Lab, Director of the Tissue/Informatics Core, University of Michigan Medical School, Department of Pathology, 1301 Catherine Street, MS1 Room 4237, Ann Arbor, MI 48109-0602. Voice: 734-936-1887; fax: 734-763-6476.
  arul@umich.edu

Ann. N.Y. Acad. Sci. 1020: 32–40 (2004). © 2004 New York Academy of Sciences.
doi: 10.1196/annals.1310.005

gene expression profiling data in the public domain, it is up to those in the field of bioinformatics to provide methods to evaluate, integrate, and make available genome-wide expression data. In this report, we will discuss bioinformatics strategies that we and others are employing to improve candidate marker selection and, ultimately, the translation of genome-wide expression analyses into clinically useful cancer markers (FIG. 1).

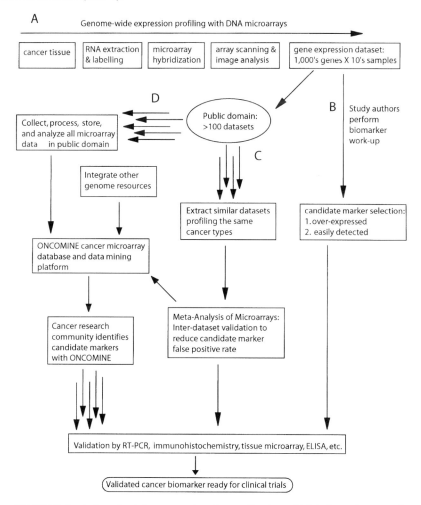

FIGURE 1. A flowchart demonstrating the application of bioinformatic strategies to the improved identification of candidate biomarkers from cancer genome-wide expression analyses. **(A)** The typical experimental procedure used to generate genome-wide expression data. **(B)** Study authors may attempt to identify and validate candidate biomarkers. **(C)** Microarray data in the public domain allows for multiple data set analysis strategies including meta-analysis of microarrays, a statistical method used to intervalidate data sets and thus reduce the candidate biomarker false-positive rate. **(D)** Furthermore, data in the public domain can be unified and made available to the cancer research community, as with the ONCOMINE cancer microarray database, so that more potential markers can be identified and validated.

MARKERS IDENTIFIED BY GENOME-WIDE EXPRESSION ANALYSIS

To date, more than 100 studies have profiled human cancer samples using DNA microarrays; however, only a fraction of these studies have demonstrated thorough validation of results and the development of clinically useful biomarkers (FIGS. 1A and 1B). Validation usually involves confirming that the protein product of a gene highly expressed in cancer is similarly overexpressed. This is necessary because most clinical tests involve measuring protein level, either by immunohistochemistry in the case of tissue biomarkers or by ELISA in the case of serum biomarkers. Furthermore, validation should be carried out on a large sample set to assure that the results can be generalized to the population of patients. This need has been addressed by the development of tissue microarrays, a technology that allows one to measure a protein's expression level in hundreds or thousands of clinical samples in a single assay.

An example of a cancer tissue marker discovered by genome-wide expression profiling and then validated by tissue microarray is alpha-methylacyl CoA racemase (AMACR), a protein specifically overexpressed in prostate cancer.[1] Multiple gene expression profiling studies,[2–5] as well as a meta-analysis,[6] found the *AMACR* gene transcript to be highly overexpressed in prostate cancer. Immunohistochemical analysis with tissue microarrays revealed that AMACR was similarly overexpressed at the protein level in 94 prostate cancer needle biopsy samples (97% sensitivity, 100% specificity). Studies are now under way evaluating the clinical utility of AMACR in uncertain diagnoses. Another example of a marker discovered in this manner is enhancer of *zeste homolog 2* (*EZH2*). *EZH2* gene transcript and protein were found to be highly expressed in metastatic prostate cancer[7] and, interestingly, were more highly expressed in tumors of patients with progressive disease. A follow-up study found that EZH2 protein level in conjunction with E-cadherin protein level significantly predicted disease recurrence following surgery in a multivariable model, which included other clinical and pathological prognostic variables.[8]

Genome-wide expression analyses have also been useful in identifying serum biomarkers that could potentially aid in the early detection of cancer. One study used microarrays to identify genes overexpressed in ovarian cancer.[9] They identified prostasin, a gene that encodes a protein thought to be secreted from cells, as one of the most highly expressed transcripts. Validation by ELISA confirmed that prostasin protein is at high levels in the serum of patients with ovarian cancer and that it may serve as a biomarker useful for the early detection of ovarian cancer (92% sensitivity, 94% specificity). Another example was the discovery of osteopontin as a potential serum biomarker for hepatocellular carcinoma.[10]

BIOINFORMATICS HURDLES SLOWING BIOMARKER DISCOVERY

While the examples highlighted in the previous section serve to illustrate the potential use of genome-wide expression data in the discovery of clinically important biomarkers, it is worth noting that these examples only represent a small minority of studies and that, in the majority of genome-wide analyses, little or no validation is performed. While the lack of validation is unfortunate, the data from these analyses are often made available to the public, so it is conceivable that those researchers interested in cancer biomarkers could further analyze published data to identify promising candidate markers for validation. This task presents a number of challenges, many of which are being addressed by the growing field of bioinformatics.

One challenge lies in coping with multiple data sets that have profiled similar cancer samples. While it is surely best to use these multiple data sets to validate one another so that the most promising candidate biomarkers can be identified, this task is challenging because microarray data exist on a variety of scales depending on the specific technological platform utilized as well as the experimental procedure. Usually, microarray data from independent laboratories are not thought to be directly comparable. Computational/statistical methods are being developed so that independent microarray data sets can be easily compared.

Another challenge lies simply in data availability and data exchange. While many genome-wide expression data sets are made freely available upon publication, the format that the data are stored in is often heterogeneous. Recently, standards have been developed for microarray data storage and exchange, designated Minimum Information about Microarray Experiments (MIAME).[11] These standards will likely facilitate use of public repositories and common data analysis tools. Multiple repositories that implement the MIAME standards are being developed, including Gene Expression Omnibus[12] and Array Express.[13] While these efforts are already beginning to prove fruitful, a mass of invaluable data in the public domain may not be deposited in these repositories. In order for these data sets to be utilized, they must be actively collected, which can be a daunting task.

A final challenge lies in microarray data analysis. This is a complex field requiring computational and statistical expertise. Moreover, because those most likely to translate genome-wide expression data into useful markers do not always possess such expertise, it is up to those in the field of bioinformatics to provide the tools necessary to analyze and visualize the data, as well as integrate the data with gene annotation resources.

META-ANALYSIS OF MICROARRAYS

While most cancer gene expression profiling studies claim to identify large sets of potential cancer markers, it is generally thought necessary to demonstrate independent experimental validations using techniques such as reverse transcriptase polymerase chain reaction (RT-PCR), Northern blots, or tissue microarrays before a gene (or a set of genes) is considered as a valid potential marker. Validation is necessary because microarray studies are known to generate falsely positive results for a number of reasons including random chance, experimental artifacts, sampling bias, cross-hybridization, etc.; therefore, it is commonplace to use the microarray as a screening tool and then to validate a few promising candidates for future study (FIGS. 1A and 1B). While this model has proved somewhat fruitful in identifying markers, it underutilizes the original microarray data set, often overlooking many other possible markers. It is likely that the best markers may have been missed or overlooked simply because of the challenge in validating many genes.

With the increasing number of publicly available gene expression data sets, we have proposed a meta-analysis of multiple data sets that addresses similar hypotheses in order to validate and statistically assess all positive results simultaneously (FIG. 1C).[6] While validating microarray data sets against one another does not offer the same confidence as validation by protein expression profiling with tissue microarrays, it does rid us of most of the causes of false positives and is sure to be void of artifacts of individual studies. Interstudy validation of microarray data sets poses unique challenges both statistically and computationally—for while the hypotheses in microarray studies are often similar (i.e., identify genes differentially expressed in cancer), individual investigators often use distinct protocols, microarray platforms, and analysis techniques, and additionally the raw gene expression measurements are often incomparable.

We developed a method, termed meta-analysis of microarrays, that compares statistical measures across studies instead of actual gene expression measurements—for while the actual expression measurements may have different meaning in different studies, P values generated for each study by a common statistical test are easily comparable. Our method begins by assigning P values to each gene in each study using the t statistic, and then the similarity of P values for each gene profiled is assessed using traditional meta-analysis methods combined with a simple correction for multiple hypothesis testing.

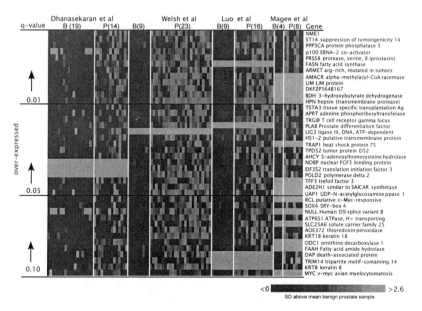

FIGURE 2. Meta-analysis of four prostate cancer gene expression data sets present in the public domain identifies *in silico* validated genes that are overexpressed in prostate cancer (P) relative to benign prostate (B). Each column represents an individual sample (number of samples is in parentheses) and each row represents a specific gene. Within each study, the data were normalized so that the mean expression level of the genes in the benign prostate specimens equaled zero and the standard deviation equaled one. Forty genes with the lowest meta-q value for overexpression are shown. Gray intensity level indicates degree of overexpression, while black indicates equal or lower expression than the mean benign sample (see scale).

The model was first implemented on four publicly available prostate cancer gene expression data sets generated by independent laboratories.[2–4,14] All four studies made comparisons between the gene expression profiles of clinically localized prostate cancer and benign prostate tissue, with the goal of identifying genes differentially expressed between the two sample groups. Two of the groups used spotted cDNA technology,[2,3] while two groups used commercial oligonucleotide-based technology.[4,14] As anticipated, a large group of genes, many more so than would be expected by chance, were significantly differentially expressed in multiple independent data sets, suggesting that they are truly differentially expressed, thus increasing the likelihood that they could serve as potential cancer markers. We found 50 genes to be reliably overexpressed and 103 genes to be reliably underexpressed in prostate cancer at a q value (i.e., meta-analysis measure of significance) of 0.10. FIGURE 2 displays the top 40 overexpressed genes. Several of the genes validated or commented on in the individual studies scored high in this analysis, including *hepsin*, *myc*, and *fatty acid synthase*, and *AMACR*, but importantly many genes that had not yet been validated scored equally high. In summary, our method for the meta-analysis of microarrays provided a statistical framework for interstudy validation, suggesting a new approach for dealing with multiple analogous microarray data sets.

We have recently extended our approach to a large compendium of public cancer microarray data sets, further defining cancer-type specific meta-profiles as well as generating meta-profiles common to multiple cancer types.[15]

THE AVAILABILITY AND INTEGRATION OF GENE EXPRESSION PROFILING DATA

In the previous section, we discussed the issues of microarray result reliability and statistical approaches for the validation of multiple analogous data sets. In this section, we will address the importance of data availability and the need for bioinformatics tools to make cancer gene expression data available and easily interpretable by the cancer research community. This issue is critical because only a fraction of laboratories are applying DNA microarrays to cancer genome-wide expression profiling, but the results from these experiments could be potentially useful to a large number of cancer researchers, both basic science and clinical. For most published microarray studies, which may comprise thousands of gene measurements across tens or hundreds of cancer specimens, the authors have usually presented one interpretation of their data and have reported on only a subset of genes that demonstrate their particular hypothesis. Furthermore, the focus is not always on developing novel cancer markers, so often times there is no validation or follow-up studies. This may be due to the fact that the researchers involved in cancer genomics are often interested in global patterns of gene expression and are not necessarily interested in translating gene expression profiles into novel cancer markers. For those interested in developing cancer markers, the complete microarray data sets are sometimes made available as supplementary data; however, even if that is the case, the data sets often sit as cryptic text files, stored and processed in an unsystematic manner, and thus difficult to interpret unless one has a fair amount of computational expertise. While the aforementioned standards and repositories have begun to ameliorate this problem, cancer microarray data will be most useful to clinical cancer researchers only when it is unified, logically analyzed, and made easily accessible.

To this end, we initiated an effort to systematically curate, analyze, and make available all public cancer microarray data via a Web-based database and data-mining platform, designated "ONCOMINE" (http://www.oncomine.org/)[16] (FIG. 1D). Our effort also includes centralizing gene annotation data from various genome resources to facilitate rapid interpretation of a gene's potential role in cancer. Furthermore, we have integrated microarray data analysis with other resources including gene ontology annotations and a therapeutic target database so that clinically interesting subsets of genes can be focused on. Currently, the ONCOMINE database houses 65 independent data sets comprising nearly 50 million gene expression measurements from more than 4700 microarray experiments. More than 100 differential expression analyses define the genes most over- and underexpressed in nearly every major cancer type as well as a number of clinical and pathology-based cancer subtypes. It is our hope that, by making these data easily accessible to the cancer research community, potential

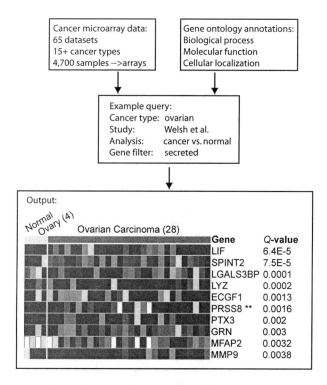

FIGURE 3. The ONCOMINE cancer microarray database used to identify potential serum biomarkers for ovarian cancer. By selecting an ovarian cancer data set generated by Welsh *et al.*,[5] specifying the differential expression analysis that identified genes overexpressed in ovarian cancer relative to normal ovary tissue, and then applying the "secreted" gene filter, which was derived from gene ontology cellular localization annotations, ONCOMINE provides a gene expression heatmap representation of the 10 genes that encode secreted proteins that are most highly expressed in ovarian cancer.

cancer markers will be easily identified, promoting an increase in validation studies and ultimately an increase in clinically useful markers.

Genes are usually considered as potential markers if they are differentially over-expressed in a particular cancer and their molecular function or localization suggests that they might be amenable to detection in serum or tissue. To provide a platform for the discovery of potential markers that are overexpressed in cancer, ONCOMINE is integrated with gene ontology annotations from the Gene Ontology Consortium.[17] Now, rather than investigating the function and localization of the genes most over-expressed in cancer to assess their potential as candidate markers, users can begin with only those genes whose function or localization suggests that they might be useful markers. For example, genes that encode proteins that are secreted from cancer cells would likely serve as candidate serum biomarkers. These include genes with a cellular localization annotation of extracellular space, extracellular matrix, or extra-cellular. With this ontology filter in place, for each cancer type in the ONCOMINE database, users can quickly identify genes that encode secreted products that are specifically overexpressed in a particular cancer. FIGURE 3 shows an analysis session as an example from ONCOMINE that highlights the genes that encode secreted proteins that are overexpressed in ovarian cancer relative to normal ovarian tissue.[5] Interestingly, the fifth most overexpressed gene, prostasin, was recently found to be a novel serum biomarker for ovarian cancer.[9] Perhaps the other genes that are more significantly overexpressed may serve as even better biomarkers. Further analysis with ONCOMINE revealed that prostasin is similarly overexpressed in prostate cancer, suggesting a broadened role for this marker.

A recent study by Welsh et al.[18] demonstrated a similar approach to serum marker discovery from genome-wide expression data. They used the gene ontology–based approach also used in ONCOMINE, as well as a sequence-based approach to define additional genes that encode secreted products. By integrating the secreted annota-tions defined by these two approaches with a large multicancer-type microarray data set, they were able to define 74 potential serum cancer markers. A number of the identified markers have been shown previously to be elevated in the serum of cancer patients, including kallikreins in ovarian carcinomas, gastrin releasing peptide in lung carcinomas, and alpha-fetoprotein in liver carcinomas. Other new markers were also identified and validated, including MIC-1, which by ELISA was found to be at high levels in a number of cancer types.

CONCLUSIONS

In summary, the field of bioinformatics is playing a critical role in beginning the translation of cancer gene expression profiling into useful cancer markers. Our approach for meta-analysis allows for the integration and validation of multiple microarray data sets so that the most promising candidate markers can be identified and followed up on. Furthermore, the development of ONCOMINE and other cancer microarray databases should promote the maximum utilization of cancer microarray data by the research community. Finally, integration of gene expression profiling data with other genome resources such as gene ontology annotations provides a powerful platform for marker discovery, as evidenced by the recent work of Welsh et al.[18]

REFERENCES

1. RUBIN, M.A. *et al.* 2002. Alpha-methylacyl coenzyme A racemase as a tissue biomarker for prostate cancer. JAMA **287:** 1662–1670.
2. DHANASEKARAN, S.M. *et al.* 2001. Delineation of prognostic biomarkers in prostate cancer. Nature **412:** 822 826.
3. LUO, J. *et al.* 2001. Human prostate cancer and benign prostatic hyperplasia: molecular dissection by gene expression profiling. Cancer Res. **61:** 4683–4688.
4. MAGEE, J.A. *et al.* 2001. Expression profiling reveals hepsin overexpression in prostate cancer. Cancer Res. **61:** 5692–5696.
5. WELSH, J.B. *et al.* 2001. Analysis of gene expression profiles in normal and neoplastic ovarian tissue samples identifies candidate molecular markers of epithelial ovarian cancer. Proc. Natl. Acad. Sci. USA **98:** 1176–1181.
6. RHODES, D.R. *et al.* 2002. Meta-analysis of microarrays: interstudy validation of gene expression profiles reveals pathway dysregulation in prostate cancer. Cancer Res. **62:** 4427 4433.
7. VARAMBALLY, S. *et al.* 2002. The polycomb group protein EZH2 is involved in progression of prostate cancer. Nature **419:** 624–629.
8. RHODES, D.R. *et al.* 2003. Multiplex biomarker approach for determining risk of prostate-specific antigen-defined recurrence of prostate cancer. J. Natl. Cancer Inst. **95:** 661–668.
9. MOK, S.C. *et al.* 2001. Prostasin, a potential serum marker for ovarian cancer: identification through microarray technology. J. Natl. Cancer Inst. **93:** 1458–1464.
10. YE, Q.H. *et al.* 2003. Predicting hepatitis B virus–positive metastatic hepatocellular carcinomas using gene expression profiling and supervised machine learning. Nat. Med. **9:** 416–423.
11. BRAZMA, A. *et al.* 2001. Minimum information about a microarray experiment (MIAME)—toward standards for microarray data. Nat. Genet. **29:** 365–371.
12. EDGAR, R., M. DOMRACHEV & A.E. LASH. 2002. Gene Expression Omnibus: NCBI gene expression and hybridization array data repository. Nucleic Acids Res. **30:** 207–210.
13. BRAZMA, A. *et al.* 2003. Array Express—a public repository for microarray gene expression data at the EBI. Nucleic Acids Res. **31:** 68–71.
14. WELSH, J.B. *et al.* 2001. Analysis of gene expression identifies candidate markers and pharmacological targets in prostate cancer. Cancer Res. **61:** 5974–5978.
15. RHODES, D.R. *et al.* 2004. Large-scale meta-analysis of cancer microarray data identifies common gene expression profiles of neoplastic transformation and progression. Under review.
16. RHODES, D.R. *et al.* 2004. ONCOMINE: a cancer microarray database and integrated data-mining platform. Neoplasia **6:** 1–6.
17. ASHBURNER, M. *et al.* 2000. Gene ontology: tool for the unification of biology—The Gene Ontology Consortium. Nat. Genet. **25:** 25–29.
18. WELSH, J.B. *et al.* 2003. Large-scale delineation of secreted protein biomarkers over-expressed in cancer tissue and serum. Proc. Natl. Acad. Sci. USA **100:** 3410–3415.

A Bayesian Hierarchical Model for the Analysis of Affymetrix Arrays

MAHLET G. TADESSE[a] AND JOSEPH G. IBRAHIM[b]

[a]*Department of Statistics, Texas A&M University, College Station, Texas 77843, USA*

[b]*Department of Biostatistics, University of North Carolina, Chapel Hill, North Carolina 27599, USA*

ABSTRACT: An area of active research in DNA microarray analysis focuses on identifying differentially expressed genes between normal and malignant tissues. The analysis is complicated by the presence of several unreliable expression readings. Here, we illustrate a methodology where the expression estimates are modeled as censored data and discriminating genes are selected using ANOVA-based criteria.

KEYWORDS: analysis of variance; censored data; DNA microarray; Gibbs sampling; gene expression; hierarchical priors

INTRODUCTION

DNA microarrays allow the parallel quantification of thousands of genes and may help improve our knowledge of cellular processes associated with different types of cancer. The identification of potential markers may help improve diagnosis and drug development efforts. The analysis, however, is complicated by the high dimensionality of the data and the sensitivity limits of the technology. Here, we address the latter issue in the context of the Affymetrix Hu6800 GeneChip arrays and use selection criteria based on analysis of variance to identify genes with distinctive patterns across different tissue types. The details of the methodology are given in reference 1.

In the next section, we give a brief description of Hu6800 arrays and the resulting data set. The third section motivates the problem of identifying differentially expressed genes and discusses the issue of quantification limits. In the fourth section, we summarize the methodology we have developed. We apply the method to the popular leukemia data set of Golub *et al.*[2] in the final section.

DESCRIPTION OF DATA FROM Hu6800 GENECHIP ARRAY

The GeneChip high-density arrays are made using light-directed *in situ* synthesis of short oligonucleotide sequences on a small glass chip. The Affymetrix Hu6800

Address for correspondence: Mahlet G. Tadesse, Department of Statistics, Texas A&M University, TAMU 3143, College Station, TX 77843-3143. Voice: 979-845-8883; fax: 979-845-3144.

mtadesse@stat.tamu.edu

Ann. N.Y. Acad. Sci. 1020: 41–48 (2004). © 2004 New York Academy of Sciences.
doi: 10.1196/annals.1310.006

arrays contain 7129 probe sets. Each probe set consists of 16–20 probe pairs of *perfect match* (PM) and *mismatch* (MM) oligonucleotide probes of length 25. The former are designed to be complementary to a fragment of the target sequence and the latter differ by a single base at the 13th position. The Affymetrix Microarray Suite 4.0 (MAS 4.0) software uses the *average difference* (AD) of PM MM intensities within a probe set to indicate the relative abundance of a transcript. Along with this expression estimate, the software provides an *absolute call* of *present, marginal,* or *absent. Present* indicates a gene designated by the algorithm as being expressed with an adequate degree of reliability. *Marginal* corresponds to a low hybridization assay. An *absent* call does not necessarily mean that the transcript is absent, but that the hybridization assay for the gene is unreliable.

The data from a microarray experiment form a $p \times n$ matrix, where the rows correspond to the expression readings associated with the p probe sets on the array and n is the sample size. The samples are collected from different tissues and, in some cases, different experimental conditions. The arrays are subject to several non-biological sources of variation that need to be reduced before further analysis. Several normalization procedures have been proposed to address this problem.[3]

MOTIVATION

In cancer research, there is often interest in identifying differentially expressed genes between normal and malignant tissues or between different subtypes of a particular malignancy. This may help identify markers for accurately diagnosing a disease without using invasive procedures. These markers may also be used to stratify patients into different risk groups and accordingly choose the appropriate treatment strategy for each individual. Various procedures have been proposed to this end. For example, Golub et al.[2] describe a selection rule to locate genes that discriminate between acute lymphoblastic and acute myeloid leukemia. Parametric methods have also received attention and have provided promising results in characterizing gene expression patterns. For example, Newton et al.[4] modeled the gene expression levels as gamma variables and used the posterior odds of change at each spot to assess differential expression. In reference 1, we have proposed two gene selection criteria based on contrasts of the interaction terms from an analysis of variance model. We describe this method in the next section.

A problem often swept under the rug in microarray data analysis relates to the quantification limits of the technology. Hu6800 GeneChip arrays, for instance, do not reliably quantify low and very high levels of expression. These problems are respectively due to sensitivity limits and spot saturation. The standard methods of analysis omit from the analysis genes whose transcripts are beyond the detection limits. As described in the previous section, processing of the image array with the MAS 4.0 software yields both expression estimates and an *absolute call* for each probe set. These calls are often used to filter genes. For example, genes not classified as *present* would be excluded from the analysis. This leads to the removal of many genes on the threshold of detection. This is problematic since some important mRNAs that may cause significant changes inside cells often have low total abundance. Another common practice is to consider genes whose transcripts are below the detection limits to be nonexpressed. Both approaches are suboptimal. The former may throw away potentially valuable data and the latter may underestimate the actual expression levels. We have proposed accounting for expression readings that are beyond the limits of reliable detection by modeling them as censored data.

METHODOLOGY

In microarray experiments, samples collected from different groups are often examined to evaluate differences in their gene expression patterns. The variation in the data can thus be assumed to arise from the effects of genes, tissue types, and their interactions. As suggested by Kerr and Churchill,[5] analysis of variance (ANOVA) is therefore a natural model for these data. Its validity, however, relies on a normality assumption that may not be justified on the raw scale.

Data Transformation

The Box-Cox[6] transformation is a particularly useful family of transformations that can be investigated to render the data close to normal. This transformation is defined as follows:

$$m(x) = \begin{cases} \dfrac{x^{\lambda} - 1}{\lambda} & \text{if } \lambda \neq 0 \\ \log(x) & \text{if } \lambda = 0 \end{cases} \tag{1}$$

where x is the random variable and λ is the transformation parameter. The Box-Cox transformation encompasses many commonly used transformations, including the log-transformation, which is popular in microarray analyses. The optimal choice of λ corresponds to the value that results in the highest correlation between the transformed data and quantiles of the standard normal density.

Model

Let $m(x_{jki})$ denote the transformed gene expression level for tissue type j ($j = 1, \ldots, J$), gene k ($k = 1, \ldots, p$), and array i ($i = 1, \ldots, n_j$). We assume that the data are randomly scattered around an established mean, which can further be decomposed as a linear combination of tissue-type effect (α_j), gene effect (β_k), and gene-tissue interactions (γ_{jk}):

$$m(x_{jki}) = \mu_{jk} + \varepsilon_{jki}, \qquad \varepsilon_{jki} \sim N(0, \sigma^2),$$

$$\mu_{jk} = \alpha_j + \beta_k + \gamma_{jk}. \tag{2}$$

Due to the quantification limits of the technology, low and high values of x_{jki} are not reliably estimated. We model these as censored data:

$$\begin{cases} y_{jki} = m(\min\{\max(x_{jki}, c_l), c_r\}) \\ l_{jki} = I\{x_{jkl} \leq c_l\} \\ r_{jki} = I\{x_{jki} \geq c_r\} \end{cases} \tag{3}$$

where l_{jki} and r_{jki} are censoring indicators taking value 1 if the corresponding expression reading is beyond the limits of detection.

The likelihood function is then given by

$$
L(\theta|D) = \prod_{j=1}^{i} \prod_{i=1}^{n_i} \prod_{k=1}^{p} \left[\Phi\left\{ \frac{y_{jki} - (\alpha_j + \beta_k + \gamma_{jk})}{\sigma} \right\} \right]^{l_{jki}}
$$

$$
\times \left(\frac{1}{\sqrt{2\pi\sigma^2}} \exp\left[-\frac{1}{2}\left\{ \frac{y_{jki} - (\alpha_j + \beta_k + \gamma_{jk})}{\sigma} \right\}^2 \right] \right)^{(1 - l_{jki})(1 - r_{jki})} \tag{4}
$$

$$
\times \left[1 - \Phi\left\{ \frac{y_{jki} - (\alpha_j + \beta_k + \gamma_{jk})}{\sigma} \right\} \right]^{r_{jki}}.
$$

Model Fitting

We specify hierarchical priors to induce correlation between gene effects as well as between tissue types for a given gene. For example, we assume that the gene effects follow a common normal distribution and the prior mean, in turn, is normally distributed:

$$
\beta_k | \beta_0, \sigma_\beta^2 \sim N(\beta_0, \sigma_\beta^2)
$$

$$
\beta_0 | b_0, v_\beta^2 \sim N(b_0, v_\beta^2). \tag{5}
$$

This leads to a prior correlation between genes k and k':

$$
\left(\begin{matrix} \beta_k \\ \beta_{k'} \end{matrix} \middle| (b_0, \sigma_\beta^2, v_\beta^2) \right) \sim N\left(\begin{bmatrix} b_0 \\ b_0 \end{bmatrix}, \begin{bmatrix} v_\beta^2 + \sigma_\beta^2 & v_\beta^2 \\ v_\beta^2 & v_\beta^2 + \sigma_\beta^2 \end{bmatrix} \right) \tag{6}
$$

$$
\Rightarrow \mathrm{corr}(\beta_k, \beta_{k'} | b_0, \sigma_\beta^2, v_\beta^2) = \frac{v_\beta^2}{\sigma_\beta^2 + v_\beta^2}
$$

which is an increasing function of the hyperprior variance v_β^2:

$$
\mathrm{corr}(\beta_k, \beta_{k'} | b_0, \sigma_\beta^2, v_\beta^2) \to 1 \text{ as } \sigma_\beta^2 \to 0 \text{ or } v_\beta^2 \to \infty.
$$

Thus, the prior correlation between gene effects can be made stronger by specifying a large value for v_β^2. The structure of the hierarchical model leads to a constant pairwise correlation. In reality, however, some genes may be acting independently or some may have negative correlations. This assumption merely represents the fact that the majority of genes will not be involved in the biological process under consideration and is a way of shrinking their posterior values toward a common value.

In the two-way ANOVA model, $y_{jki} = \alpha_j + \beta_k + \gamma_{jk} + \varepsilon_{jki}$, the data depend on the model parameters, α_j, β_k, and γ_{jk}, only through the mean $\mu_{jk} = \alpha_j + \beta_k + \gamma_{jk}$, and the map from μ_{jk} to $(\alpha_j, \beta_k, \gamma_{jk})$ is not one-to-one. The likelihood therefore does not identify these parameters. It can only identify functions of the means. Gelfand and Sahu[7] have shown that nonidentifiability does not preclude Bayesian inference as long as proper and suitably informative priors are defined. Since the strength of the prior information is controlled by the magnitude of the hyperprior variance, its specification needs to be carefully considered when attempting to draw inference on parameters that are not functions of the mean. We refer the reader to reference 1 for more details on the prior elicitation and issues of posterior propriety and model identifiability. Samples from the joint posterior distributions are drawn using Gibbs sampling. The full conditional of the model parameters do not have closed form and are not log-concave and we make use of the adaptive rejection Metropolis algorithm.[8]

Gene Selection Criteria

The interaction effects, γ_{jk}, capture differences in expression that are due to specific gene and tissue type combinations. We have proposed two selection criteria to evaluate the importance of gene k in distinguishing tissue types j and j':

$$\xi_k = \gamma_{j'k} - \gamma_{jk} - \gamma_{jr} + \gamma_{j'r} \tag{7}$$

$$\eta_k = \gamma_{j'k} - \gamma_{jk}. \tag{8}$$

Each criterion has its pros and cons. In ξ_k, the term $\gamma_{j'r} - \gamma_{jr}$ is not of interest and has to be chosen near 0. Its inclusion is needed to define a contrast in the interaction space, that is, a function of means. Posterior inference on ξ_k can therefore be drawn using weakly informative priors for all model parameters. We refer to gene r as the reference gene against which each gene k ($k = 1, \ldots, p$) is compared. With η_k, there are no extraneous parameters that complicate its interpretation. This criterion, however, does not define a contrast in the usual sense of linear models as it is not a function of means. A carefully chosen set of priors that strike a middle ground between too informative and insufficiently informative are thus needed and this requires simulation work.

Selection of differentially expressed genes is then performed based on the credible intervals. Gene k is selected if its $(1 - \lambda)\%$ credible interval for ξ_k or η_k does not contain 0.

DATA ANALYSIS

We now illustrate the methodology using the publicly available leukemia data set of Golub et al.[2] We used the training data set of 38 bone marrow samples for analysis. These consist of 27 acute lymphoblastic leukemia (ALL) and 11 acute myeloid leukemia (AML) specimens. RNA prepared from the bone marrow mononuclear cells were hybridized to the Hu6800 GeneChip arrays.

The AD values of the PM and MM probe intensities derived by the MAS 4.0 software were used to indicate transcript abundance. AD values less than $c_l = 20$ and

TABLE 1. Genes identified to be differentially expressed between AML and ALL

Probe set	GenBank	Gene Name	ξ_k	HPD
D10495_at	D10495	protein kinase C	2.35	(0.06, 4.64)
D87433_at	D87433	KIAA0246 protein	2.75	(0.33, 5.17)
D88422_at	D88422	cystatin A	2.70	(0.38, 5.03)
HG2724-HT2820_at	S62138	translocation breakpoint	2.55	(0.22, 4.88)
J04615_at	J04615	small nuclear ribonucleoprotein	-2.36	(-4.72, -0.01)
L33930_s_at	L33930	CD24 antigen	-2.80	(-5.19, -0.41)
M16336_s_at	M16336	T11 CD2 antigen	-2.85	(-5.58, -0.11)
M19507_at	M19507	myeloperoxidase	3.36	(0.93, 5.79)
M20203_s_at	M20203	neutrophil elastase	3.94	(1.19, 6.69)
M21904_at	M21904	4F2HC antigen	2.40	(0.04, 4.77)
M27783_s_at	M27783	neutrophil elastase	3.17	(0.86, 5.48)
M27891_at	M27891	cystatin C	4.21	(1.77, 6.65)
M28130_rna1_s_at	M28130	interleukin 8	3.82	(1.46, 6.18)
M30703_s_at	M30703	amphiregulin	2.63	(0.28, 4.98)
M31551_s_at	M31551	urokinase inhibitor (PAI-2)	3.07	(0.34, 5.80)
M57710_at	M57710	Epsilon-BP IgE-binding protein	3.14	(0.80, 5.47)
M57731_s_at	M57731	GRO2 oncogene	3.23	(0.85, 5.62)
M63438_s_at	M63438	Ig rearranged gamma chain	2.99	(0.70, 5.28)
M72885_rna1_s_at	M72885	GOS2 gene	2.94	(0.50, 5.40)
M83652_s_at	M83652	properdin	2.83	(0.40, 5.25)
M83667_rna1_s_at	M83667	NF-IL6-beta protein mRNA	3.75	(1.27, 6.23)
M84526_at	M84526	adipsin/complement factor D	5.21	(2.50, 7.91)
M86752_at	M86752	transformation sensitive protein	-2.56	(-5.01, -0.11)
M87789_s_at	M87789	hybridoma H210	2.63	(0.30, 4.96)
M96326_rna1_at	M96326	azurocidin	2.49	(0.08, 4.89)
U05255_s_at	U05255	glycophorin B	2.71	(0.33, 5.09)
U05259_rna1_at	U05259	MB-1 gene	-2.54	(-4.87, -0.22)
U05572_s_at	U05572	mannosidase	2.58	(0.01, 5.14)
U41813_at	U41813	homeo box A9	2.70	(0.22, 5.19)
U46499_at	U46499	MGST1 gene	2.53	(0.24, 4.82)
U60644_at	U60644	HU-K4 mRNA	2.58	(0.26, 4.89)
U70663_at	U70663	hEZF	2.80	(0.04, 5.56)
U85767_at	U85767	MPIF-1	2.46	(0.15, 4.77)
U89922_s_at	U89922	lymphotoxin beta	-2.87	(-5.42, -0.31)
X05908_at	X05908	lipocortin	2.75	(0.31, 5.19)
X52056_at	X52056	spi-1 proto-oncogene	2.84	(0.41, 5.27)
X64072_s_at	X64072	antigen CD18	2.39	(0.02, 4.77)
X82240_rna1_at	X82240	T-cell leukemia/lymphoma 1	-4.44	(-7.46, -1.42)
X95735_at	X95735	zyxin	2.60	(0.22, 4.98)
Y00339_s_at	Y00339	carbonic anhydrase II	2.89	(0.46, 5.32)
Y00787_s_at	Y00787	MDNCF	2.94	(0.45, 5.42)
Z83821_cds2_at	Z83821	aminolevulinate	2.37	(0.05, 4.70)

those above $c_r = 10,000$ were deemed censored. These thresholds are somewhat arbitrary, but have previously been used by several authors.[9] Probe sets that have unreliable expression readings in all the samples for one group were removed. This left us with 6107 probe sets for analysis.

We fitted the model described in the subsection above entitled "MODEL". The hyperprior means were set to 0 and the hyperprior variances were chosen to yield prior correlations of order 10^{-2}. We ran simulations with varying hyperprior variances to determine the appropriate ranges in controlling the strength of the prior information. For the ξ criterion, the hyperprior variances were set to 1000, a value that led to weakly informative priors. For the η criterion, the variances were set to 10, a value that yielded moderately informative priors. We used 2000 sweeps for burn-in and 10,000 iterations for the main run. For each criterion, a probe set was identified as differentially expressed if the $(1 - 10^{-6})\%$ credible interval did not contain 0. The choice of this level is arbitrary, but this magnitude ensures that we are pretty conservative in our selection.

We identified 42 differentially expressed genes between ALL and AML. These are listed in TABLE 1. Some of these match the ones selected by Golub et al.[2] MB-1, for example, was common to both results. This gene encodes cell surface proteins and has been demonstrated to be useful in distinguishing lymphoid from myeloid lineage cells. We also identified the zyxin gene, which has been shown to encode a LIM domain protein important in cell adhesion in fibroblasts, and HOXA9 oncogene, which is related to cancer pathogenesis.

Our analysis also picked genes that were not among the 50-gene list of Golub et al.[2] Some of these have known association with leukemia. For example, we picked T11 and 4F2HC antigens, which are cell surface molecules involved in T lymphocyte activation. We also selected neutrophil elastase, azurocidin, and myeloperoxidase, which are regulated during hematopoietic differentiation and are believed to promote cell-specific expression in the monocyte-myelocyte lineage.[10] Another interesting gene selected by our model is amphiregulin, which inhibits the growth of certain aggressive carcinoma cell lines and is localized to chromosomal region 4q13–4q21, a common breakpoint for ALL.[11] We also found TCL1 to discriminate between the two classes. This gene is preferentially expressed early in T and B lymphocyte differentiation, and the TCL1 locus is involved in chromosomal translocations and inversions with one of the T cell receptor loci in human T cell leukemias and lymphomas.[12]

REFERENCES

1. TADESSE, M.G., J. IBRAHIM & G. MUTTER. 2003. Identification of differentially expressed genes in high-density oligonucleotide arrays accounting for the quantification limits of the technology. Biometrics **59**: 542–554.
2. GOLUB, T.R., D. SLONIM, P. TAMAYO et al. 1999. Molecular classification of cancer: class discovery and class prediction by gene expression monitoring. Science **286**: 531–537.
3. BOLSTAD, B.M., R. IRIZARRY, M. ASTRAND & T. SPEED. 2003. A comparison of normalization methods for high density oligonucleotide array data based on bias and variance. Bioinformatics **19**: 185–193.
4. NEWTON, M.A., C. KENDZIORSKI, C. RICHMOND et al. 2001. On differential variability of expression ratios: improving statistical inference about gene expression changes from microarray data. J. Comput. Biol. **8**: 37–52.
5. KERR, M. & G. CHURCHILL. 2000. Experimental design for gene expression microarrays. Biostatistics **2**: 183–201.
6. BOX, G.E.P. & D. COX. 1964. An Analysis of Transformations. J. R. Stat. Soc. **B26**: 211–252.
7. GELFAND, A. & S. SAHU. 1999. Identifiability, improper priors, and Gibbs sampling for generalized linear models. J. Am. Stat. Assoc. **94**: 247–253.
8. GILKS, W. & P. WILD. 1992. Adaptive rejection sampling for Gibbs sampling. Appl. Stat. **41**: 337–348.
9. MUTTER, G., J. BAAK, J. FITZGERALD et al. 2001. Global expression changes of constitutive and hormonally regulated genes during endometrial neoplastic transformation. Gynecol. Oncol. **83**: 177–185.
10. ZIMMER, M., R. MEDCALF, T. FINK et al. 1992. Three human elastase-like genes coordinately expressed in the myelomonocyte lineage are organized as a single genetic locus on 19pter. Proc. Natl. Acad. Sci. USA **89**: 8215–8219.

11. PLOWMAN, G.D., J. GREEN, V. McDONALD *et al.* 1990. The amphiregulin gene encodes a novel epidermal growth factor–related protein with tumor inhibitory activity. Mol. Cell. Biol. **10:** 1969–1981.
12. VIRGILIO, L., M. NARDUCCI, M. ISOBE *et al.* 1994. Identification of the TCL1 gene involved in T-cell malignancies. Proc. Natl. Acad. Sci. USA **91:** 12530–12534.

Diagnostic Classification of Cancer Using DNA Microarrays and Artificial Intelligence

BRADEN T. GREER AND JAVED KHAN

Advanced Technology Center, National Cancer Institute, National Institutes of Health, Gaithersburg, Maryland 20877, USA

ABSTRACT: The application of artificial intelligence (AI) to microarray data has been receiving much attention in recent years because of the possibility of automated diagnosis in the near future. Studies have been published predicting tumor type, estrogen receptor status, and prognosis using a variety of AI algorithms. The performance of intelligent computing decisions based on gene expression signatures is in some cases comparable to or better than the current clinical decision schemas. The goal of these tools is not to make clinicians obsolete, but rather to give clinicians one more tool in their armamentarium to accurately diagnose and hence better treat cancer patients. Several such applications are summarized in this chapter, and some of the common pitfalls are noted.

KEYWORDS: artificial neural networks; support vector machines; artificial intelligence; microarray

INTRODUCTION

The widespread applications of cDNA and oligonucleotide microarrays, with whole-genome expression scanning at >40,000 clones in a single experiment, have heralded a new era of molecular genomics and, at the same time, are generating vast amounts of data. There is promise of accurate diagnosis and prognosis, identification of therapeutic targets, characterization of yet unknown genes, and personalized chemotherapy guided by molecular expression signatures. Classification based on gene expression signatures continues to be challenging in part due to the varied microarray platforms, labeling methods, scanners, image analysis tools, as well as classification algorithms currently available. Huge strides have been made over the past few years to increase the quantity of clones printed on an array, and the quality of RNA extraction, amplification, hybridization, and cDNA printing. Additionally, an ever-increasing array of algorithms has been reported to analyze the data produced from these high-quality, dense arrays.

Artificial intelligence (AI) is the term used to describe the ability of a computer or machine to perform activities or make decisions that normally require human

Address for correspondence: Javed Khan, Advanced Technology Center, National Cancer Institute, National Institutes of Health, Room 134F, 8717 Grovemont Circle, Gaithersburg, MD 20877. Voice: 301-435-2937; fax: 301-480-0314.
khanjav@mail.nih.gov

Ann. N.Y. Acad. Sci. 1020: 49–66 (2004). © 2004 New York Academy of Sciences.
doi: 10.1196/annals.1310.007

TABLE 1. Examples of unsupervised, supervised, and supervised learning data analysis methods

Unsupervised	Supervised	Supervised learning
k-means	t test	ANN
Self-organizing maps	ANOVA	SVM
Hierarchical clustering	Golub	
KNN	WGA	
PCA	Wilcoxon	
MDS	Kruskal-Wallis	
Reshuffling	TNoM	

intelligence. AI has been successfully applied to problems ranging from distinguishing four types of small round blue-cell tumors[1] to predicting estrogen receptor status in breast cancer[2] and a host of other applications,[3–8] several of which will be detailed later in this chapter. AI affords many significant benefits over its simplistic clustering counterparts such as hierarchical clustering, k-means clustering, and traditional statistical methods.

CLUSTERING VERSUS MACHINE LEARNING

Simple unsupervised clustering methods such as hierarchical clustering, principal component analysis (PCA), and multidimensional scaling (MDS) allow the visualization of data for the purpose of class discovery, or finding hitherto unknown relationships between samples or genes. On the other hand, supervised methods (see TABLE 1) allow for class prediction and are useful tools that can cluster data sets into meaningful groups and identify genes using a priori knowledge of the data such as stage, diagnosis, tissue type, etc. (see refs. 9 and 10 for good reviews). AI methods such as artificial neural networks (ANNs) or support vector machines (SVMs) are highly specialized forms of supervised clustering. Generally, simple clustering methods weight each input feature (or gene) the same, while ANNs and SVMs have the ability to weight input features according to their relevance to the classification scheme as determined through the learning process. The simpler methods cluster samples based on the summation of all of the inputs, while ANNs and SVMs cluster samples based on the collective effect of all of the input features. In addition, while most of the simpler methods are linear, ANNs and SVMs can learn nonlinear features of the input data. In most of the simpler clustering methods, either a sample belongs to a cluster or it doesn't; in contrast, in ANNs and SVMs, a continuous variable (i.e., an average vote) predicts whether or not a sample belongs to a particular cluster. This gives the ANN or SVM the freedom to conclude that a sample does not belong to any of the known classes if its vote lies too close to the decision boundary. This is advantageous, for example, if in a set of blinded test samples there exist samples that belong to none of the known categories and have been added to determine the specificity of the network.[1] Another limitation of most of the nonlearning methods is the way they treat more than two classification groups: in a one-verse-all manner. ANNs (but not SVMs) can simultaneously classify a sample set with more than two a priori groups directly without having to resort to a one-verse-all method. For the rest of the chapter, we will turn our attention to the technical aspects and application of two particular forms of machine learning: feed-forward ANNs and feed-forward SVMs.

ARTIFICIAL NEURAL NETWORKS

ANNs are computer algorithms that model mammalian systems of decision making using the mammalian neuron as a fundamental unit. If one thinks of "the brain [as] a complex, nonlinear, and parallel computer (information processing system)",[11] then it is logical to want to mimic the brain's capacity to learn from experience and make decisions. A neuron's ability to respond to experiences and hard-wire itself accordingly, thus adapting to its local environment, is commonly referred to as the *plasticity* of the brain.

A neural network is a massively parallel distributed processor made up of simple processing units, which has a natural propensity for storing experiential knowledge and making it available for use. It resembles the brain in two respects:

(1) knowledge is acquired by the network from its environment through a learning process;
(2) interneuron connection strengths, known as synaptic weights, are used to store the acquired knowledge.[11]

Neural networks are powerful because of their massively parallel, distributed structure and ability to learn and generalize. *Generalization* is the ability of a neural network to predict an input that was not used for training.[11] Generalization is vital to the utility of a neural network. If generalization is not possible, then AI has done little more than put known groups of samples into their corresponding groups. In this way, it offers little more than simple hierarchical or *k*-means clustering. Several properties of neural networks make them particularly powerful for the study of microarray data. The nonlinearity property of a neural network allows it to learn and adapt to nonlinear signals. This is important if the underlying signal is nonlinear, that is, the effect of one gene on another may be in a nonlinear fashion due to a positive feedback loop via a particular protein or transcriptional regulator. Input-output mapping refers to a neural network's ability to modify its synaptic weights through observing a set of training samples to minimize the error between the input classes and the predicted output classes. The concepts of *adaptivity* and *error-minimization* are what make this input-output mapping possible.

A special form of feed-forward machine learning called support vector machines (SVMs) has some interesting differences from feed-forward ANNs. In essence, the goal of an SVM is to calculate the hyperplane in *n*-dimensional feature space that optimally separates two groups of samples. Feature space is a mapping of the original data to a higher dimensional space. A sample is classified based on where it lies in relation to the hyperplane. When more than two classes are being examined, SVMs employ a one-verse-all strategy in conjunction with the hyperplane. In addition, the robustness of classification can be determined, in part, by the distance between each sample and the hyperplane in *n*-dimensional space. It has been said that SVMs can overcome the "curse of dimensionality". This is the unfavorable situation where the number of tunable parameters is much larger than the number of training samples and can lead to overfitting of the data and thus a nongeneralizable classifier. Both SVMs and ANNs have been used in various contexts for pattern recognition, including imaging, ECG, and biometric pattern recognition (e.g., voice, retina, and palm).

APPLICATIONS

Classification of Small Round Blue-Cell Tumors

Khan et al.[1] performed the proof-of-principle study for predicting unknown tumor samples using ANNs on gene expression data from a set of four small round blue-cell tumors (SRBCTs). SRBCTs are a group of tumors that are difficult to diagnose by routine histology and thus pose a significant challenge to the clinician for making an accurate diagnosis and subsequent recommendation for therapy. Accurate diagnosis is crucial because treatment, responses, and prognosis vary greatly depending on the diagnosis. In this study, the training set for the ANNs consisted of SRBCT tumors and cell lines across four tumor types: neuroblastoma (NB), rhabdomyosarcoma (RMS), a subset of non-Hodgkin lymphoma (NHL), and the Ewing's family of sarcomas (EWS).

In this paper, they suggest a schema for the application of ANN for diagnostic classification (FIG. 1a). Genes are first filtered for quality based on a quality metric calculated by the image analysis software used to extract data from the scanned microarray images. To avoid the "curse of dimensionality", PCA is employed and the first n-components can be used to train the network (in the manuscript, 10 components were used). To further ensure that the data are not overfitted, a cross-validation scheme is employed as follows. The training samples are randomly partitioned into groups, and one of these is used for validation and the rest for training. By this way, several hundred network models are trained (FIG. 1b) and an average vote can be calculated. Because a DNA microarray will typically monitor thousands of genes, and a particular disease will generally affect the expression of on the order of tens or hundreds of genes, the majority of the genes on a chip will not experience significant change in expression. This means that as much as 90% of the measurements on a chip represent noise rather than meaningful biological signal. Additionally, the decision-making process of ANNs is often considered as a "black box" with little information available as to how models determine a particular "expression signature". For these reasons, they developed a method to identify the genes that contribute most to a particular classification. After training the network as described above, the sensitivity for each gene was calculated as the derivative of the output with respect to the gene expression input. Genes with high sensitivity to the classification scheme received a high rank and genes with low sensitivity to the classification received a low rank. This can be understood functionally as the effect that a perturbation of a particular gene's expression ratio will have on the classification of each sample. If the perturbation of a particular gene affects the classification result significantly, then that gene receives a high rank. In contrast, if the perturbation of a particular

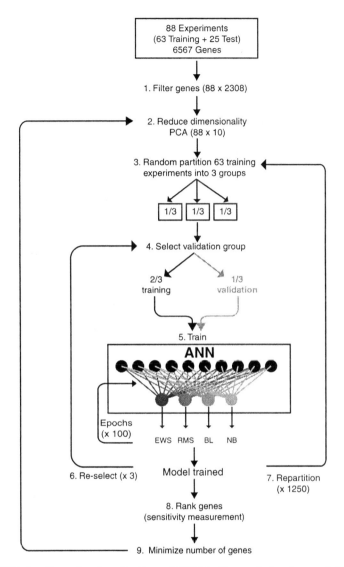

FIGURE 1a. Example of application of ANN (with permission from ref. 1). The 88 experiments were quality filtered (1) and the dimension of the data set further reduced from 2308 to 10 by PCA (2). Next, the 63 training samples were randomly partitioned into 3 groups (3) and 1 of these groups was selected for validation (4). The network was trained for 100 epochs using the 2 remaining groups (5). The samples in the validation group were tested and a different group was selected for validation (6). This process (steps 4–6) was repeated until each group was used for validation exactly one time. Then, the data were repartitioned into 3 new random groups (3) and steps 4–6 repeated again. In total, the data were repartitioned 1250 times (7), generating 3750 trained models. After this procedure, the genes were ranked using the sensitivity measurement (8), increasing numbers of the top-ranking genes were used for training (steps 2–6), and the gene set that produced the minimal number of errors (9) was used to calibrate the ANNs for testing the 25 blinded samples.

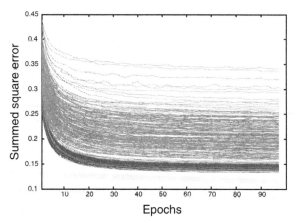

FIGURE 1b. Training error results from step 5 of FIGURE 1a. A plot of the classification error with increasing training epochs. The *light gray lines* represent the error of the validation samples and the *darker lines* represent the classification error of the training samples. The consistent decrease in error over increasing epochs implies that overfitting of the data did not occur.

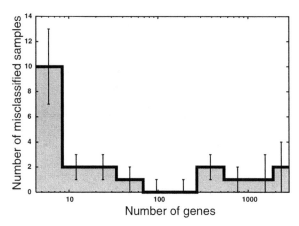

FIGURE 1c. Gene minimization results from step 9 of FIGURE 1a. This is a plot of the average number of misclassifications when increasing numbers of genes were used: the number of misclassifications minimized at 96 and 192 genes. The top-ranking 96 genes were used to calibrate the neural networks for subsequent training and testing of the 25 blinded test samples.

gene has a minimal effect on the classification result, then it receives a low rank. Then, in order to determine the best number of high-ranking genes, a gene minimization strategy was employed in which the network was trained with increasing numbers of the top genes (i.e., 6, 12, 24, 48, 96, 192, 384, 768, 1536, and 2308 genes) and the performance of the network determined using the a priori information about the training samples. When the network was trained using the top 96 genes, the average number of misclassifications was near zero (<0.5) (FIG. 1c). They clas-

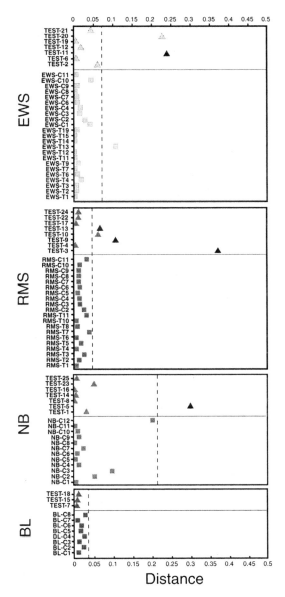

FIGURE 2. Classification and diagnosis of the SRBCT samples (with permission from ref. 1). The *x-axis* is the Euclidean distance between an ideal ANN output vote and the observed average vote. The *vertical dashed line* represents the empirical 95 percentile boundary beyond which diagnosis is not confident. Testing samples are represented by *triangles*, and training samples are shown as *squares*. *Black triangles* are the non-SRBCT samples not associated with any of the diagnostic categories. Two testing samples are correctly diagnosed, but lie outside the 95 percentile boundary (Test20-EWS and Test10-RMS). Only one training sample (EWS-T13) lies outside the 95 percentile boundary. All 5 non-SRBCT samples lie outside the 95 percentile boundary as they should.

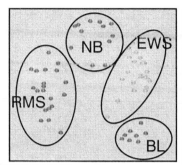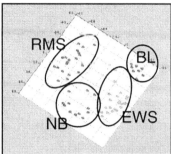

FIGURE 3a. MDS using the top 96 discriminating genes (with permission from ref. 1). Two views of the MDS results depicting the difference in gene expression of the four SRBCT classes.

sified all the training samples correctly with >98% accuracy and correctly diagnosed >90% of the blind test samples, which included 5 non-SRBCT samples (see FIG. 2). Based on all training and testing samples, the sensitivity of the network was 93% for EWS, 96% for RMS, and 100% for both NB and BL. The specificity was 100% for all four SRBCT categories. Many of these 96 genes were not previously known to be associated to the four cancers examined. MDS using these 96 genes is shown in FIGURE 3a. Hierarchical clustering of the samples and the top 96 genes is shown in FIGURES 3b and 3c. One gene, *FGFR4*, a tyrosine kinase receptor, is highly expressed in RMS and could be useful as a therapeutic target. Thus, they demonstrated that a diagnostically sound classifier of cancer could be achieved using microarray technology and ANNs and that meaningful biology could be extracted through ANN gene ranking. Since this study was published, it is worth noting that the microarray technology used, from the RNA preparation to the cDNA printing to the image scanning, has been significantly improved upon. cDNA chips, for example, have gone from parallel monitoring of ~6k clones to ~40k–100k clones. In addition, the improvement of microarray scanner technology has brought much greater consistency to the scanning process. This study marks the first successful attempt at using ANNs to classify cancers according to their gene expression profiles.

Estrogen Receptor Status in Breast Cancer

In another study, a very similar ANN approach (see FIG. 4a) was used to classify breast cancers based on their estrogen receptor status.[2] In this study, Gruvberger *et al.* analyzed the gene expression profiles of 58 node-negative breast carcinomas using a 6.7k cDNA microarray: 47 samples were used to train the network and 11 samples were used as test samples to verify the universality of the classifier. They were able to predict all 47 training and 11 testing samples with 100% accuracy using the top 100 genes (FIG. 4b and TABLE 2). When they repeated the classification procedure excluding the ER gene, 1 of the 47 training samples was incorrectly classified, but all of the 11 test samples remained correctly classified. This led them to look at how far down the list of discriminating genes they could go and still obtain accurate sample prediction. When they used the genes that ranked between 301 and 400, the

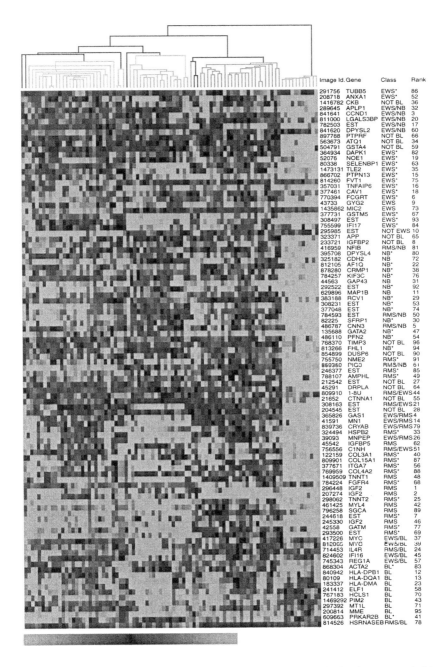

FIGURE 3b. Hierarchical clustering using the top 96 discriminating genes (with permission from ref. 1). Hierarchical clustering and heatmap of genes and samples with dendrogram colored according to clinical diagnosis.

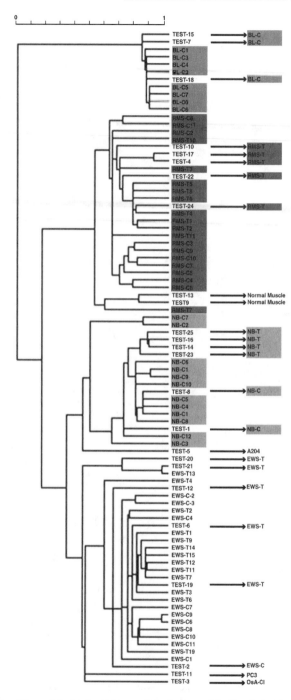

FIGURE 3c. Hierarchical clustering using the top 96 discriminating genes (with permission from ref. 1). Enlargement of the sample dendrogram in FIGURE 3b. All 63 training samples were correctly clustered within their diagnostic categories.

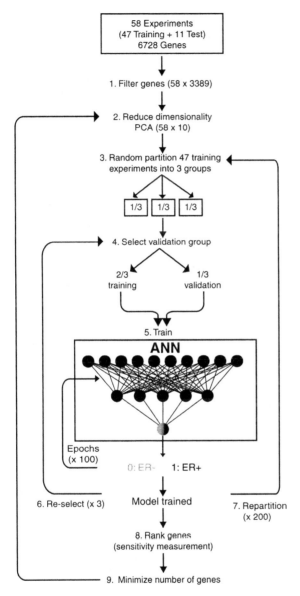

FIGURE 4a. ER status ANN work flow (with permission from ref. 2): 6728 genes from 58 experiments were filtered for quality, reducing the number of genes to 3389 (1). Dimensionality was reduced by using the top 10 components from PCA (2). The 47 training samples were randomly partitioned into 3 groups (3). Two groups were used for training, while the third was held aside for validation (4). The multilayer perceptron ANN was trained with 5 nodes in the hidden layer for 100 epochs (5). A different third (see step 4) was selected for validation, and training (5) was performed again. Steps 4–6 were performed one more time such that each third was chosen for validation once. After this, steps 3–6 were repeated 199 more times, making a total of 200 random partitions (7). The genes were ranked for their sensitivity to the classification scheme (8). Next, the number of top-ranking genes required to classify accurately was determined through a gene minimization process using increasing numbers of the top-ranking genes (9). Finally, these selected genes were taken through steps 2–7.

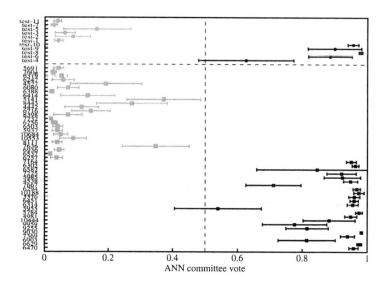

FIGURE 4b. ER status ANN results (with permission from ref. 2): ANN average voting results and standard deviations (*solid lines*) using the top 100 genes. An average vote (*x-axis*) of 1 represents the ideal vote for ER+ (*black*) and an average vote of 0 represents the ideal vote for ER− (*gray*). The decision threshold is 0.5. The 47 training samples are below the *dashed black horizontal line*, and the 11 test samples are located above this line.

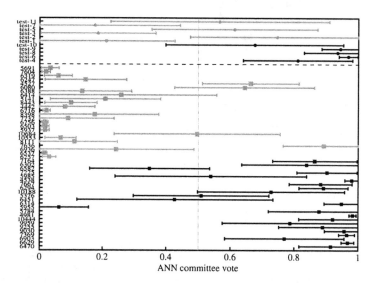

FIGURE 4c. ER status ANN results (with permission from ref. 2): ANN average voting results and standard deviations (*solid lines*) using the top 301–400 genes. An average vote (*x-axis*) of 1 represents the ideal vote for ER+ (*black*) and an average vote of 0 represents the ideal vote for ER− (*gray*). The decision threshold is 0.5. The 47 training samples are below the *dashed black horizontal line*, and the 11 test samples are located above this line.

TABLE 2. Prediction of ER status

Genes	Validation ($n = 47$)		Test ($n = 11$)	
	Correct	ROC area	Correct	ROC area
Top 100	47	100.00%	11	100.00%
51–150	43	97.80%	9	100.00%
101–200	45	99.30%	11	100.00%
151–250	44	97.50%	9	100.00%
201–300	41	93.70%	11	100.00%
251–350	39	95.30%	9	93.30%
301–400	41	93.10%	8	96.70%
Random	38.8 ± 0.2	$91.8 \pm 0.2\%$	5.5 ± 0.2	$53.0 \pm 2.6\%$

NOTE: Adapted with permission from ref. 2.

classification still had ROC areas of 93.7% for the training set and 96.7% for the test set (FIG. 4c and TABLE 2). They did report, however, that the ANN committee votes when using this list of genes were closer to the decision boundary and thus should be invested with less confidence. By this experiment, they demonstrated that some of the information content was found in the 301–400 range of discriminators. Using the weighted-gene analysis (WGA) method,[12] the authors discovered a set of 113 genes that were able to classify the samples with 96% accuracy using hierarchical clustering (FIG. 5b). The MDS of the samples using the 113 genes is also shown in FIGURE 5a. Using ANNs, this study showed that ER+ and ER– tumors have very different gene expression profiles with the ability to accurately predict even when the ER gene and the top-ranking genes are removed from the analysis.

Other Applications of Machine Learning to Cancer Classification

West et al.[6] used Bayesian regression modeling to develop a classifier to predict both the estrogen receptor status and the categorized lymph node status of primary breast tumors. Bayesian modeling does not assign a sample to a particular class, but rather assigns a probability that each sample belongs to each output class. Lymph node status is the single most important prognostic indicator for breast cancer,[13] and estrogen receptor status has received attention as a factor in breast cancer development and progression.[4,6,14,15] This study was published only one month after Gruvberger's ER paper[2] and represents further proof that both ER and clinical status can be predicted using gene expression profiling.

Van't Veer et al.[5] used a leave-one-out supervised correlation-based method to predict clinical outcome of breast cancer. They defined "poor prognosis" ($n = 34$) as patients who were lymph node–negative, but developed distant metastases within 5 years (mean time to metastasis was 2.5 years), and "good prognosis" ($n = 44$) as patients that were lymph node–negative and did not develop distant metastases within 5 years (mean follow-up time of 8.7 years). The authors first selected ~5000 genes from the 25,000 genes measured using an unsupervised selection method (i.e., two-fold regulation and P value of less than .01 in more than 5 tumors). In one of their

TABLE 3. Breast cancer patients eligible for adjuvant systemic therapy

	Patient group		
Consensus	Total patient group ($n = 78$)	Metastatic disease at 5 years ($n = 34$)	Disease-free at 5 years ($n = 44$)
St. Gallen	64/78 (82%)	33/34 (97%)	31/44 (70%)
NIH	72/78 (92%)	32/34 (94%)	40/44 (91%)
Prognosis profile[a]	43/78 (55%)	31/34 (91%)	12/44 (27%)
			[18/44 (41%)[b]]

NOTE: The conventional consensus criteria are as follows: tumor $\geq$2 cm, ER–, grade 2–3, patient < 35 years (either one of these criteria; St. Gallen consensus); tumor >1 cm (NIH consensus). Table adapted with permission from ref. 5.

[a]Number of tumors having a poor prognosis signature using microarray profile, defined by the optimized sensitivity threshold in the 70-gene classifier.

[b]Number of tumors with a poor prognosis signature in the group of disease-free patients when the cross-validated classifier is applied.

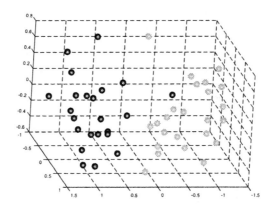

FIGURE 5a. ER+ (*black*) and ER– (*gray*) clustering using the 113 genes selected by weighted-gene analysis (WGA) (with permission from ref. 2): MDS plot of the 47 training samples. The distance between each of the samples represents their approximate degree of correlation.

FIGURE 5b. ER+ (*black*) and ER– (*gray*) clustering using the 113 genes selected by weighted-gene analysis (WGA) (with permission from ref. 2): Hierarchical clustering of the samples (*in columns*) and genes (*in rows*). The cluster of genes denoted "ER Cluster" are those genes that clustered with the ER gene (*ESR1*).

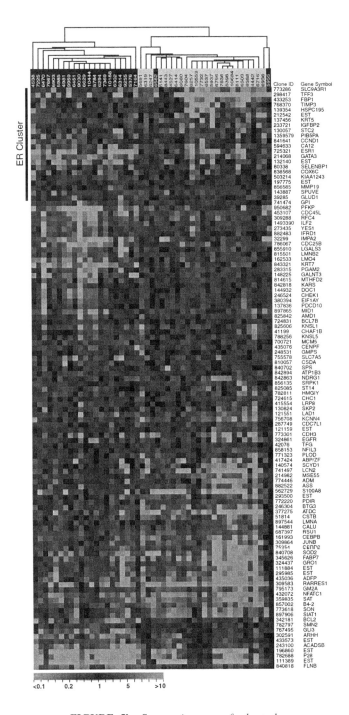

FIGURE 5b. *See previous page for legend.*

analyses, they performed 78 leave-one-out classifications, each time using the 77 training samples to select the discriminatory gene list and predict the left out 78th sample. With this validation scheme, they successfully predicted the left out samples between 56 and 68 times out of 78 depending on the correlation threshold used. In addition, they correctly predicted 17 out of 19 tumors from an independent test set using a 70-gene classifier. Van't Veer et al. compared their classifier to the St. Gallen and NIH consensus conference guidelines for eligibility for adjuvant chemotherapy. These guidelines are based on histological and clinical observations. The comparison is detailed in TABLE 3. For patients who developed metastatic disease and should receive adjuvant systemic therapy, van't Veer's classifier was slightly less sensitive than both the St. Gallen and NIH consensuses. Of the patients who remained disease-free, however, van't Veer's classifier was significantly more specific than either of the two consensuses. The findings of this and similar subsequent studies may significantly change the way a breast cancer patient is determined to be eligible for adjuvant chemotherapy. Disease-free patients may be more accurately diagnosed and suffer much less in the way of harmful side effects.

Furey et al.[4] used SVMs and the expression of 97,802 clones to discriminate between 16 ovarian cancers and 15 normal tissues (mixed ovarian tissue and other normal tissue). With various optimization attempts of the SVM parameters and the number of genes used as input, they achieved between 71% and 84% accuracy using leave-one-out cross-validation. Interestingly, their analysis misclassified a normal ovarian tissue sample as ovarian cancer and, upon further investigation, the sample was discovered to be mislabeled. This study demonstrates the power of SVMs to (1) predict whether a tissue sample is cancerous and (2) validate sample information based on gene expression data.

Other studies include that of Xu et al.,[3] who used ANNs to distinguish between Barrett's esophagus (BA) ($n = 14$) and esophageal cancer (CA) (3 squamous cell carcinomas and 5 adenocarcinomas). They selected the 160 most relevant genes using SAM (Statistical Analysis of Microarray).[16] After training the network with 12 samples (8 BAs and 4 CAs), it correctly predicted 10 test samples (6 BAs and 4 CAs).

Shipp et al.[7] used a supervised learning approach to predict the outcome of diffuse large B cell lymphoma (DLBCL) using oligonucleotide arrays with 6817 probes and tumor samples from 58 DLBCL patients. The 58 patients were separated into two groups: cured disease ($n = 32$) and fatal or refractory disease ($n = 26$). The 5-year overall survival (OS) rate of the 58 patients was 54%. Their supervised learning algorithm employed a leave-one-out cross-validation procedure that generated 58 sets of 13 discriminatory genes. Seven of the 13 genes were common to all of the 58 sets of 13. Using these 58 sets of 13 genes and testing on the single sample that was left out, they generated a prognosis prediction for each patient. Recalculating the 5-year OS for the two prediction classes produced the following: predicted to be cured, 5-year OS = 70%; predicted to have fatal/refractory disease, 5-year OS = 12% (nominal log rank $P = .000004$). Thus, using a supervised learning approach, Shipp et al. demonstrated that there is likely to be a gene expression profile at time of diagnosis that can help clinicians predict the outcome of DLBCL patients and proceed accordingly.

Another application of ANNs to DLBCL was performed by O'Neill and Song,[8] who achieved improved classification accuracy using ANNs on the data of Alizadeh et al.[17] Alizadeh et al. performed cluster analysis and achieved 93% diagnostic accuracy and were not able to successfully predict prognosis with their methods. O'Neill and Song, using the same data set, were able to achieve 99% diagnostic accuracy and 100% prognostic accuracy. Thus, they demonstrate the significant superiority of ANNs over cluster analysis.

OUTLOOK

It is clear that AI is bringing to reality some of the promises made by proponents of microarray. AI can accurately predict tumor subtype, metastatic state, and estrogen receptor status. Studies are starting to emerge that demonstrate the power of ANNs to predict clinical outcome. One of the keys to unlocking the power of AI to predict clinical outcome is identifying the misregulated genes in each cancer type. Using this information, we can develop custom arrays containing on the order of 10 to 100 unique genes (and replicates of these genes) that have been implicated in a particular cancer's prognosis profile. We predict that, once a set of diagnostic/prognostic specific genes are identified for all human diseases, handheld computers with an embedded or hard-coded, trained neural network could scan this gene chip, combine the acquired transcriptional data with known clinical parameters such as age, sex, date of presentation, etc., and output a diagnosis or prognosis prediction and a suggested course of treatment. Personalized medicine such as this may sound futuristic, but the fundamental building blocks are already a reality.

REFERENCES

1. KHAN, J. *et al.* 2001. Classification and diagnostic prediction of cancers using gene expression profiling and artificial neural networks. Nat. Med. **7:** 673–679.
2. GRUVBERGER, S. *et al.* 2001. Estrogen receptor status in breast cancer is associated with remarkably distinct gene expression patterns. Cancer Res. **61:** 5979–5984.
3. XU, Y. *et al.* 2002. Artificial neural networks and gene filtering distinguish between global gene expression profiles of Barrett's esophagus and esophageal cancer. Cancer Res. **62:** 3493–3497.
4. FUREY, T.S. *et al.* 2000. Support vector machine classification and validation of cancer tissue samples using microarray expression data. Bioinformatics **16:** 906–914.
5. VAN'T VEER, L.J. *et al.* 2002. Gene expression profiling predicts clinical outcome of breast cancer. Nature **415:** 530–536.
6. WEST, M. *et al.* 2001. Predicting the clinical status of human breast cancer by using gene expression profiles. Proc. Natl. Acad. Sci. USA **98:** 11462–11467.
7. SHIPP, M.A. *et al.* 2002. Diffuse large B cell lymphoma outcome prediction by gene-expression profiling and supervised machine learning. Nat. Med. **8:** 68–74.
8. O'NEILL, M.C. & L. SONG. 2003. Neural network analysis of lymphoma microarray data: prognosis and diagnosis near-perfect. BMC Bioinformatics **4:** 13.
9. RINGNER, M., C. PETERSON & J. KHAN. 2002. Analyzing array data using supervised methods. Pharmacogenomics **3:** 403–415.
10. QUACKENBUSH, J. 2001. Computational analysis of microarray data. Nat. Rev. Genet. **2:** 418–427.
11. HAYKIN, S. 1999. Neural Networks: A Comprehensive Foundation. Prentice–Hall. Upper Saddle River, NJ.
12. BITTNER, M. *et al.* 2000. Molecular classification of cutaneous malignant melanoma by gene expression profiling. Nature **406:** 536–540.
13. SHEK, L.L. & W. GODOLPHIN. 1988. Model for breast cancer survival: relative prognostic roles of axillary nodal status, TNM stage, estrogen receptor concentration, and tumor necrosis. Cancer Res. **48:** 5565–5569.

14. OSBORNE, C.K. 1998. Steroid hormone receptors in breast cancer management. Breast Cancer Res. Treat. **51:** 227–238.
15. PARL, F.F. 2000. Estrogens, Estrogen Receptor, and Breast Cancer. IOS Press. Amsterdam.
16. TUSHER, V.G., R. TIBSHIRANI & G. CHU. 2001. Significance analysis of microarrays applied to the ionizing radiation response. Proc. Natl. Acad. Sci. USA **98:** 5116–5121.
17. ALIZADEH, A.A. *et al.* 2000. Distinct types of diffuse large B-cell lymphoma identified by gene expression profiling. Nature **403:** 503–511.

Application of Bioinformatics in Cancer Epigenetics

HOWARD H. YANG AND MAXWELL P. LEE

Laboratory of Population Genetics, National Cancer Institute,
Bethesda, Maryland 20892, USA

ABSTRACT: With the completion of the human genome sequence and the advent of high-throughput genomics-based technologies, it is now possible to study the entire human genome and epigenome. The challenge in the next decade of biomedical research is to functionally annotate the genome, epigenome, transcriptome, and proteome. High-throughput genome technology has already produced massive amounts of data including genome sequences, single nucleotide polymorphisms, and microarray gene expression. Our ability to manage and analyze data needs to match the speed of data acquisition. We will summarize our studies of allele-specific gene expression using genomic and computational approaches and identification of sequence motifs that are signature of imprinted genes. We will also discuss about how bioinformatics can facilitate epigenetic researches.

KEYWORDS: genomics; bioinformatics; cancer; epigenetics; genomic imprinting

INTRODUCTION

Genetic variation in humans is largely caused by DNA polymorphism and differences in gene expression. A biological role has been identified for differential allelic expression associated with X-inactivation and genomic imprinting. Mendelian inheritance assumes that genes from maternal and paternal chromosomes contribute equally to human development. X chromosome inactivation silences gene expression from one of the two X chromosomes, thus providing an exception to Mendelian inheritance.[1] In addition, approximately 50 human autosomal genes are known to be imprinted and thus are expressed from only one chromosome.[2] However, it is unknown whether variations in allelic gene expression affect only the X chromosome and imprinted genes or whether they affect human genes generally. Recently, a group from Johns Hopkins University reported that 6 out of 13 genes show significant difference in gene expression between the two alleles and that this variation in allelic gene expression was transmitted by Mendelian inheritance.[3] They had previously shown that the allelic variation in the APC gene expression plays a critical role in colon cancer.[4] It will be interesting to know if genetic variations, especially

Address for correspondence: Maxwell P. Lee, Laboratory of Population Genetics, National Cancer Institute, 41 Library Drive D702C, Bethesda, MD 20892. Voice: 301-435-1536; fax: 301 402-9325.
  leemax@mail.nih.gov

Ann. N.Y. Acad. Sci. 1020: 67–76 (2004). © 2004 New York Academy of Sciences.
doi: 10.1196/annals.1310.008

regulatory single nucleotide polymorphisms (SNPs), contribute to common diseases including cancer.

Genomic imprinting is an unusual mechanism of gene regulation that results in preferential expression of one specific parental allele of a gene. Abnormal imprinting can cause human diseases such as Beckwith-Wiedemann syndrome, Prader-Willi syndrome, or Angelman's syndrome.[5–7] Loss of imprinting (LOI) is often associated with human cancers.[8,9] Although the exact mechanism of genomic imprinting is still largely unknown, differentially methylated CpG islands, imprinted antisense transcripts, and insulators may play important roles in the regulation of imprinting.[10–12] Most of the imprinted genes are located in the imprinting domains.[13] However, some genes in the imprinting domain can escape imprinting regulation.[14] Many imprinted genes are scattered throughout the human genome. Therefore, it is likely that local cis-elements as well as chromatin structure control genomic imprinting. Since patterns of gene regulation and the corresponding regulatory elements are often conserved across species, sequence comparison between human and mouse is a powerful approach to identify regulatory sequences.[15] Such comparative sequence analysis has already identified a number of conserved sequences and novel imprinted genes in human 11p15[16] and Dlk1-Gtl2 loci.[17,18]

The current release of human Unigene (build #162) contains 4,472,210 EST clones that are in 123,995 clusters: 16,069 of these Unigene clusters contain at least 33 EST clones. Genes with multiple ESTs can be used to deduce information about digital gene expression.[19] Computational methods have been used to identify SNPs in redundant EST clones.[20–22] We have also used EST database to mine allele-specific gene expression.[23]

GENOME-WIDE ANALYSIS OF ALLELE-SPECIFIC GENE EXPRESSION

A biological role has been identified for differential allelic expression associated with X-inactivation and genomic imprinting; however, a large-scale analysis of differential allelic expression of human genes has not been carried out. The HuSNP chip was designed for simultaneous typing of 1494 SNPs of the human genome. We adapted the HuSNP chip system to study allele-specific gene expression.[24]

Affymetrix only provided software for genotyping using the HuSNP chip. We decided to develop the following computational method to quantify allele-specific gene expression. We extracted the intensity values for each probe from the .CEL files generated by Affymetrix MAS 4.0. The .CEL files contain the fluorescent intensity values for each of the probes. The HuSNP chip contains 16 probes for each SNP locus. Four of the 16 probes match perfectly to allele A, 4 to allele B, 4 have 1 mismatch to allele A, and the other 4 have 1 mismatch to allele B. Allele A and allele B represent the two alleles of the SNP. Each probe contains 20 nucleotides. The centers of the nucleotide probes are located at positions $-4, -1, 0$, and 1 relative to the SNP. The 4 mismatch probes are identical to the perfect match probes, except for 1 mismatched base, which is always located in the center of the probe. The value for each probe pair was computed by subtracting the mismatch intensity from the perfect match intensity. A t test was used to calculate a P value for the presence of signal (intensity greater than 0) for each allele of each SNP. We considered a signal to be present if at least one allele had signal ($P < .01$, t test). Affymetrix defines a miniblock as a group of 4 probes that include a perfect match probe for allele A (PMA), a mismatch probe for allele A (MMA), a perfect match probe for allele B (PMB), and a mismatch probe for allele B (MMB). We set (PMA − MMA) = 50 if (PMA − MMA) is less than 50 for each miniblock. Similarly, baseline for allele B was set at 50. An allele A fraction, defined as f = (PMA − MMA)/(PMA − MMA + PMB − MMB), was computed for each miniblock, and the mean of the allele A fraction f from miniblocks was computed for each SNP. The gene expression difference between the two alleles from a heterozygous individual can be quantified using the ratio of allele A/allele B, computed from $f/(1 − f)$. For each chip, we have intensities from two scans called scan A and scan B. Generally, we used the intensity values from scan A. We used the intensity values from scan B if the t test showed that both alleles have no signal in scan A, while at least one of the alleles from scan B had signal. The ratio was further normalized by the ratio of genomic DNA for the SNP. We analyzed a set of HuSNP chip data from 7 individuals and found that 39 SNPs were heterozygous in at least 5 individuals. We computed the 95% confidence interval for the allelic ratio of genomic DNA for each of these 39 SNPs, and the average confidence interval was between 0.5 and 2.0. This value was used to select those genes that show significant difference in the expression between the two alleles.

In order to measure allele-specific gene expression quantitatively, we first needed to find out (1) which of the SNPs on the chip are located in transcribed regions and (2) whether the system can measure allele-specific expression accurately. Using blast searches and annotations in dbSNP, we found that 1063 of the SNPs are located in transcribed regions. To address the second issue, we used our computational method to extract the fluorescent intensity for each probe from an Affymetrix output file and quantify the ratio of expression of the two alleles. To assess the precision of the system, we performed experiments in duplicate for both genomic DNA and for polyA RNA from 3 fetuses. We found that the correlation between the repeated experiments was very high, with average Pearson correlation coefficients of 0.98 ($P < .001$) for genomic DNA and 0.95 ($P < .001$) for RNA. We then performed genotyping and allele-specific gene expression in kidney and liver from 7 fetuses. Genotype calls were obtained using the Affymetrix MAS 4.0 software, and quantitative allele-specific gene expression was computed using the method that we have developed. To be included in our analysis, each SNP had to meet the following criteria: (1) at least one fetus is heterozygous for the SNP; (2) the SNP is among the 1063 mapped within a transcribed region; and (3) the gene containing the SNP is expressed in kidney or liver. We found that 603 SNPs met all three criteria and 326 (54%) of which showed preferential expression of one allele; for 170 genes, there was at least a 4-fold difference in expression between the two alleles in at least one sample. Some of these 170 genes are imprinted (i.e., *SNPRN*, *IPW*, *HTR2A*, and *PEG3*). The genomic locations of all SNPs on the Affymetrix HuSNP chip were identified. Some of the genes showing differential allelic expression are clustered in the same genomic region, and some are in imprinted domains. *HTR2A*, *LOC51131*, and *FLJ13639* are located at 13q14, and all three show mono-allelic expression. *SNPRN*, *IPW*, and *LOC145622* are in the imprinted domain at 15q12, and all three genes preferentially express one allele. However, the majority of the genes that show preferential expression of one allele are scattered on different chromosomes, indicating that allelic variation is very common throughout the human genome. Our studies demonstrate that allele-specific gene expression is common and thus may play a significant role in human genetic variation.

COMPUTATIONAL ANALYSIS OF ALLELE-SPECIFIC GENE EXPRESSION

We developed a computational method by data mining of Unigene database to predict differential allelic gene expression and imprinted genes.[23] A schematic diagram of the computational method is shown in FIGURE 1.

For each SNP in a cDNA library, we could observe ESTs containing either allele A, allele B, or both alleles. D1 designates data that only allele A is observed in the cDNA library. If only allele A was observed, we can calculate the probability of genotype of the cDNA library as $P_{AA} = 1/(1 + 0.5^{n-1})$, $P_{AB} = 0.5^n \ ^1/(1 + 0.5^{n-1})$, and $P_{BB} = 0$. Similarly, D3 designates data that only allele B is observed in the cDNA library. If only allele B was observed, we can calculate the probability of genotype of the cDNA library as $P_{BB} = 1/(1 + 0.5^{n-1})$, $P_{AB} = 0.5^{n-1}/(1 + 0.5^{n-1})$, and $P_{AA} = 0$. If both allele A and allele B were observed, $P_{AB} = 1$ and $P_{AA} = P_{BB} = 0$. For the population allele frequency, $Q_A = P_{AA} + 0.5P_{AB}$. From Hardy-Weinberg equilibrium, we obtained $Q_{AB} = 2Q_A(1 - Q_A)$. A significant reduction in observed heterozygosity (P_{AB}) compared to the expected heterozygosity (Q_{AB}) is computed using the Z-statistics.

Imprinted genes and mono-allelic genes differentially express one allele. To model allele-specific gene expression, it is assumed that each cDNA library represents an individual and all libraries (or the sum of available libraries) constitute a population. If both A and B alleles of an SNP in a gene X are represented in a cDNA library, the individual is heterozygous at the SNP in the gene X. If only allele A is represented in the cDNA library (FIG. 1), the genotype for that individual could be either AA or AB. The probability that the individual is AA or AB can be inferred using Bayes' rule.

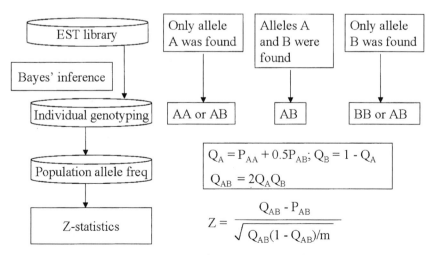

FIGURE 1. Computational analysis of genes preferentially expressing one allele.

We consider the following three kinds of allele observations D for an SNP from a library:

D1: the allele A appeared n times in the library, or

D2: the alleles A and B appeared $n1$ and $n2$ times, respectively, in the library, or

D3: the allele B appeared n times in the library.

With the uniform prior, the posterior probability of genotypes AA and AB with the observation of n EST clones containing the allele A was calculated as

$$P_{AA|D1} = 1/(1 + 0.5^{n-1}) \text{ and } P_{AB|D1} = 0.5^{n-1}/(1 + 0.5^{n-1}).$$

Similarly, the posterior probability of genotypes BB and AB with the observation of n EST clones containing the allele B was calculated as

$$P_{BB|D3} = 1/(1 + 0.5^{n-1}) \text{ and } P_{AB|D3} = 0.5^{n-1}/(1 + 0.5^{n-1}).$$

When both alleles appeared at least once in the library,

$$P_{AB|D2} = 1, P_{AA|D2} = 0, \text{ and } P_{BB|D2} = 0.$$

Genotype frequencies, P_{AA}, P_{AB}, and P_{BB}, were estimated from individual genotypes. The allele frequency in the population is calculated as $Q_A = P_{AA} + 0.5P_{AB}$ and $Q_B = 1 - Q_A$. The expected heterozygote frequency based on the Hardy-Weinberg equilibrium distribution is calculated as $Q_{AB} = 2Q_AQ_B$. P_{AB} tends to be lower than Q_{AB} for imprinted genes and genes displaying mono-allelic expression. This behavior can be analyzed using Z-statistics described in FIGURE 1. Bayes' inference of genotypes and the computation of Z-statistics are two different procedures. The computational results from Bayes' inference are used in computing Z-statistics. The approach was applied to a data set based on SNP data from Buetow et al.[20] We have taken several steps to ensure that high-quality EST clones are used in our data set. The EST clones and SNPs must meet the following three criteria to be included in our data set: (1) Phred quality score of an EST clone is equal to or greater than 20; (2) SNP score is equal to or greater than 0.99;[20] (3) SNPs are mapped to Locuslink. This data set consists of 112,812 records for 19,312 unique SNPs.

The difference between P_{AB} and Q_{AB} was calculated for each SNP using Z-statistics. The probability of differential allele-specific expression is indicated by the P value for each SNP. Fifty of 19,312 SNPs in the data set are in known imprinted genes. The validity of the computational method was tested by determining if SNPs in imprinted genes had small P values, that is, within the top 1% (194 out of 19,312) of SNPs ordered according to increasing P value. Four SNPs in imprinted genes were in the top 1% of the data set: 3 in IGF2 and 1 in PEG3. This finding is highly significant ($P = .0016$ in one-sided Fisher's exact test). Interestingly, when ESTs in tumor tissue libraries were used to populate the data set, only 1 of these 4 SNPs was in the top 1% of differentially expressed genes. This is consistent with the hypothesis that LOI occurs during tumorigenesis. Bayes' rule was used to infer the individual genotype frequencies. As a comparison, we consider the following non-Bayesian rule in the inference:

$$P_{AA|D1} = 1, P_{AB|D1} = P_{BB|D1} = 0, \text{ and }$$

$$P_{AB|D2} = 1, \ P_{AA|D2} = P_{BB|D2} = 0, \text{ and}$$

$$P_{BB|D3} = 1, \ P_{AA|D3} = P_{AB|D3} = 0.$$

When we replaced the Bayes' rule by the non-Bayesian rule, the SNPs in known imprinted genes had higher P values and were not in the top 1% of SNPs in the data set.

An alternative method for identifying imprinted genes was also developed. In this case, allele-specific gene expression is analyzed in libraries from heterozygotes. This approach identified 165 SNPs with differential allele-specific expression ($P < .05$, binomial test) and 2 of them were in known imprinted genes ($P = .0681$ in one-sided Fisher's exact test). Thus, this alternative method performs less well than the former method, although it may seem more intuitive.

An initial validation experiment demonstrated that 2 of 18 genes selected from the top 1% showed mono-allelic gene expression in fetal kidney and fetal liver using MALDI-TOF. Thus, we demonstrated the potential utility of this computational method in identifying differential allelic gene expression and novel imprinted genes.

SEQUENCE MOTIFS OF IMPRINTED GENES

We set out to identify novel sequence motifs that are associated with imprinted genes. Regulatory elements tend to locate on the conserved sequences.[15] Thus, we searched conserved sequences between human and mouse imprinted genes using PipMaker program.[25] Genomic sequences of 41 imprinted genes (including their 10-kb upstream and 10-kb downstream sequences) were retrieved from ftp://ftp.ncbi.nih.gov/genomes/. We were able to find both human and mouse sequences for 36 imprinted genes, 24 of which were used as a training set and 12 of which were used as a testing set. The PipMaker program was used to align human and mouse genomic DNA sequences. We used the MEME program[26] to search motifs in the conserved noncoding sequences among the human imprinted genes. This analysis identified 16 motifs. Motifs 1–4 are located in the upstream regions of the imprinted genes, while motifs 5–8 and motifs 9–16 are located in the downstream and intron regions of the imprinted genes, respectively. We then used MAST program[27] to search the presence of these motifs in the 24 imprinted genes as well as 128 non-imprinted genes, which were identified in our previous study.[24] Fifteen of the 16 motifs were found to be significantly associated with the 24 imprinted genes ($P < .05$, Fisher's exact test).

It has been suggested that imprinted genes share some common features.[16,28] Based on the distribution of the motifs among the 24 imprinted genes and the 128 nonimprinted genes, we developed a logistic regression model that was able to distinguish imprinted genes from nonimprinted genes. We initially had 16 motifs as predictor variables for the model. However, when all 16 motifs were used to build a logistic regression model, the iteration process to find the coefficients of the model was not convergent. We excluded motifs 4, 5, and 15 because their P values in Fisher's exact test were greater than 0.01. We also excluded motif 11 since it was underrepresented in the imprinted genes. We started a model with 12 motifs. An input vector to the model is a feature vector for a gene indicating whether each of these 12 motifs is associated with this gene. The response of the model is the probability of the gene being an imprinted gene. We performed the stepwise model selection by minimizing the AIC criterion and found the optimal 6 motifs (motifs 3, 7, 10, 12, 13, and 16) as input variables for a logistic regression model to score imprinted genes. As we reduce the number of the predictor variables from 12 to 6, the AIC of the corresponding model drops from 43.2 to 34. The minimum AIC for the model with 5 motifs is 37. Thus, the 6 motifs are optimal predictors from the AIC point of view. In fact, we computed AIC for every possible subset of the 12-motif set. The 6-motif set (3, 7, 10, 12, 13, 16) has the minimum AIC. The estimated model is as follows:

$$P = 1/[1 + \exp(7.1 - 4.8*M3 - 12.2*M7 - 4.2*M10 - 4.9*M12 - 12.1*M13 - 12*M16)].$$

Our model correctly assigned 127 out of the 128 nonimprinted genes and 22 out of the 24 imprinted genes in the training set. The accuracy, sensitivity, and specificity of the model are 98%, 92%, and 99%, respectively. To further validate the model, we performed an open test on the 12 imprinted genes, which were set aside as a testing set as described. The model is able to assign high probability scores to 8 of the 12 imprinted genes.

BIOINFORMATICS APPROACH TO EPIGENOME RESEARCH

Extensive bioinformatics infrastructure is needed to fully integrate data from genome sequences, epigenome, experiments, analysis, and knowledge, and to apply these data to improve our understanding of cancer. We have built software tools and databases to support information-driven cancer research (FIG. 2). We have been developing robust software pipelines that can seamlessly integrate heterogeneous data from external and internal sources. Object-oriented programming has been used for the pipelines, which are implemented using Perl and Java. We stored data either in flat files or in a relational database such as Oracle to allow efficient storage, retrieval, and updating of the data. We built our bioinformatics system by leveraging

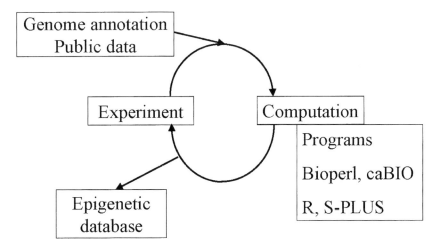

FIGURE 2. An integrated system to study cancer epigenetics.

the existing infrastructures such as Bioperl (http://bio.perl.org/), NCBI (http://www.ncbi.nlm.nih.gov/), and caBIO (http://ncicb.nci.nih.gov/core/caBIO/). Our primary focus is to build a computation engine for biological knowledge discovery and bioinformatics system to manage the data and computation. We use statistical packages such as R, SPLUS, and SAS as the core, complemented by customized programs. We develop modules that automatically fetch data from external sources, preprocess the data, and format the input and output. Preprocessing data include data filtering, normalization, and merging relevant properties. Some examples of the application of statistical computation have been described in the previous sections. We are interested in extracting patterns, trends, and relationships of molecular activities in five levels from massive data sets using cluster analysis, classification, and regression techniques. The five levels are genome (sequence, SNP, and mutation), epigenome (methylation, imprinting, and chromatin), RNA (gene expression and RNA splicing), protein (protein expression and biochemical properties), and functions (cancer phenotype and cellular functions). It is critical to choose the correct features and models to quantify molecular processes in these levels. The learning problems for these models can be either unsupervised or supervised. The unsupervised learning methods such as clustering methods and self-organization maps will enable us to verify the existing functions and to discover new functions of genes. We can apply unsupervised learning methods to extract useful features that characterize the molecular activities. On the other hand, the supervised learning methods such as linear or nonlinear regression models, artificial neural networks, ensemble methods, and support vector machines will enable us to code biological knowledge into the models. A successful modeling depends critically on the strategy used for model selection when a huge number of factors are related to the process that we are trying to quantify. We can use Akaike's information criterion (AIC) (an example was shown in the previous section), Bayesian information criterion (BIC), Minimum Message Length (MML), and Minimum Description Length (MDL) methods for model selection. With the advanced machine learning methods and the model selection strategies, we will find better models for biological knowledge discovery.

SUMMARY

In conclusion, challenge in the next decade of biomedical research lies in the functional annotation of the genome, epigenome, and proteome in interaction networks. The success of this mission critically depends on integration between experiments and data management. The experimental design and execution should fully utilize existing data and knowledge, while computational analysis should be based on experimental data and supported by the data and should suggest new experiments. The continued cycles of experiments and computations will be the approach to study cancer in the systems biology era.

ACKNOWLEDGMENTS

We wish to thank Dr. Ying Hu for many stimulating discussions about the application of computation and statistics to cancer epigenetics.

REFERENCES

1. GARTLER, S.M. & M.A. GOLDMAN. 2001. Biology of the X chromosome. Curr. Opin. Pediatr. **13**: 340–345.
2. TYCKO, B. & I.M. MORISON. 2002. Physiological functions of imprinted genes. J. Cell. Physiol. **192**: 245–258.
3. YAN, H., W. YUAN, V.E. VELCULESCU et al. 2002. Allelic variation in human gene expression. Science **297**: 1143.
4. YAN, H., Z. DOBBIE, S.B. GRUBER et al. 2002. Small changes in expression affect predisposition to tumorigenesis. Nat. Genet. **30**: 25–26.
5. NICHOLLS, R.D., J.H. KNOLL, M.G. BUTLER et al. 1989. Genetic imprinting suggested by maternal heterodisomy in nondeletion Prader-Willi syndrome. Nature **342**: 281–285.
6. CLAYTON-SMITH, J. & M.E. PEMBREY. 1992. Angelman syndrome. J. Med. Genet. **29**: 412–415.
7. MANNENS, M., J.M. HOOVERS, E. REDEKER et al. 1994. Parental imprinting of human chromosome region 11p15.3-pter involved in the Beckwith-Wiedemann syndrome and various human neoplasia. Eur. J. Hum. Genet. **2**: 3–23.
8. RAINIER, S., L.A. JOHNSON, C.J. DOBRY et al. 1993. Relaxation of imprinted genes in human cancer. Nature **362**: 747–749.
9. OGAWA, O., M.R. ECCLES, J. SZETO et al. 1993. Relaxation of insulin-like growth factor II gene imprinting implicated in Wilms' tumour. Nature **362**: 749–751.
10. SUTCLIFFE, J.S., M. NAKAO, S. CHRISTIAN et al. 1994. Deletions of a differentially methylated CpG island at the SNRPN gene define a putative imprinting control region. Nat. Genet. **8**: 52–58.
11. WUTZ, A., O.W. SMRZKA, N. SCHWEIFER et al. 1997. Imprinted expression of the Igf2r gene depends on an intronic CpG island. Nature **389**: 745–749.
12. LEE, M.P., M.R. DEBAUN, K. MITSUYA et al. 1999. Loss of imprinting of a paternally expressed transcript, with antisense orientation to KVLQT1, occurs frequently in Beckwith-Wiedemann syndrome and is independent of insulin-like growth factor II imprinting. Proc. Natl. Acad. Sci. USA **96**: 5203–5208.
13. FEINBERG, A.P. 1999. Imprinting of a genomic domain of 11p15 and loss of imprinting in cancer: an introduction. Cancer Res. **59**: 1743s–1746s.
14. LEE, M.P., S. BRANDENBURG, G.M. LANDES et al. 1999. Two novel genes in the center of the 11p15 imprinted domain escape genomic imprinting. Hum. Mol. Genet. **8**: 683–690.
15. WASSERMAN, W.W., M. PALUMBO, W. THOMPSON et al. 2000. Human-mouse genome comparisons to locate regulatory sites. Nat. Genet. **26**: 225–228.
16. ONYANGO, P., W. MILLER, J. LEHOCZKY et al. 2000. Sequence and comparative analysis of the mouse 1-megabase region orthologous to the human 11p15 imprinted domain. Genome Res. **10**: 1697–1710.
17. CHARLIER, C., K. SEGERS, D. WAGENAAR et al. 2001. Human-ovine comparative sequencing of a 250-kb imprinted domain encompassing the callipyge (clpg) locus and identification of six imprinted transcripts: DLK1, DAT, GTL2, PEG11, antiPEG11, and MEG8. Genome Res. **11**: 850–862.
18. PAULSEN, M., S. TAKADA, N.A. YOUNGSON et al. 2001. Comparative sequence analysis of the imprinted Dlk1-Gtl2 locus in three mammalian species reveals highly conserved genomic elements and refines comparison with the Igf2-H19 region. Genome Res. **11**: 2085–2094.
19. STRAUSBERG, R.L., K.H. BUETOW, M.R. EMMERT-BUCK & R.D. KLAUSNER. 2000. The cancer genome anatomy project: building an annotated gene index. Trends Genet. **16**: 103–106.
20. BUETOW, K.H., M.N. EDMONSON & A.B. CASSIDY. 1999. Reliable identification of large numbers of candidate SNPs from public EST data. Nat. Genet. **21**: 323–325.
21. IRIZARRY, K., V. KUSTANOVICH, C. LI et al. 2000. Genome-wide analysis of single-nucleotide polymorphisms in human expressed sequences. Nat. Genet. **26**: 233–236.
22. MARTH, G.T., I. KORF, M.D. YANDELL et al. 1999. A general approach to single-nucleotide polymorphism discovery. Nat. Genet. **23**: 452–456.

23. YANG, H.H., Y. HU, M. EDMONSON *et al.* 2003. Computation method to identify differential allelic gene expression and novel imprinted genes. Bioinformatics **19:** 952–955.
24. LO, H.S., Z. WANG, Y. HU *et al.* 2003. Allelic variation in gene expression is common in the human genome. Genome Res. **13:** 1855–1862.
25. SCHWARTZ, S., Z. ZHANG, K.A. FRAZER *et al.* 2000. PipMaker—a Web server for aligning two genomic DNA sequences. Genome Res. **10:** 577–586.
26. BAILEY, T.L. & C. ELKAN. 1994. Fitting a mixture model by expectation maximization to discover motifs in biopolymers. Proc. Int. Conf. Intell. Syst. Mol. Biol. **2:** 28–36.
27. BAILEY, T.L. & M. GRIBSKOV. 1998. Combining evidence using *P*-values: application to sequence homology searches. Bioinformatics **14:** 48–54.
28. GREALLY, J.M. 2002. Short interspersed transposable elements (SINEs) are excluded from imprinted regions in the human genome. Proc. Natl. Acad. Sci. USA **99:** 327–332.

Pathway Databases

CARL F. SCHAEFER

Center for Bioinformatics, National Cancer Institute, Rockville, Maryland 20852, USA

ABSTRACT: Network representations of biological pathways offer a functional view of molecular biology that is different from and complementary to sequence, expression, and structure databases. There is currently available a wide range of digital collections of pathway data, differing in organisms included, functional area covered (e.g., metabolism vs. signaling), detail of modeling, and support for dynamic pathway construction. While it is currently impossible for these databases to communicate with each other, there are several efforts at standardizing a data exchange language for pathway data. Databases that represent pathway data at the level of individual interactions make it possible to combine data from different predefined pathways and to query by network connectivity. Computable representations of pathways provide a basis for various analyses, including detection of broad network patterns, comparison with mRNA or protein abundance, and simulation.

KEYWORDS: bioinformatics; pathway; database

INTRODUCTION

High-throughput methods for sequence identification and mRNA expression are making it possible to define molecular profiles of diseases and to identify molecular targets for diagnosis and therapy. However, in many cases, the real target is not an individual protein, but a biological process, such as uncontrolled cell proliferation; the individual protein identified in an expression profile may be only one of many molecules on which the process depends. Increasingly, understanding of biochemical processes (pathways) is recognized as key to future advances in biomedical research in the understanding of cancer and the development of molecularly targeted therapies.[1] Further, as the amount of information grows, digital representations of pathways will be essential to convert data into useful information.[2]

A "pathway" is a biochemical process that can be partitioned into component steps. The term is not commonly used to describe processes that are either very small and simple (e.g., the mere formation of the MDM2:p53 complex) or very large and complex (e.g., the death of a multicellular organism). However, between these extremes lie a great many processes that are normally described as pathways, from small metabolic processes involving a handful of reactants to macroprocesses involving hundreds of molecular species and the cooperation of multiple cells.

Address for correspondence: Carl F. Schaefer, Center for Bioinformatics, National Cancer Institute, 6116 Executive Boulevard, Suite 403, Rockville, MD 20852. Voice: 301-435-1535; fax: 301-480-4222.
    schaefec@mail.nih.gov

Ann. N.Y. Acad. Sci. 1020: 77–91 (2004). © 2004 New York Academy of Sciences.
doi: 10.1196/annals.1310.009

Since there exists a consensus of sorts on what types of processes are pathways, one might assume, naively, that there is also consensus on the naming of pathways and on the inventory of their component steps. However, this is far from the truth. One source might treat "valine, leucine, and isoleucine biosynthesis" as a single process, while another source might treat these as three separate processes. Likewise, one source might identify the "caspase cascade in apoptosis" as a separate pathway, while another source might not award separate pathway status to this sequence of steps at all. Again, one source might include the deactivation of AKT by PP2A to be part of apoptosis, while another source might consider this step to fall outside the bounds of apoptosis.

COMPUTABLE REPRESENTATIONS OF PATHWAY INFORMATION

The sequence of steps comprising a pathway is rarely a simple linear sequence.[3] A single step may rely on multiple inputs and may create multiple outputs. The pathway may contain redundancy; that is, there may be multiple parallel chains of events that achieve what appears to be the same result. Conversely, an individual step may be multifunctional; that is, it may play a role in two different pathways achieving different effects. Further, pathways may be competitive; that is, one pathway's being active may render a second pathway inactive because the first consumes, binds, or inactivates a resource on which the second pathway depends.

Given this complexity, a natural representation for a pathway is a directed graph. Mathematically, a graph is a set of nodes and a set of connecting edges. At a high level of interpretation, edges in a pathway graph represent cause/effect dependencies holding among molecular species. It is worth noting that a digital representation of a pathway that looks like a network may fail to be a computable graph. For example, one can visually infer cause/effect relationships from the digitized version of the extraordinarily detailed Boehringer Mannheim Biochemical Pathways wall chart,[4] but an automated query cannot compute dependencies from this representation of biological processes. The BioCarta pathway diagrams[5] represent a further step toward computability since individual molecular species are hyperlinked; however, the various graphic arrows that connect molecules in the BioCarta diagrams are not available to computation.

In graph representations of biological pathways, it has been more common to represent only molecular species as nodes and to represent underlying events (reaction, modification, translocation, transcription) as edges. This is the general usage, for example, in the BioCarta diagrams, the Boehringer Mannheim Biochemical Pathways wall chart, and the automatically drawn EcoCyc diagrams.[6] It is also the practice in KEGG metabolic pathway diagrams,[7] where an edge may represent not only the event (reaction), but also the molecular species that catalyzes the event. If one chooses to model events as edges, one must employ a generalization of the directed graph, a *hypergraph*, to capture the biological reality.[8] An edge in a hypergraph can connect not just one source node with one destination node, but a set of source nodes with a set of destination nodes (FIG. 1a). This allows one to distinguish two cases: (a) either A or B is a sufficient cause of X; (b) both A and B are necessary causes of X. Alternatively, one can model both molecular species and events as nodes; an edge then represents the role that a molecule plays in an event. In this case,

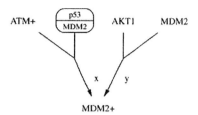

FIGURE 1a. Hypergraph representation of two processes ("x" and "y"). In a hypergraph, the source and destination of an edge may each be a set of nodes.

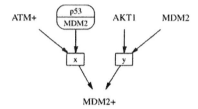

FIGURE 1b. Directed graph with explicit representation of event nodes, equivalent to FIGURE 1a. In a simple directed graph, each edge has one source node and one destination node.

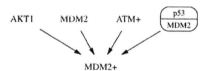

FIGURE 1c. Directed graph without explicit representation of events. Semantics of FIGURES 1a and 1b are lost in this version. It is no longer clear that MDM2 interacts with AKT and that ATM+ interacts with the p53:MDM2 complex.

a simple directed graph is sufficient to distinguish multiple sufficient causes from multiple necessary causes (FIG. 1b). In contrast, in FIGURE 1c, a representation with neither hyperedges nor event nodes, information is lost.

The bare nodes and edges of a pathway graph can be labeled with any amount of additional information. For example, a node can be labeled to indicate the location of a molecule within the cell (nucleus, cytoplasm, etc.), and a process node (or edge in a hypergraph) can be labeled with references to the literature and equations describing the kinetics of the reaction.

SOURCES OF PATHWAY DATA

Pathway databases are populated with data obtained from a variety of sources.

Data Curated from Literature

In many cases, expert curators have encoded their knowledge of particular biological processes, backed by small-scale experiments. In some cases, the detailed representations are supplemented with new descriptions synthesized by the curator (e.g., as in the Genome KnowledgeBase[9]); in other cases, literature references may be added to the database at the level of the pathway or the individual interaction (e.g., BIND[10]). There have been attempts to construct databases by automatically mining the literature.[11,12] This requires text analysis tools that can recognize identifiers of molecular species and words that designate interactions ("interacts", "inhibits", "catalyzes", "produces", etc., as well as their nominalizations "interaction", "inhibition", "catalysis", "production", etc.). Precise identification of proteins, complexes, and small molecules is notoriously difficult; even when the participating molecules are correctly identified, determining the correct relationship entails dealing with all the ambiguities and complexities of natural language. Consequently, raw output of text mining is not sufficiently precise or complete to be entered directly into a pathway database. Nevertheless, automated text mining can be a useful first step in identifying candidate interactions.

Orthologous Pathways

Some databases rely on assumed conservation of pathways across organisms to fill in missing data. The KEGG database contains abstract "reference" pathways that can be instantiated for any of several particular organisms;[13] the instantiation relies on the mapping between organism-specific proteins and enzyme function (EC number). Similarly, the WIT database reconstructs or predicts metabolic pathways from the genomic sequence of an organism and the organism-specific metabolic data in the EMP database.[14,15] The construction of reference pathway signaling processes is more problematic since these are less well conserved than the metabolic pathways.

High-Throughput Techniques

High-throughput techniques for uncovering protein/protein interactions, for example, yeast two-hybrid screens, are being used to populate some databases (e.g., DIP[16]). Unfortunately, while these techniques can show that two proteins are able to interact, they do not show the effect of the interaction (e.g., phosphorylation, complex association, etc.). In addition, the protein/protein interactions uncovered in a yeast two-hybrid screen may have little overlap with interactions uncovered by more traditional small-scale experiments and may contain false positives (i.e., the proteins may interact *in vitro*, but they may never be coexpressed in a real cell type).[17]

Reverse-Engineering of Networks

It is not unreasonable to assume that genes that are coregulated are more likely to be functionally related; that is, they are likely to be participants in the same biological process, and some members of the coregulated cluster are likely to interact directly with each other. This is the basis for studies that attempt to infer network structure from gene perturbation data. Wagner[18] attempts to reconstruct only statistical properties of the genetic network in *Saccharomyces cerevisiae*, concluding that the transcription regulatory interaction graph is sparse and (in contrast with the metabolic network) diffuse, having a large number of small subnetworks. However, there have been more ambitious efforts to reverse-engineer the detailed structure of genetic networks, reviewed by D'Haeseleer et al.,[19] de Jong,[20] and van Someren.[21] Various mathematical models have been proposed: discrete (Boolean) and continuous; deterministic and stochastic; spatial and nonspatial. However, efforts at finergrained (i.e., high-resolution) reverse-engineering of genetic networks on the basis of expression data are bedeviled by two facts: expression data are notoriously noisy and the number of parameters to be estimated is usually far greater than the number of observations. Consequently, there are simply too many models that are consistent with the data. At present, it appears that detailed modeling efforts are more likely to prove useful in forward-engineering of pathways (i.e., simulation) than in reconstructing the cause/effect network.

PATHWAY QUERY AND CONSTRUCTION

Static Pathway Retrieval

Many digital collections of pathway information contain representations of predefined pathways corresponding to well-known biological processes. The simplest query against such a collection is to retrieve the set of interactions in a single-named pathway, presented as a predrawn graphic or interaction list. The name of the pathway may be indexed (and queried) in various ways: keyword, GO Biological Process term, involvement of a particular compound or protein, etc. However, the result of this simple query is still the representation of a single predefined pathway or a list of pointers to separate predefined pathways.

Dynamic Pathway Construction

A database of pathway interactions allows one to construct pathways dynamically through a set of operations. Fundamental to dynamic pathway construction is the assumption that two interactions may be joined into a connected pathway if they share a molecular species. Dynamic pathway construction operations include basic retrieval by sets of predefined pathways or participating molecular species, retrieval by graph adjacency (connectedness), and graph simplification.

Basic retrieval operations include retrieving sets of interactions by named pathways or by participating molecular species:

(1) Retrieval of a set of predefined pathways, merging sets of interactions and joining interactions on molecular identity: The result may be a single connected graph or, if the predefined pathways failed to share molecular species, a set of disjoint graphs.

(2) Retrieval of all interactions that involve any of a set of molecular species as immediate participants: Again, the result may be a single connected graph or a set of disjoint graphs.

A basic query can be modified to include additional interactions that are (direct or indirect) predecessors or successors of an initially specified set of interactions:

(1) Retrieval of all the successors and/or predecessors of a set of interactions: An interaction A is a predecessor of interaction B if a molecular species output from A is input to B. Successor is defined analogously. As an example, a query might specify an initial set of all interactions involving RAS and all first- and second degree predecessors of those initial interactions.

(2) Retrieval of a *connected* graph that includes a set of specified interactions: As an example, a query might specify retrieving a connected graph that includes interactions involving p15, p16, p21, and p27. Since the SMAD3 complex plays a role in the transcription of all of these genes, this query might return a connected graph without any additional searching. On the other hand, a query to retrieve a connected graph that includes any interaction involving ERK2 and any interaction including RAS would probably involve searching for additional interactions to build a connected path. A path through interactions involving MEKK1 and MEK1 (RAS → MEKK1 → MEK1 → ERK2) (FIG. 2a) would satisfy the query. In general, there is not a unique way to satisfy a query to construct a connecting path, and a search for an optimal solution (i.e., a connecting path of mimimal length) is equivalent to the NP-complete traveling salesman problem.

Finally, a pathway graph can be modified by eliminating certain nodes or by treating two nodes that are distinct in the database as equivalent:

(1) Pruning molecular species from a set of interactions: It is important to be able to construct a model of a pathway that abstracts the essence of a process by discarding detail that holds less information value. A good example of this is pruning ubiquitous cofactors such as water, carbon dioxide, and ATP from representations of metabolic reactions. In the KEGG predrawn metabolic diagrams, these molecular species are commonly omitted. The ability to prune molecular species becomes essential when querying by adjacency: a query for third-degree predecessors of a single metabolic interaction may end up including thousands of interactions unless common cofactors are pruned.

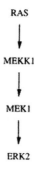

FIGURE 2a. RAS → MEKK1 → MEK1 → ERK2 cascade.

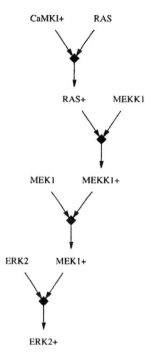

FIGURE 2b. Detailed view of RAS → MEKK1 → MEK1 → ERK2 cascade, showing individual activation steps.

(2) Collapsing molecule variants: It is often useful to ignore certain distinctions between variants of a molecular species. This is most obviously true in the case of proteins that are products of splice variants of a single gene. In fact, since so little in known about the functional differences of splice variants, pathway databases routinely ignore these distinctions. However, it is occasionally useful to abstract a simpler model by ignoring better-understood functional distinctions. For example, if one is interested merely in analyzing the structural patterns of protein/protein interactions, it may be desirable to ignore posttranslational modifications. The path that connects RAS with ERK2, noted above, is actually an abstraction of a longer path that takes explicit account of the active and inactive forms of RAS, MEKK1, and MEK1: RAS → RAS+ → MEKK1 → MEKK1+ → MEK1 → MEK1+ → ERK2 → ERK2+ (FIG. 2b).

PATHWAY ANALYSIS

Computable representations of pathway information can support a variety of analyses.

Analysis of Structural Patterns

Purely graph-theoretic analysis techniques may be applied to biochemical inter-action networks, with interesting results. It has been shown, for example, that meta-bolic networks tend to resemble the hub-and-spoke networks of air transportation more than they resemble the more evenly interconnected network of the Interstate Highway system.[22] Furthermore, there exists a positive correlation between the metabolic "hubs" and lethality to the cell.[23] More speculatively, Nurse[24] suggests it might be possible to identify biological functional "modules" that are analogous to the functional modules (feedback loops, switches, timers, oscillators, and amplifiers) of electronic design.

Comparison with mRNA or Protein Abundance

As already noted, it is reasonable to assume that genes that are coregulated are more likely to be functionally related. Pathway models can thus be used to generate hypotheses regarding the effects of anomalies and then test these hypotheses on expression data. Ideker *et al.*[25] propose a four-step iterative process for refining knowledge of a particular pathway on the basis of expression data. The four steps are as follows:

(1) Identify the molecular species involved in a pathway and propose a model of their interaction.
(2) Perturb each component of the pathway—for example, by deleting a gene or introducing an environmental factor.
(3) Analyze mRNA and protein expression data for the genes in the pathway as well as for other genes in the genome, identifying clusters of apparently coregulated genes.
(4) Refine the model of interaction to account for the observed variations in expression and apparent coregulation. For example, the expression data may suggest that a set of interactions thought to represent one temporally and spatially coherent process may in fact fall into two separable processes. Conversely, the data may suggest that additional interactions be considered an integral part of the initial pathway model.

Simulation

Given (a) the basic network topology of a pathway, (b) a mathematical model for evaluating the network, and (c) the necessary constants (kinetic parameters, initial concentrations, etc.), it is possible to simulate the behavior of the pathway. The simplest model is Boolean: each node and edge assumes one of two values ("0" or "1", "high" or "low", "on" or "off"), with output values being computed as Boolean functions of inputs. While clearly oversimplified, Boolean pathway models can be useful in developing hypotheses about the effects of anomalies (overexpression, silencing, mutation, etc.) on biological function. In principle, higher fidelity models could support *in silico* studies of candidate therapeutic agents; however, at present, high-fidelity simulation is limited to small networks that are already well under-stood. There is evidence that deterministic models do not fit some biological pro-cesses as well as stochastic models; McAdams and Arkin[26] have show this to be true of transcription, where the number of copies of a particular transcription factor is small in a given cell.

SOME PATHWAY DATABASES

TABLE 1 presents basic information on 10 of the better-known databases. The databases may differ from each other in many respects:

(1) Most contain data for multiple organisms, in varying degrees of completeness, while others are limited to one or two organisms.
(2) Many contain data on all types of cellular processes (metabolism, signal transduction, transport, transcription regulation), while others are limited to one type (e.g., metabolism).
(3) Some contain low-level quantitative data such as kinetic and binding constants, while others are limited to higher-level qualitative data.
(4) Some include only predefined pathways, while others allow the dynamic construction of interaction networks.
(5) Some use hand-drawn diagrams for visualization, while others use automatically constructed diagrams.
(6) Some rely on interaction data curated from the literature, while others import high-throughput experimental data.

DATA EXCHANGE

From a cursory look at some of the better-known pathway databases, it is clear that none of these databases claims to provide a complete picture of human cellular process (or of mouse or rat, the best-developed cancer model organisms). While there is some overlap among the various databases, each has a unique emphasis. To construct an integrated view—a view, for example, that includes metabolic, signaling, and transcription processes—one might attempt to combine data drawn from several sources. However, one is immediately confronted by the variety of ways in which data are represented in the different databases. The dimensions of difference include not only the type of information a database covers (types of processes, coverage of kinetic parameters, etc.), but also the way in which that information is structured. A common representation of pathway data, built on unambiguous syntax and semantics, would facilitate the integration of data from diverse sources.

One might approach the problem of a common data exchange language from two directions. Suppose the goal in mind is the repeated application of a well-defined analytic or visualization task, such as the display of expression data in a pathway context. In this case, one could define a data representation that met exactly the requirements of the particular piece of software that performed the task. All users of this software would then be able to exchange and reuse pathway data among themselves. Such is the direction followed by the GenMAPP project, which combines a freely available tool for constructing pathway diagrams and displaying microarray data on the resulting diagrams with a simple, compact data exchange format.[27]

TABLE 1. Selected pathway databases

Acronym	Name	Ref.	URL	Scope	Notes
aMAZE	Protein Function and Biochemical Pathways (PFBP) Project	36	http://www.ebi.ac.uk/research/pfbp	Metabolism, signal transduction, transport, transcription regulation. Multiorganism.	5200 interactions. Dynamic query to find a path connecting molecular species.
BIND	Biomolecular Interaction Network Database	10	http://www.bind.ca	Metabolism, signal transduction, transport, transcription regulation. Multiorganism.	22,000 interactions. 8 predefined pathways.
BRENDA	Braunschweig Enzyme Database	33	http://www.brenda.uni-koeln.de	Metabolism. Multiorganism.	50,000 interactions. No predefined pathways. Molecular and functional parameters (e.g., Michaelis constant). Interactions organized by EC number
DIP	Database of Interacting Proteins	16	http://dip.doe-mbi.ucla.edu	Protein-protein interactions. Multiorganism.	19,000 interactions. Records region involved in the interaction, dissociation constant, and experimental methods. Includes data from high-throughput experiments (e.g., yeast two-hybrid screens).
EcoCyc	Encyclopedia of *E. coli* Genes and Metabolism	6	http://ecocyc.org	Metabolism, transport, transcription regulation. *E. coli*.	165 predefined pathways (automatically drawn diagrams). 2600 reactions.
EMP	Enzymes and Metabolic Pathways	15	http://www.empproject.com/about	Metabolism. Multiorganism.	3000 predefined, hand-drawn pathway diagrams. Enzyme data include kinetics, structure, physical chemistry.

TABLE 1. (*continued*) Selected pathway databases

Acronym	Name	Ref.	URL	Scope	Notes
GeneNet	GeneNet	34	http://www.mgs.bionet.nsc.ru/mgs/systems/genenet	Metabolism, signal transduction, transport, transcription regulation. Multiorganism.	23 predefined pathways. 1900 interactions. Automated construction of diagrams.
GK	Genome KnowledgeBase	9	http://www.genomeknowledge.org	Metabolism, signal transduction, transport, transcription regulation. Multiorganism.	1800 events. Events (e.g., a pathway) can contain subevents (e.g., a reaction). Distinguishes concrete and abstract entities. Events may be annotated with descriptive text. Explicit links to preceding/following events.
KEGG	Kyoto Encyclopedia of Genes and Genomes	7, 13	http://www.genome.ad.jp/kegg	Metabolism. Multiorganism.	143 predefined pathways (hand-drawn diagrams), containing 2700 interactions. Dynamic query to find a path connecting molecular species. Interactions organized by EC number.
MINT	Molecular Interaction Database	35	http://cbm.bio.uniroma2.it/mint/index.html	Metabolism, signal transduction, transport, transcription regulation. Multiorganism.	4600 interactions, largely curated from literature. No predefined pathways. Allows the specification of indirect interactions (e.g., suppression). Kinetic and binding constants recorded where available.

Developing a data exchange format that is independent of a particular software application is a more ambitious task. There are at least two contenders for standardization. Systems Biology Markup Language (SBML)[28] and CellML.[29] Both SBML and CellML are strongly oriented to the requirements of model simulation. Thus, they each have features enabling one to specify units of measurement, kinetic parameters, and complex mathematical formulae, including differential equations, and to associate these quantitative specifications with individual reactions. CellML has a more systematic way of associating model metadata with a model. Metadata, such as the name of the modeler, citations, and additional descriptive information, are useful in constructing searchable catalogues of models. CellML also offers the ability to declare model subcomponents and connections among subcomponents. This is analogous to the hardware designer's ability to declare wired connections among components built from lower-level circuitry in hardware description languages like VHDL[30] and Verilog.[31] Both SMBL and CellML use XML to define their syntax.

A more recent effort to develop a standard exchange format for pathway data is BioPAX (Biopathway Exchange Language, URL: http://www.biopax.org/). While the BioPAX model is still evolving, it appears that BioPAX will be oriented less toward the specification of simulation models and more toward the inclusion of a broad range of data sources, including high-throughput protein/protein interaction data, and genetic interactions such as epistasis and suppression.

DISCUSSION

Pathway databases provide a view of biology that is distinct from that offered by sequence, expression, or structure databases, or collections of encyclopedic gene/protein pages such as LocusLink (www.ncbi.nih.gov/LocusLink), GeneCards (bioinfo.weizmann.ac.il/cards), and the Cancer Genome Anatomy Project (cgap.nci.nih.gov). By describing individual events and their aggregation into networks of events, pathway databases make it possible to query by connectivity, to trace effects to necessary or sufficient causes, and (given the appropriate mathematical model and kinetic parameters) to simulate the progress of a biological process. Consequently, pathway databases can support *in silico* investigations central to cancer research. They can further the identification of interactions that, if perturbed singly or in combination, could affect processes known to be important in tumorigenesis and metastasis. Also, they can identify possible unintended effects of a candidate therapeutic agent.

It would be a mistake, however, to equate the value of a pathway database with simulating the effects of molecular abnormalities or therapeutic agents. Apart from an ability to support simulation, pathway databases provide a powerful way of organizing and representing knowledge about cancer biology.

In particular, a pathway database's linking of molecules and interactions can bring into proximity independent observations about molecular abnormalities. For example, one study might find a mutated form of ATR in tumor samples and a separate study might find that ATM was significantly underexpressed in a different batch of tumor tissue. If these observations are recorded in a knowledge representation that exposes pathway connectivity, it will become evident that the two abnor-

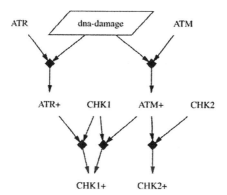

FIGURE 3. Redundant paths leading to activation of CHK1 and CHK2 in the presence of DNA damage. Abnormalities or underexpression of either ATR or ATM might be expected to be a factor in accumulation of DNA defects.

malities are closely related in effect since each activates the checkpoint proteins, CHK1 and CHK2 (FIG. 3). Clustering of genes by expression profile is also a technique for bringing observations in proximity. However, clustering is not a substitute for a network representation. The membership of genes in an expression cluster depends heavily on the choice of clustering algorithm and thresholds and on the original set of probes; an expression-defined cluster is thus a transient entity, not suited to play the role of persistent locus for the accumulation of knowledge. In contrast, the makeup of a signaling interaction based on curated data is far more stable. Furthermore, in our hypothetical example, clustering of genes by expression would not have related a mutation in one gene to underexpression of another gene, while the pathway network framework is flexible enough to relate these different sorts of anomalies.

The advances of the 1990s in high-throughput sequencing have made it possible to identify many of the proteins that drive cellular processes. As a result, we now can draw up reasonably complete biological "parts lists" for a number of organisms.[32] Further, with high-throughput expression analysis, we can create specialized parts lists that describe different cell types. However, just as a parts list of transistors, capacitors, and resistors reveals little of the overall function of a radio, so a list of proteins does not define biological function very clearly. The key to both electronic and biological function is in the wiring of the components.

REFERENCES

1. HANAHAN, D. & R.A. WEINBERG. 2000. The hallmarks of cancer. Cell **100:** 57–70.
2. KARP, P.D. 2001. Pathway databases: a case study in computational symbolic theories. Science **293:** 2040–2044.
3. BHALLA, U.S. & R. IYENGAR. 1999. Emergent properties of networks of biological signaling pathways. Science **283:** 381–387.
4. ROCHE APPLIED SCIENCE. [No date.] Boehringer Mannheim Biochemical Pathways (digitized version of the Roche Applied Science "Biochemical Pathways" wall chart). URL: http://www.expasy.org/cgi-bin/search-biochem-index/.

5. BIOCARTA. [No date.] Pathway diagrams. URL: http://www.biocarta.com/.
6. KARP, P.D., M. RILEY, M. SAIER et al. 2002. The EcoCyc Database. Nucleic Acids Res. **30:** 56–58. URL: http://ecocyc.org/.
7. KANEHISA, M., S. GOTO, S. KAWASHIMA et al. 2002. The KEGG databases at GenomeNet. Nucleic Acids Res. **30:** 42–46. URL: http://www.genome.ad.jp/kegg/.
8. KRISHNAMURTHY, L., J. NADEAU, G. OZSOYOGLU et al. 2003. Pathways Database System. an integrated system for biological pathways. Bioinformatics **19:** 930–937.
9. COLD SPRING HARBOR LABORATORY, EUROPEAN BIOINFORMATICS INSTITUTE & GO CONSORTIUM. [No date.] Genome KnowledgeBase. URL: http://www.genomeknowledge.org/.
10. BADER, G.D., D. BETEL & C.W. HOGUE. 2003. BIND: the Biomolecular Interaction Network Database. Nucleic Acids Res. **31:** 248–250.
11. ONO, T., H. HISHIGAKI, A. TANIGAMI et al. 2001. Automated extraction of information on protein-protein interactions from the biological literature. Bioinformatics **17:** 155–161.
12. DONALDSON, I., J. MARTIN, B. DE BRUIJN et al. 2003. PreBIND and Textomy—mining the biomedical literature for protein-protein interactions using a support vector machine. BMC Bioinformatics **4:** 11.
13. KANEHISA, M. & S. GOTO. 2000. KEGG: Kyoto Encyclopedia of Genes and Genomes. Nucleic Acids Res. **28:** 27–30.
14. OVERBEEK, R., N. LARSEN, G.D. PUSCH et al. 2000. WIT: integrated system for high-throughput genome sequence analysis and metabolic reconstruction. Nucleic Acids Res. **28:** 123–125.
15. SELKOV, E., S. BASMANOVA, T. GAASTERLAND et al. 1996. The metabolic pathway collection from EMP: the enzymes and metabolic pathways database. Nucleic Acids Res. **24:** 26–28.
16. XENARIOS, I., L. SALWINSKI, X.J. DUAN et al. 2002. DIP, the Database of Interacting Proteins: a research tool for studying cellular networks of protein interactions. Nucleic Acids Res. **30:** 303–305.
17. DEANE, C.M., L. SALWINSKI, I. XENARIOS & D. EISENBERG. 2002. Protein interactions: two methods for assessment of the reliability of high throughput observations. Mol. Cell. Proteomics **1:** 349–356.
18. WAGNER, A. 2002. Estimating coarse gene network structure from large-scale gene perturbation data. Genome Res. **12:** 309–315.
19. D'HAESELEER, P., S. LIANG & R. SOMOGYI. 2000. Genetic network inference: from coexpression clustering to reverse engineering. Bioinformatics **16:** 707–726.
20. DE JONG, H. 2002. Modeling and simulation of genetic regulatory systems: a literature review. J. Comput. Biol. **9:** 67–103.
21. VAN SOMEREN, E.P., L.F.A. WESSELS, E. BACKER et al. 2002. Genetic network modeling. Pharmacogenomics **3:** 507–525.
22. JEONG, H., B. TOMBOR, R. ALBERT et al. 2000. The large-scale organization of metabolic networks. Nature **407:** 651–654.
23. JEONG, H., S.P. MASON, A-L. BARABASI et al. 2001. Lethality and centrality in protein networks. Nature **411:** 41–42.
24. NURSE, P. 2003. Systems biology: understanding cells. Nature **424:** 883.
25. IDEKER, T., V. THORSSON, J.A. RANISH et al. 2001. Integrated genomic and proteomic analyses of a systematically perturbed metabolic network. Science **292:** 929–934.
26. MCADAMS, H. & A. ARKIN. 1997. Stochastic mechanisms in gene expression. Proc. Natl. Acad. Sci. USA **94:** 814–819.
27. DAHLQUIST, K.D., N. SALOMONIS, K. VRANIZAN et al. 2002. GenMAPP, a new tool for viewing and analyzing microarray data on biological pathways. Nat. Genet. **31:** 19–20. URL: http://www.genmapp.org/.
28. HUCKA, M., A. FINNEY, H.M. SAURO et al. 2003. The Systems Biology Markup Language (SBML): a medium for representation and exchange of biochemical network models. Bioinformatics **19:** 524–531. URL: http://www.sbml.org/.
29. HEDLEY, W. & M. NELSON. 2001. CellML 1.0 specification. URL: http://www.cellml.org/.
30. IEEE. 2002. IEEE Standard VHDL Language Reference Manual (IEEE Std 1076-2002).
31. IEEE. 2001. IEEE Standard Verilog Hardware Description Language (IEEE Std 1364-2001).

32. IDEKER, T., T. GALITSKI & L. HOOD. 2001. A new approach to decoding life: systems biology. Annu. Rev. Genomics Hum. Genet. **2:** 343–372.
33. SCHOMBURG, I., A. CHANG & D. SCHOMBURG. 2002. BRENDA, enzyme data and metabolic information. Nucleic Acids Res. **30:** 47–49.
34. KOLPAKOV, F.A., E.A. ANANKO, G.B. KOLESOV *et al.* 1998. GeneNet: a gene network database and its automated visualization. Bioinformatics **14:** 529–537.
35. ZANZONI, A., L. MONTECCHI-PALAZZI, M. QUONDAM *et al.* 2002. MINT: a Molecular INTeraction database. FEBS Lett. **513:** 135–140.
36. VAN HELDEN, J., A. NAIM, R. MANCUSO *et al.* 2000. Representing and analyzing molecular and cellular function using the computer. Biol. Chem. **381:** 921–935.

Microarrays and the Gene Expression Profile of a Single Cell

ERNEST S. KAWASAKI

Advanced Technology Center, National Cancer Institute, National Institutes of Health, Bethesda, Maryland 20892, USA

ABSTRACT: With completion of the human genome sequence, it is now possible to study the expression of the entire human gene complement of ~30,000–35,000 genes. To accomplish this goal, microarrays have become the leading methodology for the analysis of global gene expression. Improvements in technology have increased the sensitivity of microarrays to the point where it is feasible to study gene expression in a small number of cells and *even at the single cell level*. A summary of developments in the area of expression profiling in single cells will be described, and the rationale for these types of studies will be presented. In addition, from a biologist's point of view, some bioinformatic challenges of expression analysis of single cells will be discussed.

KEYWORDS: single cell; microarray; expression profile; laser capture; cancer cell

INTRODUCTION

The advent of microarrays as a research tool is approaching the decade mark,[1,2] and its widespread use and technological maturation have paralleled the large-scale genomic sequencing of hundreds of organisms. Whole genome expression profiling is now being carried out in bacteria, humans, mice, plants, and other organisms. The "Holy Grail" of many of these studies is to determine the exact number and type of genes being expressed in a given tissue or organ, and the expression level and regulation of these genes under a variety of conditions, both normal and pathological. Until recently, a large number of cells have been required to obtain enough material for complete expression profiles using, for example, gene expression arrays. Thus, by necessity, most expression profile studies to date of complex organisms have used samples that were composed of a mixture of cell types. Although cells may appear morphologically and anatomically identical, they may have different gene expression phenotypes and quite distinct functions. This mixture invariably leads to obtaining an average expression of genes for a tissue or organ and may have very little correlation with the actual expression in any single cell type. While these types of data are important, true physiologic levels of expression require that a synchro-

Address for correspondence: Ernest S. Kawasaki, Advanced Technology Center, National Cancer Institute, 8717 Grovemont Circle, Bethesda, MD 20892. Voice: 301-435-2891; fax: 301-402-3134.
  kawasake@mail.nih.gov

Ann. N.Y. Acad. Sci. 1020: 92–100 (2004). © 2004 New York Academy of Sciences.
doi: 10.1196/annals.1310.010

nized, homogeneous sample of cells be used or that a *single cell be the ultimate source* of material for microarray analysis. Advances in several fronts such as laser capture microdissection of cells, RNA amplification schemes, and other areas have now made it possible to carry out studies at this ultraminiaturized level. Below, we describe the technological aspects of single cell array work, some applications, the rationale behind these studies, and a few bioinformatic challenges related to this level of expression profiling, and finish with a summary and some thoughts on the future of this technology. For further information on single cell microarray technologies, the reader is referred to several excellent reviews on this topic.[3–17]

TECHNOLOGICAL ASPECTS

Single Cell Isolation

The first step in single cell isolation is obviously to be able to identify the cells of interest amidst the mixture of contaminating cells. Cells may be characterized by morphology, differential staining, and immunohistochemistry, but details of this will not be discussed here as it is beyond the scope of this article. Once the cell type is identified, there are several methods by which to isolate individual cells. Advances in flow sorting of cells in suspension enable the isolation of a single cell population as well as a single cell.[18] A single cell population is defined in this case as cells that can be recognized and sorted as single entities, but may be heterogeneous with respect to other aspects of gene expression. For instance, certain leukemias may be identified by surface receptors and sorted to great purity, but individual cells within the population may be very diverse by other criteria such as leukemogenicity, metastatic potential, and so on. Thus, it may be still desirable in many cases to resort to single cell sorting rather than analyzing a population of cells. Fluorescence activated cell sorting (FACS) works well for cells in suspension, but does not lend itself easily to purifying cells from solid tissues such as found in tumors.

For purification of single cells from solid tissues, some form of microdissection is required. Mechanical methods involving microscopy and micromanipulators enable the dissection of single cells from tissues mounted on slides, but require a major investment in time and labor. The slow pace may also interfere with the isolation of undegraded RNAs required for probe labeling and array analysis. Recently, methods involving the use of laser-assisted microdissection have greatly facilitated obtaining single cells from tissues. The most common laser microdissection methods are the laser "catapult"[19,20] and the laser "capture"[21,22] techniques. In the catapult system, a focused UV laser is used to burn or ablate an area around the cell(s) of interest on a tissue section contained on a glass slide. The UV laser beam is small enough that it can ablate an area around a single cell. The laser is then defocused and positioned directly below the cell of interest. The cell is then "catapulted" off the slide into a collecting cap via light pressure from the defocused beam. In the laser capture method, an infrared laser beam is positioned above tissue section that is sandwiched between a plastic film and glass slide. When the laser beam is focused on a cell of interest, the plastic melts and penetrates the area around the cell. When the beam is turned off, the plastic solidifies and sticks to the cell, which can then be removed or "captured" from the tissue section. The cells removed by both the laser "capture" and "catapult" systems can be stored or used immediately for the isolation of RNA, DNA, or protein. For further excellent discussion of methods and applications of laser-assisted microdissection, the reader is referred to the following publications.[23–28] Most microarray studies using laser microdissection techniques utilize hundreds to thousands of cells for labeling purposes as the amount of RNA from a single cell is not sufficient for probe production. To overcome this problem, several RNA amplification strategies, although not entirely new, requiring only picogram quantities of RNA are being adapted to single cell studies as described below.

RNA Amplification Schemes

Originally, protocols for labeling of probes for microarrays specified the use of 100–200 μg of total RNA, and this amount contains approximately 3–6 μg of mRNA. To obtain this quantity, several million cells would have to be processed. A single cell has ~25 pg of total RNA, with 2% of this mass as mRNA. This is equivalent to about 0.5 pg of mRNA or ~500,000 mRNAs of average size. Thus, to obtain a sufficient amount of RNA from a single cell for probe production, the messenger fraction would have to be amplified more than a millionfold. To accomplish this, a modification of two methods is being used to amplify mRNA from single cells: polymerase chain reaction (PCR)[29] and amplified antisense (aRNA) technologies.[30] The PCR approach has been used to obtain cDNA clones from single cells,[31] to amplify subpicogram quantities of mRNA up to 3×10^{11}–fold,[32] to study the transcriptome of single micrometastatic cells,[33] to analyze pancreas development,[34] and to profile single cells of neuronal progenitors.[35] In the PCR method, mRNA is first converted to double-stranded (ds) cDNA and, in the process, sequences for PCR priming are incorporated at both ends. The ds cDNA is then amplified exponentially to the desired level, and the amplified products are used to make probes for array analysis. Theoretically, 20–30 cycles of PCR will amplify the cDNA a millionfold or more, so there should not be any difficulty in obtaining sufficient material for probe labeling. However, there may be problems associated with this protocol such as differential amplification of the genes, and this will discussed in the section on bioinformatics.

The aRNA method is called a linear amplification procedure as there is not an exponential increase, but a theoretical linear increase in product over time. Briefly, cDNA is synthesized with an oligo-dT primer containing the T7 promoter sequence at its 5′ end. After ds cDNA is made, T7 RNA polymerase is used to linearly synthesize large quantities of antisense RNA, which can be used as a probe itself or used as a template to make a sense cDNA probe. One advantage of this protocol is that the RNA polymerase is not generally affected by template sequences or the concentration of templates in a complex mixture. In other words, there should be no differential amplification of different mRNA sequences that are present at widely different concentrations in a normal cell. A disadvantage is that the maximum amplification of one cycle is about 1000-fold so that two or more cycles are required to approach the level necessary for sampling single cells, and this is somewhat a cumbersome procedure. Perhaps, a combination of PCR with aRNA synthesis will work the best for probe amplification as described in several recent publications.[36–39] For further thoughts and ideas on amplification strategies and optimization, the following articles may prove useful.[40–49]

RATIONALE/APPLICATIONS

Why use a single cell for whole genome expression profiling studies? There are a number of fascinating publications in this area, and a few examples will serve to illustrate applications and provide a firm rationale for studying expression at the single cell level.

Neurosciences

The neurosciences have been a fertile field for single cell transcriptional analysis. The mammalian nervous system is a highly complex and heterogeneous organ that consists of hundreds or thousands of different cell types and neurons.[35,50] To study this complex system, both micromanipulation and laser capture methods are being employed, and single cell mRNA has been amplified by PCR or RNA amplification. The variety of cell types studied include olfactory sensory neurons,[34] hippocampus CA1 neurons,[50,51] entorhinal cortex stellate cells,[51] and isolated dendrites.[52] The single cell studies have enabled the investigators to identify hundreds of transcriptional differences between olfactory progenitor cells and mature sensory neurons. Expression studies in the rat hippocampus revealed for the first time two different types of neurons within the hippocampus and even demonstrated a difference among the same cell types. In human hippocampal cells, significant age-related decreases were found in dopamine receptor mRNAs, but not in the entorhinal cortex stellate cells. It is obvious that none of these findings would have been possible without resorting to single cell microarray analysis.

Development

One of the goals of developmental biologists is to determine the timing and order of gene expression during development. At certain stages, cells are not distinguishable morphologically, but their "fate" is determined. The mouse was used as a model system to study single cell transcript analysis during development of the pancreas.[34] In this case, the authors demonstrated that morphologically uniform cells were distinguishable by single cell microarray analysis and found the expression of unique combinations of genes. With these data, they were able to identify subtypes of developing pancreatic cells. With these results, along with known genetic and biochemical data, they were able to propose a pathway for pancreatic cell development, details of which were not possible without their single cell studies.

Immunology

Immune cells may be grouped into T cells, B cells, macrophages, granulocytes, and so on. Although the total number of cell types is not large, their complexity is increased by many subtypes found within each cell category. A good example is illustrated by a study[53] that perfectly illustrates the necessity of using single cells to characterize expression in seemingly uniform batches of cells. Human natural killer (NK) cells express different NK receptors per cell. A population of resting NK cells was collected via FACS and tested for 9 NK receptors by RT-PCR. None of the 38 cells tested was found to contain exactly the same pattern of receptors on their surface. These findings point to a unique facet of NK cell biology that would not have been found if a mixture of cells were tested.

Cancer

The "war on cancer" has been raging for well over 50 years, yet we are far from able to claim any clear-cut victory over it. Why is this? A major contributing factor for this depressing fact is simply that we do not yet have a precise understanding or definition of what a cancer cell is. Without knowledge of the basic biology of the tumor cell, efficacious and relatively nontoxic therapies are difficult to design and develop. This will hopefully change as we now can design experiments to determine the expression of every gene in a cancer cell, and this knowledge will eventually enable us to defeat this disease. Tumors and their component cells are heterogeneous in nature. Common biopsy methods yield samples that are mixture of normal and tumor types,[54] and some type of careful microdissection is essential to obtain meaningful expression profiles from clinical samples.[55] A study designed to characterize these cells must by necessity examine the tumors at a single cell level. A good example of this is the fact that, like other cancers, breast cancer may proceed or metastasize not by the bulk of the tumor, but by a very small population of cells.[56–58] It is entirely plausible that present therapies are directed against the wrong group of cells and that microarray analysis at the single cell level of the stem cells will point the way to a more effective, long-lasting therapy. Another example illustrates this point. A major microarray study of several different types of cancers found that a metastatic expression signature was present in the primary tumor of all the patients, indicating that the metastatic potential was already encoded in the bulk of the primary tumor.[59] This finding could have major impact in the area of diagnostics and could have important clinical and therapeutic applications. However, as noted by a reviewer of the article,[60] two of the upregulated genes important for metastasis were, in fact, derived from normal tissue, providing further impetus for the necessity of the use of single cells in the analysis of cancer.

BIOINFORMATIC/STATISTICAL CHALLENGES OF SINGLE CELL EXPRESSION ANALYSIS

Advances and convergence of several cutting edge technologies have enabled the researcher to analyze global gene expression at the single cell level. Before this methodology becomes more commonplace, several questions of a bioinformatic/ statistical nature should be answered regarding the overall validity of this procedure.

Do You Lose mRNAs That Are Present in Low Copy Number?

This is basically a question alluding to the possibility of sampling error. If an "average" cell contains about 500,000 mRNAs and you wish to detect a gene expressed at one copy per cell, is there a possibility that you will lose this sequence during the processing steps? How many cells do you need to sample to ensure the detection of the lowest copy number mRNAs? As a test, one might use "spiking" experiments to demonstrate that one added copy of a defined sequence can be added to a "real life" sample and be detected by microarrays at the end of the procedure. This has been done with large-scale RNA isolation using hundreds of thousands or millions of cells, and single copy equivalents can be detected. In an elegant single cell study, 1, 2, 10, and 100 RNA copies of a control bacterial RNA were spiked into lysed solutions of single olfactory neurons.[35] After amplification and array analysis, the authors were able to consistently detect 100 and 10 copies, and the 1 and 2 copy spikes were detectable in two of four experiments. These results provide assurance that low copy number mRNAs are not lost during the protocol. One may object to the fact that the 1 and 2 copy number spikes were detected in only two out of four experiments, but this result would be acceptable even if microgram amounts of RNA were used versus the picogram amounts found in a single cell. Additional evidence for the robustness of the single cell procedure can be found by the fact that rare transcripts down to 0.7 copies per cell can be detected in single hippocampal CA1 neurons.[50] Quantitative RT-PCR was used confirm this finding and indicated that detection of low copy number mRNAs is not a problem using this protocol.

How Many Cells Should Be Sampled to Get an Average Expression Value?

This is somewhat of a basic biology question whose answer will vary from tissue to tissue and organ to organ. It is probable that every cell of a "homogeneous" set will have a different expression profile due to differences of position in the cell cycle, influence by proximity to other cell types, and so on. Studies to determine this have not been carried out yet. Almost all array analyses to date have tested the "average cell" population, and the single cell studies will shed light on how heterogeneous the homogeneous populations really are.

Does Probe Amplification Distort the Original Cellular mRNA Ratios?

For studying expression at the single cell level, the mRNA must be amplified a millionfold or more; a picogram of messenger is amplified to a microgram or more. As described above, this can be done by two rounds of linear amplification using the T7 RNA polymerase technique, by >20 cycles of RT-PCR, or by a combination of the two protocols. Any differential amplification of the mRNA species will distort their original ratios and can invalidate the data. The effects of mRNA amplification on gene expression ratios were estimated by analysis of variance (ANOVA).[61] Two rounds of amplification were carried out and the impact of amplification on gene expression ratios was estimated. They found that 10% of the genes investigated showed significantly different expression ratios. However, the amplified probes gave a better signal-to-noise ratio and allowed detection of more genes with lower expression than unamplified RNAs. These types of results have been found in numerous RNA amplification studies where, although some of the ratios may be changed slightly,[62] the results of amplification are highly reproducible and provide improved quality of data with higher sensitivity for the lower expressing genes.[44,45,47,49,63–66] Many of these studies, but not all, use quantitative RT-PCR to verify their findings. In general, the results are comparable and, thus, the amplification schemes do not seem to affect the original mRNA ratios to a significant degree.

Conclusions

Most of the bioinformatic questions will center around sampling issues of single cells and probable biases in amplification of mRNA sequences. Studies are showing that mRNA ratios obtained from single cells are indicative of their "true" values.

SUMMARY/THE FUTURE

Whole genome expression profiling of single cells is still in a developmental stage. The clean isolation of cells, purification of representative RNA, and equal amplification of the typical mRNA populations are crucial factors to consider when working with single cells for microarray analysis. All these steps require further optimization and this work is well under way in many laboratories at this time. The literature has already shown that single cell analysis is a very fruitful approach for investigating basic biological phenomena in neurons, immune cells, plant cells, cancer, etc. The future is bright as the human and other genome sequences are being fully annotated and the technology for whole genome expression profiling on single chips becomes commonplace. Finally, it is hoped that expression profiling of single cells will provide unique insights into the basic biology of cells and, concomitantly, the knowledge required to fully diagnose and treat cancer and other diseases.

REFERENCES

1. SCHENA, M. *et al.* 1995. Quantitative monitoring of gene expression patterns with a complementary DNA microarray. Science **270:** 79–92.
2. LOCKHART, D.J. *et al.* 1996. Expression monitoring by hybridization to high-density oligonucleotide arrays. Nat. Biotech. **14:** 1675–1680.
3. HINKLE, D.A. & J.H. EBERWINE. 2003. Single-cell molecular biology: implications for diagnosis and treatment of neurologic disease. Biol. Psychiatry **54:** 413–417.
4. KEHR, J. 2003. Single cell technology. Curr. Opin. Plant Biol. **6:** 617–621.
5. KAMME, F. & M.G. ERLANDER. 2003. Global gene expression analysis of single cells. Curr. Opin. Drug Discov. Dev. **6:** 231–236.
6. LEVSKY, J.M. & R.H. SINGER. 2003. Gene expression and the myth of the single cell. Trends Cell Biol. **13:** 4–6.
7. DIXON, A.K. *et al.* 2002. Single cell expression analysis—pharmacogenomic potential. Pharmacogenomics **3:** 809–822.
8. TODD, R. & D.H. MARGOLIN. 2002. Challenges of single-cell diagnostics: analysis of gene expression. Trends Mol. Med. **8:** 254–257.
9. BRANDT, S. *et al.* 2002. Using array hybridization to monitor gene expression at the single cell level. J. Exp. Botany **53:** 2315–2323.
10. TODD, R., M.W. LINGEN & W.P. KUO. 2002. Gene expression profiling using laser capture microdissection. Expert Rev. Mol. Diagn. **2:** 497–507.
11. COHEN, C.D. & M. KRETZLER. 2002. Gene expression analysis in microdissected renal tissue: current challenges and strategies. Nephron **92:** 522–528.
12. KELZ, M.B. *et al.* 2002. Single-cell antisense RNA amplification and microanalysis as a tool for studying neurological degeneration and restoration. Sci. Aging Knowledge Environ. **1:** 1.
13. EBERWINE, J. *et al.* 2002. Analysis of subcellularly localized mRNAs using *in situ* hybridization, mRNA amplification, and expression profiling. Neurochem. Res. **27:** 1065–1077.
14. EBERWINE, J. 2001. Single-cell molecular biology. Nat. Neurosci. Suppl. **4:** 1155–1156.

15. DIXON, A.K. *et al.* 2000. Gene-expression analysis at the single-cell level. Trends Pharmacol. Sci. **21**: 65–70.
16. BRADY, G. 2000. Expression profiling of single mammalian cells—small is beautiful. Yeast **17**: 211–217.
17. FREEMAN, T.C., K. LEE & P.J. RICHARDSON. 1999. Analysis of gene expression in single cells. Curr. Opin. Biotech. **10**: 579–582.
18. ORMEROD, M. 2000. Flow Cytometry: A Practical Approach. Oxford University Press. Oxford, United Kingdom.
19. SCHUTZE, K. & G. LAHR. 1998. Identification of expressed genes by laser-mediated manipulation of single cells. Nat. Biotech. **16**: 737–742.
20. WESTPHAL, G. *et al.* 2002. Noncontact laser catapulting: a basic procedure for functional genomics and proteomics. Methods Enzymol. **356**: 80–99.
21. EMMERT-BUCK, M.R. *et al.* 1996. Laser capture microdissection. Science **274**: 998–1001.
22. WITTLIFF, J.L. & M.G. ERLANDER. 2002. Laser capture microdissection and its application in genomics and proteomics. Methods Enzymol. **356**: 12–25.
23. LUZZI, V. *et al.* 2003. Accurate and reproducible gene expression profiles from laser capture microdissection, transcript amplification, and high density oligonucleotide microarray analysis. J. Mol. Diagn. **5**: 9–14.
24. MORA, J., M. AKRAM & W.L. GERALD. 2002. Comparison of normal and tumor cells by laser capture microdissection. Methods Enzymol. **356**: 240–247.
25. BURGESS, J.K. & B.E. MCPARLAND. 2002. Analysis of gene expression. Methods Enzymol. **356**: 259–270.
26. OHYAMA, H. *et al.* 2002. Use of laser capture microdissection–generated targets for hybridization of high-density oligonucleotide arrays. Methods Enzymol. **356**: 323–333.
27. MIKULOWSKA-MENNIS, A. *et al.* 2002. High-quality RNA from cells isolated by laser capture microdissection. BioTechniques **33**: 176–179.
28. LUO, L. *et al.* 1999. Gene expression profiles of laser-captured adjacent neuronal subtypes. Nat. Med. **5**: 117–122.
29. SAIKI, R.K. *et al.* 1985. Enzymatic amplification of beta-globin genomic sequences and restriction site analysis for diagnosis of sickle cell anemia. Science **230**: 1350–1354.
30. VAN GELDER, R.N. *et al.* 1990. Amplified RNA synthesized from limited quantities of heterogeneous cDNA. Proc. Natl. Acad. Sci. USA **87**: 1663–1667.
31. DULAC, C. & R. AXEL. 1995. A novel family of gene encoding putative pheromone receptors in mammals. Cell **83**: 195–206.
32. ISCOVE, N.N. *et al.* 2002. Representation is faithfully preserved in global cDNA amplified exponentially from sub-picogram quantitites of mRNA. Nat. Biotech. **20**: 940–943.
33. KLEIN, C.A. *et al.* 2002. Combined transcriptome and genome analysis of single micrometastatic cells. Nat. Biotech. **20**: 387–392.
34. CHIANG, M-K. & D.A. MELTON. 2003. Single-cell transcript analysis of pancreas development. Dev. Cell **4**: 383–393.
35. TIETJEN, I. *et al.* 2003. Single-cell transcriptional analysis of neuronal progenitors. Neuron **38**: 161–175.
36. PETALIDIS, L. *et al.* 2003. Global amplification of mRNA by template-switching PCR: linearity and application to microarray analysis. Nucleic Acids Res. **31**: 142.
37. AOYAGI, K. *et al.* 2003. A faithful method for PCR-mediated global mRNA amplification and its integration into microarray analysis on laser-captured cells. Biochem. Biophys. Res. Commun. **300**: 915–920.
38. SAGHIZADEH, M. *et al.* 2003. Evaluation of techniques using amplified nucleic acid probes for gene expression profiling. Biomol. Eng. **20**: 97–106.
39. SETH, D. *et al.* 2003. SMART amplification maintains representation of relative gene expression: quantitative validation by real time PCR and application to studies of alcoholic liver disease in primates. J. Biochem. Biophys. Methods **55**: 53–66.
40. WANG, E. *et al.* 2000. High-fidelity mRNA amplification for gene profiling. Nat. Biotech. **18**: 457–459.
41. LISS, B. 2002. Improved quantitative real-time RT-PCR for expression profiling of individual cells. Nucleic Acids Res. **30**: 89.
42. SHUSTOVA, V.I. & S.J. MELTZER. 2002. Amplified RNA for gene array hybridizations. Methods Mol. Biol. **193**: 227–236.

43. FELDMAN, A.L. *et al.* 2002. Advantages of mRNA amplification for microarray analysis. BioTechniques **33:** 906–914.
44. ZHAO, H. *et al.* 2002. Optimization and evaluation of T7 based linear amplification protocols for cDNA microarray analysis. BMC Genomics **3:** 31.
45. ATTIA, M.A. *et al.* 2003. Fidelity and reproducibility of antisense RNA amplification for the study of gene expression in human CD34⁺ haemopoietic stem and progenitor cells. Br. J. Haematol. **122:** 498–505.
46. POLACEK, D.C. *et al.* 2003. Fidelity and enhanced sensitivity of differential transcription profiles following linear amplification of nanogram amounts of endothelial mRNA. Physiol. Genomics **13:** 147–156.
47. XIANG, C.C. *et al.* 2003. Probe generation directly from small numbers of cells for DNA microarrays. BioTechniques **34:** 386–393.
48. WANG, J. *et al.* 2003. RNA amplification strategies for cDNA microarray experiments. BioTechniques **34:** 394–400.
49. SCHERER, A. *et al.* 2003. Optimized protocol for linear RNA amplification and application to gene expression profiling of human renal biopsies. BioTechniques **34:** 546–556.
50. KAMME, F. *et al.* 2003. Single-cell microarray analysis in hippocampus CA1: demonstration and validation of cellular heterogeneity. J. Neurosci. **23:** 3607–3615.
51. HEMBY, S.E., J.Q. TROJANOWSKI & S.D. GINSBERG. 2003. Neuron-specific age related decreases in dopamine receptor subtype mRNAs. J. Comp. Neurol. **456:** 176–183.
52. EBERWINE, J. *et al.* 2001. mRNA expression analysis of tissue sections and single cells. J. Neurosci. **21:** 8310–8314.
53. HUSAIN, Z. *et al.* 2002. Complex expression of natural killer receptor genes in single natural killer cells. Immunology **106:** 373–380.
54. SYMMANS, W.F. *et al.* 2003. Total RNA yield and microarray gene expression profiles from fine-needle aspiration biopsy and core-needle biopsy samples of breast carcinoma. Cancer **97:** 2960–2971.
55. SUGIYAMA, Y. *et al.* 2002. Microdissection is essential for gene expression profiling of clinically resected cancer tissues. Am. J. Clin. Pathol. **117:** 109–116.
56. REYA, T. *et al.* 2001. Stem cells, cancer, and cancer stem cells. Nature **414:** 105–111.
57. DICK, J.E. 2003. Breast cancer stem cells revealed. Proc. Natl. Acad. Sci. USA **100:** 3547–3549.
58. AL-HAJJ, M. *et al.* 2003. Prospective identification of tumorigenic breast cancer cells. Proc. Natl. Acad. Sci. USA **100:** 3983–3988.
59. RAMASWAMY, S. *et al.* 2003. A molecular signature of metastasis in primary solid tumors. Nat. Genet. **33:** 49–54.
60. LIOTTA, L.A. & E.C. KOHN. 2003. Cancer's deadly signature. Nat. Genet. **33:** 10–11.
61. NYGAARD, V. *et al.* 2003. Effects of mRNA amplification on gene expression ratios in cDNA experiments estimated by analysis of variance. BMC Genomics **4:** 11.
62. PUSKAS, L.G. *et al.* 2002. RNA amplification results in reproducible microarray data with slight ratio bias. BioTechniques **32:** 1330–1340.
63. MA, X-J. *et al.* 2003. Gene expression profiles of human breast cancer progression. Proc. Natl. Acad. Sci. USA **100:** 5974–5979.
64. GOMES, L.I. *et al.* 2003. Comparative analysis of amplified and nonamplified RNA for hybridization in cDNA microarray. Anal. Biochem. **321:** 244–251.
65. LI, Y. *et al.* 2003. Direct comparison of microarray gene expression profiles between non-amplification and a modified cDNA amplification procedure applicable for needle biopsy tissues. Cancer Detect. Prev. **27:** 405–411.
66. HU, L. *et al.* 2002. Obtaining reliable information from minute amounts of RNA using cDNA arrays. BMC Genomics **3:** 16.

Bioinformatics Tools for Single Nucleotide Polymorphism Discovery and Analysis

ROBERT J. CLIFFORD, MICHAEL N. EDMONSON, CU NGUYEN, TITIA SCHERPBIER, YING HU, AND KENNETH H. BUETOW

Laboratory of Population Genetics, Center for Cancer Research, National Cancer Institute, Bethesda, Maryland 20892, USA

ABSTRACT: Single nucleotide polymorphisms (SNPs) are a valuable resource for investigating the genetic basis of disease. These variants can serve as markers for fine-scale genetic mapping experiments and genome-wide association studies. Certain of these nucleotide polymorphisms may predispose individuals to illnesses such as diabetes, hypertension, or cancer, or affect disease progression. Bioinformatics techniques can play an important role in SNP discovery and analysis. We use computational methods to identify SNPs and to predict whether they are likely to be neutral or deleterious. We also use informatics to annotate genes that contain SNPs. To make this information available to the research community, we provide a variety of Internet-accessible tools for data access and display. These tools allow researchers to retrieve data about SNPs based on gene of interest, genetic or physical map location, or expression pattern.

KEYWORDS: bioinformatics; single nucleotide polymorphisms; SNPs

INTRODUCTION

Advances in information technology and bioinformatics have revolutionized biological research. DNA and protein homology searches, identification of protein motifs, and measurement of global gene expression using SAGE or microarrays are standard tools used by the research community. The World Wide Web (WWW) allows instant access to centralized databases containing a wealth of information about the human genome, chromosome aberrations, gene and protein sequences, protein motifs and three-dimensional structures, genetic polymorphisms, gene expression profiles, and biochemical pathways. It is now possible to search the vast research literature through a desktop computer. These advances have hastened the pace of scientific discovery and have facilitated an integration of genetics, molecular biology, cell biology, and biochemistry.

Bioinformatics provides powerful approaches for investigating the molecular basis of disease. These tools include both computational procedures for data analysis as well as methods to efficiently store and retrieve information. The mission of the Cancer Genome Anatomy Project (CGAP) is to catalog the gene expression patterns

Address for correspondence: Robert J. Clifford; NCI/CCR/LPG, MSC8302, 8424 Helgerman Court, Bethesda, MD 20892. Voice: 301-435-1527; fax: 301-402-9325.
clifforr@mail.nih.gov

Ann. N.Y. Acad. Sci. 1020: 101–109 (2004). © 2004 New York Academy of Sciences.
doi: 10.1196/annals.1310.011

of normal, precancerous, and cancer cells to enhance our ability to detect, diagnose, and treat cancer.[1] Within this large-scale effort, the Genetic Annotation Initiative (CGAP-GAI) uses bioinformatics to identify genetic variations in genes important for cancer. Our focus is on single nucleotide polymorphisms (SNPs), the most common form of genetic variation in humans.

SNPs are valuable tools for cancer research. Because of their prevalence, they can serve as markers for mapping genetic traits. SNPs may be used in positional cloning studies designed to map disease loci in pedigrees or populations. Alternatively, these variants can be used as markers in genome-wide association studies.[2] The International HapMap Project is currently developing an SNP-based haplotype map for use in disease gene discovery; the goal is to develop a minimal set of SNPs that serve as signatures for the most common haplotype blocks in humans.[3] SNPs may themselves represent genetic variants that affect disease susceptibility or progression. Producing a catalogue of variants in a disease-associated gene is an important resource for identifying alleles responsible for development of disease susceptibility.

Members of the CGAP-GAI project have created a variety of tools for SNP discovery, analysis, and display. We identify novel variants through computational methods, validate SNPs with mass spectroscopy, and use bioinformatics tools to predict whether SNPs are likely to alter gene function. We provide detailed annotation for SNPs. We have created WWW-based tools that allow researchers to search for SNPs by gene, by cytogenetic or physical map location, or by expression pattern.

RESULTS

SNP Discovery

A key area of investigation by the CGAP-GAI is the discovery of novel SNPs in transcripts. We search for SNPs among publicly available mRNA and expressed sequence tag (EST) sequences;[4] the basic unit of this analysis is the UniGene cluster.[5] SNP detection has been the focus of intense effort in the past several years. The SNP Consortium (TSC), for example, has identified 1.79 million SNPs by examining high-quality genome sequences. Putative variants are validated using a panel of 24 ethnically diverse individuals.[6,7] Several features of our approach distinguish our work from the TSC project. First, we focus on SNPs in transcripts. Our collection of SNPs consists exclusively of variants in exons. Second, sequences used in our analysis come from a larger set of individuals than that used for the genome sequence, so we may find SNPs not represented in the 48 chromosomes examined by the TSC. Third, we examine transcripts from healthy individuals, individuals with diseases, tumor tissue, and cell lines. As a result, CGAP-GAI SNPs likely include rare disease-causing mutations in addition to variants that occur at a high frequency in healthy populations.

Because ESTs are high-throughput, low-quality sequences, false positives arising from sequencing artifacts are a serious concern. To distinguish bona fide SNPs from the background of false positives, our analysis is based on the examination of sequencing traces rather than the ASCII representations of sequences. Traces are reanalyzed with the Phred package,[8,9] which allows us to measure the quality of each base call. Next, sequences from each UniGene cluster are reassembled into contigs using Phrap (P. Green; http://www.phrap.org/) and then contigs are further refined using PHYLIP (J. Felsenstein; http://evolution.genetics.washington.edu/phylip.html/). Rebuilding the clusters reduces the chance that we compare sequences derived from highly homologous genes, another source of false positives. Last, when two alternative bases are observed at a position in a sequence alignment, we use a statistical analysis that takes into account sequence trace quality and whether the variant is observed in traces derived from both DNA strands to calculate the probability that the candidate SNP is genuine.

To validate candidate SNPs identified *in silico*, we use MALDI-TOF mass spectrography.[10] Pooled DNA prepared from a panel of 94 individuals is screened for the presence of variants. As a further step, a subset of validated SNPs have been confirmed by segregation analysis.[11] Confirmation involves typing the SNP locus in human pedigrees from the CEPH collection of extended families and using the CRI-MAP program[12] to genetically map the marker. This step establishes whether the variant is transmitted from parent to child in a Mendelian fashion and can provide conclusive evidence that the SNP is genuine.

SNP Annotation

Our SNP prediction method is rooted in UniGene clusters. Over time, UniGenes are refined. New sequences may be added to a cluster. When a cluster is rebuilt, some of its sequences may be reassigned to another cluster, or sequences from other clusters may be assigned to it. Occasionally, a cluster may merge with another UniGene or may be split into a set of new clusters. In addition to changes in the sequence composition of UniGene clusters, gene names and descriptions can change over time. Given the evolving nature of UniGenes, it is critical that annotation be kept up to date. At each UniGene release, we reannotate SNPs. To account for sequence reassignments and the merging and splitting of clusters, SNPs are remapped to UniGenes via the sequences used to detect the polymorphism. We then annotate the cluster using data files for the current UniGene build provided by the National Center for Biotechnology Information (NCBI).

Based on their assignments to UniGene clusters, we determine the genetic, physical, and cytogenetic positions of SNPs.[11] Cytogenetic positions are from the annotation of UniGenes provided by the NCBI. Locations of genes containing SNPs on integrated genetic/physical maps are determined using radiation hybrid map markers from the UniGenes. The genetic portion of the map is the CHLC/ABI version 2 recombination map; the physical map is the NCBI Genebridge 4 radiation hybrid map.

We also collect information about the expression patterns of genes with SNPs.[11] These data are obtained from the CGAP, which maintains a database of gene expression patterns with respect to tissue type and histology. Patterns are based on the tissue type and histology of the EST libraries used to isolate transcripts from UniGenes.

Analysis of Coding Region SNPs

In addition to updating the mapping of SNPs to genes and UniGene annotation, we determine location of SNPs with respect to mRNA coding regions of mRNAs, protein motifs, and three-dimensional protein structures.[13] SNPs that lead to amino acid substitutions are of particular interest because they have the obvious potential to alter protein stability or activity. For this work, we examine not only SNPs discovered by the CGAP-GAI project, but also those submitted to the dbSNP database[14] by other laboratories. The initial stage in this analysis is to map SNPs onto mRNA sequences by BLAST. These sequences include NCBI RefSeqs,[15] which are curated "virtual" mRNAs whose structures are derived from public domain mRNA and EST sequences, and Mammalian Gene Collection (MGC) full-length transcripts,[16] which are high-quality sequences obtained from IMAGE Consortium clones. If an SNP lies in a coding region, the variant form of the transcript is translated to determine whether an amino acid substitution occurs. Additionally, we use the Pfam set of protein motif models[17,18] and the HMMER suite of tools[19] to identify conserved domains in gene products.

If an SNP maps to a conserved protein domain, we perform additional analysis. First, if a crystal structure of the domain is known, we determine the location of the amino acid residue within that motif. The domain of interest in the human protein is aligned with the sequence whose structure has been determined, allowing a translation of the affected residue onto the three-dimensional structure. If the variant alters an amino acid, we use computational methods to predict whether these alterations are likely to affect protein function.

The approach we have taken is to assay how the introduction of a new amino acid affects the fit of a protein sequence to a domain model. Our reasoning is that there should be a correlation between the magnitude of this change and the effect of the substitution on protein function. To measure this fit, we use the HMMER "hmmsearch" program. Two statistics are produced by this program. The score is the log 2 probability that the target sequence was produced by the motif model rather than a model that generates random sequences. The E-value is the number of randomly generated sequences expected to fit the domain model as well as or better than the target sequence. Using a set of biochemically analyzed mutations in T4 lysozyme, HIV-1 protease, and HIV-1 reverse transcriptase as benchmarks, we find that the log 10 ratio of the variant sequence and canonical sequence E-values is a good predictor of whether an amino acid alteration is deleterious. Our "LogR.E-value" method outperforms amino acid conservation based on amino acid substitution matrices and is robust—the prediction is not highly dependent on the sequences used to construct the domain model. We have generated predictions for 7391 variants lying in 2683 loci.

Display Tools

To make data accessible to the research community, the GAI has developed a variety of WWW-based tools for displaying information about SNPs.

As an adjunct to our SNP discovery efforts, we provide a Java-based viewer that displays SNPs in the context of the sequence assemblies from which they were predicted. The SNP Launcher applet provides two views of an assembly: a sequence alignment (FIG. 1A) and an assembly overview (FIG. 1B). In the sequence alignment, the quality of each base call is indicated by case and shading. Clicking on a nucleotide launches a sequencing trace viewer. From the assembly viewer, users can also get an SNP report that shows the sequences flanking the polymorphism, which alternate base occurs in each sequence in the alignment, and the sequence trace quality scores of those residues. Links are also provided to the GenBank records for

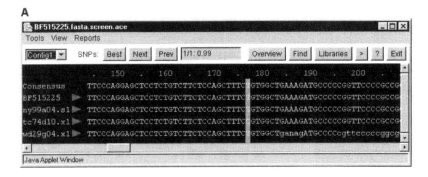

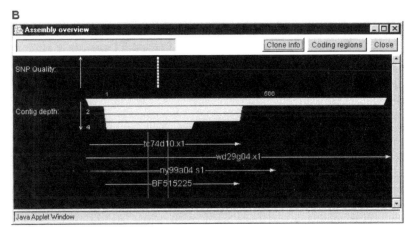

FIGURE 1. SNP Launcher. **(A)** The sequence viewer window. The position of the SNP is indicated by vertical shading. High-quality base calls are in uppercase; low-quality base calls are in lowercase. **(B)** The assembly overview window.

sequences and the contig consensus sequence. A BLAST client and software for designing PCR primers for SNP assays is accessed through the tools menu. The assembly overview shows a graphical representation of the sequence assembly, along with clone coverage along the length of the consensus sequence. If the assembly contains mRNAs, the predicted open reading frame can be displayed as well. A button is provided for generating a report of coding region SNPs. The entry point for the SNP Launcher is http://lpgws.nci.nih.gov/perl/snpbr/. This search engine allows searching for SNPs by gene name, keyword, DNA sequence accession, UniGene cluster number, or GCAP-GAI SNP identification number. Users can also search for SNPs in a sequence of interest via BLAST.

We provide a set of tools for map-based searches. To search by an interval of the integrated genetic/physical map, we provide a graphical search tool. Form-based tools allow searching by radiation hybrid map coordinates, marker-delimited physical map intervals, or cytogenetic location. A novel feature of the SNP maps and associated search engines is that we have integrated expression data with gene mapping.

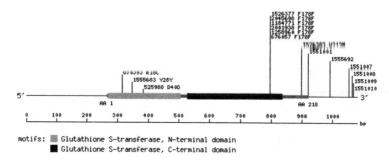

FIGURE 2. Gene Viewer. SNPs in the GSTM4 gene. This gene has nonsynonymous cSNPs, silent cSNPs, and noncoding single nucleotides. The multiple SNP IDs for the F178F variant indicate that it has been observed in independent experiments.

Thus, it is possible to perform searches for SNPs in genes that are expressed in particular tissue types or histologies (e.g., SNPs in genes on the X chromosome that are expressed in colon cancer, but not normal colon tissue). Map-based search tools are accessed through http://lpgws.nci.nih.gov/html-snp/imagemaps.html/.

Finally, we have developed a number of resources for retrieving information about SNPs in the context of mRNA sequences. First, a search page that returns a table of SNPs in mRNAs is http://lpgws.nci.nih.gov/perl/snp2ref/. Results can be limited to validated SNPs. A graphical view of these data is provided by the Gene Viewer (http://lpgws.nci.nih.gov/cgi-bin/GeneViewer.cgi/) (Fig. 2). This script displays SNPs mapped onto a schematic diagram of a transcript. Coding regions and protein motifs are shown as well. This display page contains a link to more detailed information about coding region SNPs. The Motif set of tools provides detailed information about cSNPs. SNPs are displayed in the context of conserved protein motifs. For SNPs that cause amino acid alterations, we show how the amino acid substitution changes the fit of the domain to the Pfam motif model as is measured by score and E-value, making it apparent which SNPs are most likely to affect protein function. In addition, this display shows whether the affected residue is invariant or variable in the Pfam motif model. Last, we provide a Java-based viewer for visualizing the location of the altered amino acid in the context of a three-dimensional protein structure (Fig. 3). The residue is displayed on both side-chain and backbone models. The structure viewer has zoom and rotation features. The structure viewer makes it easy to see whether the affected residue is located in an enzyme active site, a protein-protein interaction surface, or the structural core of a domain.

Data Repositories

Our WWW-based tools are designed for searching for SNPs within a specific gene or a defined genetic, physical, or cytogenetic map location. For researchers who wish to perform whole genome analyses using SNPs as reagents, we provide a portion of our data in text files. Data dumps include basic information about SNPs (alternative bases, flanking sequences, probability scores, consensus sequences for alignments used to predict SNPs), SNP validation status, map locations and expres-

NM_000850.1				LPG id: R10755	
Domain #1					
PF02798	GTA1_HUMAN		2	to	82
pdb1gsd	Chain: A		3	to	76

Molecule-View   **Backbone-View**

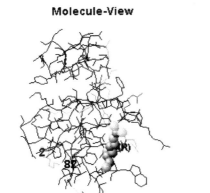 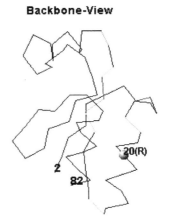

Drag mouse to rotate;
Drag mouse while holding the Shift key to zoom in or out.

Snp ID	Refseq/MGC		3D Residue	
	Pos	AA change	Pos	AA
870393	18	R-> C	20	R

FIGURE 3. Structure viewer. Coding region SNPs in the GST_N domain of GSTM4. Since the crystal structure of GSTM4 has not been determined, SNPs are projected onto side-chain and backbone views of the GST_N domain of human GSTA1. The Arg residue at position 18 of GSTM4, which is changed to Cys by a cSNP, corresponds to the Arg residue at position 20 of GSTA1.

sion patterns of genes with SNPs, and lists of cSNPs that alter amino acids. Files are available via anonymous FTP from ftp1.nci.nih.gov/pub/GAI-SNP/.

Public Accessibility of SNP Discovery Tools

Our set of SNP discovery tools are freely available to the research community. Researchers may submit their own sets of DNA sequences to be analyzed for the presence of SNPs. Users should contact Kenneth Buetow (buetowk@mail.nih.gov) to obtain an account for using our tools.

CONCLUSIONS

Single nucleotide polymorphisms are a powerful resource for cancer research. We have used bioinformatics for SNP discovery and analysis and provide a variety of WWW-accessible tools to display information about SNPs. Two use cases for our tools are as follows:

- Use Case 1: A researcher has mapped a locus involved in a hereditary cancer to a small cytogenetic location. She uses the cytogenetic search engine to retrieve SNPs in genes from the cytoband of interest and then chooses validated SNPs in these loci for use as markers for fine-scale linkage disequilibrium mapping in affected families. When a candidate gene is identified, she sequences exons from the gene in cancer patients. She then uses CGAP-GAI SNP detection tools to analyze this collection of sequences for polymorphisms that may represent disease alleles.

- Use Case 2: A worker is investigating the role of a signaling pathway in tumor metastasis. He takes the approach of searching for genetic variants that occur more frequently in patients with aggressive forms of cancer. To perform the association study, he retrieves a list of SNPs in genes encoding components of the molecular pathway. From these, he selects a set of validated SNPs for use in the association study. Priority is given to variants that alter amino acids in conserved protein domains and are likely to affect protein function.

Future Directions

The mouse is a versatile model organism for studying cancer development. In addition to SNP prediction for humans, we also have used our tools to discover murine SNPs. At present, these variants are accessible through a subset of our tools. We are modifying the Gene Viewer and the scripts that generate chromosome maps to display mouse SNPs. In addition, we are mapping SNPs onto the draft human and mouse genome sequences, which will allow the direct physical mapping of SNPs rather than indirect mapping through the genes in which they lie. Finally, we will catalog "protein haplotypes" by determining which cSNPs are observed together on mRNA and EST sequences. We will use our analysis tools to determine how multiple changes affect the fit of protein sequences to domain models.

REFERENCES

1. STRAUSBERG, R.L., S.F. GREENHUT, L.H. GROUSE *et al.* 2001. *In silico* analysis of cancer through the Cancer Genome Anatomy Project. Trends Cell Biol. **11:** S66–S71.
2. BOTSTEIN, D. & N. RISCH. 2003. Discovering genotypes underlying human phenotypes: past successes for Mendelian disease, future approaches for complex disease. Nat. Genet. **33:** 228–237.
3. CARDON, L.R. & G.R. ABECASIS. 2003. Using haplotype blocks to map human complex trait loci. Trends Genet. **19:** 135–140.
4. BUETOW, K.H., M.N. EDMONSON & A.B. CASSIDY. 1999. Reliable identification of large numbers of candidate SNPs from public EST data. Nat. Genet. **21:** 323–325.
5. SCHULER, G.D., M.S. BOGUSKI, E.A. STEWART *et al.* 1996. A gene map of the human genome. Science **274:** 540–546.

6. ALTSHULER, D., V.J. POLLARA, C.R. COWLES *et al.* 2000. An SNP map of the human genome generated by reduced representation shotgun sequencing. Nature **407:** 513–516.
7. THORISSON, G.A. & L.D. STEIN. 2003. The SNP Consortium Website: past, present, and future. Nucleic Acids Res. **31:** 124–127.
8. EWING, B., L. HILLIER, M.C. WENDL & P. GREEN. 1998. Base-calling of automated sequencer traces using Phred: I. Accuracy assessment. Genome Res. **8:** 175–185.
9. EWING, B. & P. GREEN. 1998. Base-calling of automated sequencer traces using Phred: II. Error probabilities. Genome Res. **8:** 186–194.
10. BUETOW, K.H., M. EDMONSON, R. MACDONALD *et al.* 2001. High-throughput development and characterization of a genomewide collection of gene-based single nucleotide polymorphism markers by chip-based matrix-assisted laser desorption/ionization time-of-flight mass spectrometry. Proc. Natl. Acad. Sci. USA **98:** 581–584.
11. CLIFFORD, R., M. EDMONSON, Y. HU *et al.* 2000. Expression-based genetic/physical maps of single-nucleotide polymorphisms identified by the Cancer Genome Anatomy Project. Genome Res. **10:** 1259–1265.
12. GREEN, P. 1992. Construction and comparison of chromosome 21 radiation hybrid and linkage maps using CRI-MAP. Cytogenet. Cell Genet. **59:** 122–124
13. CLIFFORD, R., M. EDMONSON, C. NGUYEN & K.H. BUETOW. 2003. Large-scale analysis of non-synonymous coding region single nucleotide polymorphisms. Bioinformatics. In press.
14. SHERRY, S.T., M. WARD & K. SIROTKIN. 1999. dbSNP—database for single nucleotide polymorphisms and other classes of minor genetic variation. Genome Res. **9:** 677–679.
15. PRUITT, K.D. & D.R. MAGLOTT. 2001. RefSeq and LocusLink: NCBI gene-centered resources. Nucleic Acids Res. **29:** 137–140.
16. STRAUSBERG, R.L., E.A. FEINGOLD, R.D. KLAUSNER & F.S. COLLINS. 1999. The Mammalian Gene Collection. Science **286:** 455–457.
17. BATEMAN, A., E. BIRNEY, R. DURBIN *et al.* 1999. Pfam 3.1: 1313 multiple alignments and profile HMMs match the majority of proteins. Nucleic Acids Res. **27:** 260–262.
18. BATEMAN, A., E. BIRNEY, L. CERRUTI *et al.* 2002. The Pfam protein families database. Nucleic Acids Res. **30:** 276–280.
19. EDDY, S.R. 1998. Profile hidden Markov models. Bioinformatics **14:** 755–763.

Numerical Deconvolution of cDNA Microarray Signal

Simulation Study

SIMON ROSENFELD,[a] THOMAS WANG,[b] YOUNG KIM,[c] AND JOHN MILNER[c]

[a]Biometry Research Group, Division of Cancer Prevention, National Cancer Institute, National Institutes of Health, Department of Health and Human Services, Rockville, Maryland 20892, USA

[b]Phytonutrients Laboratory, USDA, Beltsville, Maryland 20705, USA

[c]Nutritional Sciences Research Group, Division of Cancer Prevention, National Cancer Institute, National Institutes of Health, Department of Health and Human Services, Rockville, Maryland 20892, USA

ABSTRACT: A computational model for simulation of the cDNA microarray experiments has been created. The simulation allows one to foresee the statistical properties of replicated experiments without actually performing them. We introduce a new concept, the so-called bio-weight, which allows for reconciliation between conflicting meanings of biological and statistical significance in microarray experiments. It is shown that, for a small sample size, the bio-weight is a more powerful criterion of the presence of a signal in microarray data as compared to the standard approach based on t test. Joint simulation of microarray and quantitative PCR data shows that the genes recovered by using the bio-weight have better chances to be confirmed by PCR than those obtained by the t test technique. We also employ extreme value considerations to derive plausible cutoff levels for hypothesis testing.

KEYWORDS: microarray data analysis; numerical simulation; polymerase chain reaction (PCR); replicated experiment

INTRODUCTION

DNA microarray technology is a revolutionary advance in experimental biology allowing scientists to simultaneously monitor expression levels of thousands of genes.[1,2] Despite rapid progress in the technology, extracting useful information from microarray data has not yet become a straightforward task. Genomic response is usually obscured by noise from numerous sources, and application of elaborate statistical techniques is required at all steps of data analysis. During the last several

Address for correspondence: Simon Rosenfeld, Biometry Research Group, Division of Cancer Prevention, National Cancer Institute, National Institutes of Health, Department of Health and Human Services, EPN 3136, 6130 Executive Boulevard, Rockville, MD 20892. Voice: 301-496-7748; fax: 301-402-0816.
  sr212a@nih.gov

Ann. N.Y. Acad. Sci. 1020: 110–123 (2004). © 2004 New York Academy of Sciences.
doi: 10.1196/annals.1310.012

years, microarray data analysis has become an arena of active statistical experimentation with dozens of notable publications.[3–6] This surge of activity is motivated not only by the flood of new data, but also by a novelty of the problem in a statistical sense. Classical statistics usually deals with the situation when the number of parameters to be estimated is smaller, or even substantially smaller, than the number of the subjects in the study. This is not the case in the microarray data analysis where, usually, the expression profiles of many thousands of genes have to be estimated from experiments with several dozen subjects at best. This new statistical paradigm, termed as the "curse of dimensionality",[7] stimulated development of a wide range of innovative ideas whose pros and cons are currently being scrutinized by the statistical and biological communities. Although it is obvious that dimensionality reduction is impossible without adequate modeling of the error and signal structures, it is necessary to maintain a parsimonious balance between the data quality and the model complexity.

A popular idea widely used in microarray data analysis is the assumption that the cDNA expression levels are approximately log-normally distributed, thus producing approximate normality of logarithms of intensities. This assumption makes it possible to employ numerous statistical techniques such as ANOVA,[8] cluster analysis,[9] mixed-effects models,[10] etc. Albeit the consequences of this assumption are plentiful and powerful, its justification is often vague and almost never goes far beyond the considerations of simplicity and mathematical convenience. However, in our experience, even a preliminary inspection of the empirical distributions of the microarray intensities reveals drastic violations of the log-normality assumption. The first goal of this paper is to create a more realistic simulation model for the cDNA intensities without the assumptions of log-normality. The second goal is to introduce a new concept for determination of significant genes. This concept, termed further as the "bio-weight", is designed to overcome the conflict between a tendency to declare significant only the genes with high observed differential expression versus strict statistical requirements that recognize as significant only the genes with high between-replicates reproducibility. It will be shown through simulation experiments that, for a small number of replicates, the bio-weight produces a higher true positive rate compared to traditionally used methods based on *t* test *P* values. A useful by-product of our simulation study is the determination of plausible cutoff values for hypothesis testing using extreme value considerations.

MODEL STRUCTURE AND FITTING

The data available in this study resulted from hybridization experiments with the human prostate cancer cell LNCaP treated by the garlic component diallyl disulfide (DADS). The hybridization experiments were replicated three times under four different experimental conditions, thus producing 12 slides with wide variations in expression profiles. Each NCI cDNA slide contained 10,368 spots, including genes, ESTs, and empty wells. Preprocessing included several standard steps, such as correction for background intensity, correction for nonlinearity of dependence of intensity versus expression level using the local optimal regression estimator (LOESS), adjustment for slide-to-slide variability (median and interquartile adjustment), and adjustment for within-slide variability.[2,11] FIGURE 1 shows the sample

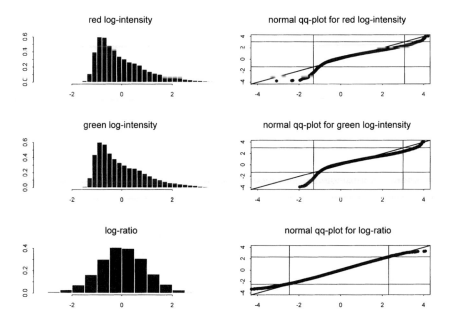

FIGURE 1. Distributions and qq-plots for logarithms of channel intensities and log-ratio.

distributions and normal quantile-quantile plots of log-intensities and log-ratio obtained from the DADS 25 μM/24 h experiment. Similar distributions were observed under other experimental conditions. Interesting features of these distributions are strong asymmetry and presence of a characteristic "hump" in the distributional shapes, indicating strong deviations from normality. Nevertheless, the difference of log-intensities (i.e., log-ratio) is seemingly very close to normality. This observation suggests the idea that the red and green log-intensities may be modeled as a pair of interrelated additive models with independent normal error terms and highly dependent nonnormal signal terms. This structure is capable of producing the desirable effect of strong nonnormality of log-intensities and approximate normality of their difference. We now elaborate this premise in more detail.

We assume the mixed-effects model for log-intensities:

$$\log(y_{i,j,k}) = \mu + x_{i,k} + \varepsilon_{i,j,k} \quad [i = 1,\dots,N; j = 1,\dots,M; k = 1, 2] \tag{1}$$

where $y_{i,j,k}$ are intensities, and i, j, and k are the indices of genes, replicates, and Cy5/Cy3 channels, respectively. We also assume that the error terms $\varepsilon_{i,j,k}$ are independent normal identically distributed random variables with the expectations 0 and variances σ^2. The random effect term $x_{i,k}$ represents a pair of channel-specific random variables, each of which may be in turn represented as a sum of two parts, $x_{i,k} = \xi_i + \eta_{i,k}$, where ξ_i is the log-intensity in the control channel (Cy5) and $\eta_{i,k}$ values are the random deviations of this log-intensity in the treatment channel (Cy3) arising from the differences in gene activity. It is often assumed that all of the $\eta_{i,k}$ are zero for $k = 1$ and nonzero for a certain comparatively small group of differentially expressed genes for $k = 2$. This kind of clear-cut dichotomy between the differentially expressed and nonexpressed genes never takes place in reality. Even if the mRNA samples are taken from the same specimen, they still may differ due to random spatial variations of biological conditions within the specimen, uncontrollable variations in the protocol implementation, and even subtler effects such as waiting times between the slide preparations and scanning, for example.[12] In such an experimental environment with many uncertainties, it seems more reasonable to characterize a model in more general terms, assuming that all of the genes in the treatment and control groups are more or less differentially expressed and that there is a continuous distribution of these differences. In our model, we characterize the differential expression by a continuous distribution with the probability P_L of over/under-expression above level L. An exact form of this distribution is not of any importance because we are mostly interested only in the quantiles of this distribution. As mentioned above, the distributions of $x_{i,k}$ are expected to be strongly nonnormal. In order to parsimoniously capture both nonnormality and covariance between the channels, we assume that random variable X is a polynomial transformation of the bivariate standard normal random variable Z with correlation coefficients between the components ρ_z: $X = BZ + CZ^2 + DZ^3$. The choice of the third-order polynomial is motivated by the considerations of simplicity coupled with flexibility, allowing one to simulate a wide variety of distributional shapes.

The difference between the log-intensities, that is, log-ratio

$$R_{i,j} = \log(y_{i,j,2}/y_{i,j,1}) = \eta_{i,2} + \varepsilon_{i,j,2} - \varepsilon_{i,j,1}, \tag{2}$$

would be purely normal except for a comparatively small distortion provided by the term $\eta_{i,2}$. Reproducibility of the microarray experiment is determined by the statistical properties of this term. We can measure this reproducibility by the average pairwise correlation coefficient, λ, between the expression profiles in different replicates. In the DADS data, for example, $\lambda \approx 0.35$. As a matter of fact, the combination of two parameters, that is, the between-channels correlation coefficient, ρ, and the between-replicates correlation coefficient, λ, reflects the quality of the microarray experiment. Other than simplicity, the motivation behind the choice of the third-order polynomials for representing nonnormal microarray signal is that, by having at our disposal four free coefficients, we can always find the distributions possessing the prespecified four first cumulants, that is, mean, variance, skewness, and kurtosis. This four-parameter family can in turn be presented through the Pearson system, which is known to encompass a wide range of distributions commonly used in statistical practice. We rewrite the above introduced model as

$$y_1 = \varepsilon_1 + A + Bz_1 + Cz_1^2 + Dz_1^3, \quad y_2 = \varepsilon_2 + A + Bz_2 + Cz_2^2 + Dz_2^3, \tag{3}$$

assuming now that $y_{1,2}$ values are the log-intensities and $z_{1,2}$ is the bivariate standard normal random variable with the correlation coefficient between components ρ_z. We first express means and variances of u and v through the coefficients A, B, C, D:

$$E(y_{1,2}) = A + C; \quad var(y_{1,2}) = \sigma^2 + A^2 + B^2 + 2C^2 + 6BD + 15D^2. \tag{4}$$

Then, we compute the variance of the difference between the red and green log-intensities:

$$var(y_2 - y_1) = 2\sigma^2 + 2B^2(1 - \rho_z) + 4C^2(1 - \rho_z^2) +$$

$$[30 - 2(9\rho_z + 6\rho_z^3)]D^2 + 12BD(1 - \rho_z). \tag{5}$$

The correlation coefficient between red and green log-intensities is

$$\rho = [B^2\rho_z + 2C^2\rho_z^2 + 6BD\rho_z + (9\rho_z + 6\rho_z^3)D^2]/[\sigma^2 + B^2 + 2C^2 + 6BD + 15D^2]. \tag{6}$$

Equation 6 is a cubic equation with respect to the unknown correlation coefficient ρ_z. Solving it, we obtain ρ_z, which provides a required between-channels correlation coefficient ρ.

In order to specify the model, we need to estimate six parameters: σ^2, A, B, C, D, and ρ. The first five parameters may be obtained by taking into account the above shown shapes of distributions of log-intensities. For this purpose, in addition to the already determined means and variances of the marginal distributions, we also compute the skewness and kurtosis. Because y_1, z_1 as well as y_2, z_2 are pairwise independent, their cumulants are additive and therefore

$$\gamma_3(y_{1,2}) = \{\sigma^2(x_{1,2})/[\sigma^2(x_{1,2}) + \sigma^2(z_{1,2})]\}^{3/2}\gamma_3(x_{1,2}),$$

$$\gamma_4(y_{1,2}) = \{\sigma^2(x_{1,2})/[\sigma^2(x_{1,2}) + \sigma^2(z_{1,2})]\}^2\gamma_4(x_{1,2}), \tag{7}$$

where γ_3 and γ_4 denote skewness and kurtosis, respectively. Identification of the model is split into three steps. First, we estimate marginal cumulants of log-intensities from the actual DADS data. Then, we numerically fit the coefficients A, B, C, D of the polynomial transformation for producing the random variables with these cumulants. Numerical solution of nonlinear equations for the determination of coefficients is performed using the smooth nonlinear optimizer *nlminb* of S-PLUS.[13] The final step is solving equation 6 with respect to correlation coefficient ρ of the parent bivariate normal distribution. After this step, all of the parameters are in place that are necessary for simulation. The qq-plots in FIGURE 2 show the results of comparison of the simulated data versus the observed ones. As seen from this figure, the simulated and observed samples are almost indistinguishable in terms of their distributional properties, thus demonstrating the adequacy of the model. TABLE 1 shows the parameters resulting from the model fitting. These parameters are further used as a basis for numerical experiments. Standard deviations in the second row of TABLE 1 demonstrate a reasonable stability of the model parameters across different experimental conditions.

TABLE 1. Parameters of the polynomial model for log-intensities derived from the DADS data

	SE(ε)	A	B	C	D	SE(x)	ρ
Mean	0.245	0.452	0.792	0.181	−0.061	0.685	0.973
SD	0.031	0.129	0.097	0.058	0.007	0.114	0.008

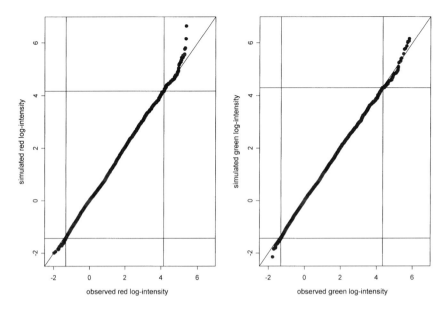

FIGURE 2. Quantile-quantile plots comparing observed and simulated microarray data.

CONFLICTING MEANINGS OF SIGNIFICANCE IN MICROARRAY DATA ANALYSIS: THE CONCEPT OF BIO-WEIGHT

FIGURE 3 represents the so-called volcano plot, which is frequently used in micro-array data analysis. In this plot (computed from the DADS 25 μM/24 h experiment), the horizontal axis represents the average across-replicates binary logarithm of the ratio of green to red intensities. The vertical axis is the negative decimal logarithm of P values for the gene-specific t tests, with the null hypotheses that the average log-ratios are zero (i.e., there is no difference between DADS-treated and untreated bio-assays). The most statistically significant genes (i.e., corresponding to the smallest P values) are located on the top of the volcano plot. The leftmost and rightmost genes correspond to a large average across-the-replicates absolute fold change. The volca-no plot vividly shows a conflict between the notions of the "biological" and "statis-tical" significance. A biologist seeks the over/underexpressed genes with the reservation that any substantial finding can and must be validated in independent experimental settings. On the contrary, a statistician seeks the statistically significant genes, that is, those corresponding to the smallest P values. Unfortunately, simultaneous application of both of these criteria results in a very small number (if any) of significant genes. Due to the multiple comparison problem, the traditional significance levels of 5% or 1% are not applicable to microarray data, and much more stringent criteria should be imposed to minimize the false-positive findings.[14] The simplest known approach to obtaining the P values adjusted for multiple comparisons is the Bonferroni adjustment, which requires, roughly speaking, dividing the individual P values by the number of genes. This criterion is excessively

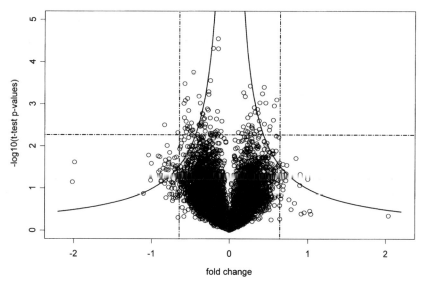

FIGURE 3. Selection of significant genes using bio-weight.

conservative because individual testing at the significance level of 10^{-6} almost for sure would produce no significant genes. Even if we impose much milder criteria by declaring "statistically" significant all the genes with P values only below 0.1% and "biologically" significant the genes with the absolute fold change only above 1.5, we will still find no significant genes.

Recognizing an equal importance of the gene selection based on fold changes as well as on P values, we introduce a new measure of significance that is further referred to as "bio-weight" and is defined as the product of absolute average fold change and negative logarithm of the P value. The concept of bio-weight is illustrated by the volcano plot in FIGURE 3, where the horizontal and vertical dashed lines represent 99% quantiles of P values and fold changes, respectively. As mentioned above, several approaches to selecting significant genes are conceivable. We may apply the criterion of smallest P values and declare significant all the genes above the horizontal dashed line. Alternatively, we may apply the criterion of largest fold change and declare significant all the genes to the right and to the left of the vertical dashed lines. Applied separately, these two rules result in two groups of genes that are drastically different in terms of their statistical properties. Applied jointly, these rules would reveal either a very small number of significant genes or none at all. Yet another approach is to declare significant the union of the above two groups. This rule, however, would impose unjustifiably abrupt bounds in the selection criteria without corresponding abrupt changes in the gene properties. This conflict is resolved by application of the bio-weight because, in contrast to the above three approaches, this criterion declares significant all the genes above the hyperbolic solid lines in FIGURE 3, representing 0.99-quantile of bio-weight. The advantage of such an approach is that it pays attention to both small P values and large fold changes and provides a smooth transition between these two, generally conflicting, groups.

The principal motivation for introducing the criterion of bio-weight comes from the considerations of validation. Whatever instrument is used for this purpose, it always has its own sensitivity and specificity. The genes that are declared to be highly significant in a microarray experiment may turn out to be intractable for independent validation due to a very small over- or underexpression. Currently, the most common experimental methodology for validating microarray data is the quantitative PCR.[15] The major limitation of the q-PCR is the necessity to keep the amplification curve within the exponential growth limits.[16] These limits, as well as the PCR amplification efficiency, are generally unknown and often require sophisticated algorithms and additional calibration efforts for reducing errors in the quantitation.[17] The bottom line is that the genes with relative abundances too close to 1 are not reliably discernable by PCR; therefore, the genes declared significant solely because of the smallness of their P values have little chance to be independently validated due to low over- or underexpression. In the above cited work by Rajeevan *et al.*,[15] for example, only the genes with fold change 2 or greater are considered as differentially expressed (as seen from FIGURE 3, none of such genes are statistically significant in the DADS experiment). As a result, an experimental biologist faces a difficult choice between reliance solely on the microarray data on the one hand and relaxing the requirements of statistical significance in exchange for higher probability of independent validation on the other hand. The criterion of bio-weight attempts to reconcile these conflicting requirements and retains those genes that are the most likely candidates for the follow-up validation.

These intuitive considerations of interplay between microarray experiment and PCR validation may be confirmed by direct numerical simulation. Let s_i be the number of mRNA copies after the i-th cycle of PCR amplification and let E_i be the PCR efficiency in this cycle. We suggest the following simple stochastic model for the dynamics of PCR amplification:

$$s_{i+1} = s_i(1 + E_i) + \theta_i, \quad E_{i+1} = 1/(1 + \beta s_i^{\gamma}), \tag{8}$$

where θ_i is the random term with statistical characteristics dependent on s_i. Equations 8 realistically reproduce the basic features of PCR amplification, such as exponential growth during the first cycles and tendency to saturation and fluctuations when the cycle number exceeds a certain limit.[15,18] FIGURE 4 shows several examples of the PCR growth curve computed using equations 8 with parameters $\beta = 10^{-11}$, $\gamma = 1.2$, and θ_i normally distributed with expectation 0 and standard deviation $0.13s_i$. In these examples, the model is fitted in such a way as to maintain the PCR efficiency approximately constant and the amplification curves approximately exponential up to the 20th cycle, as usually takes place in practice.

Assuming that the number of mRNA copies in the treatment and control samples is proportional to the corresponding microarray intensities, we may now apply the model (1–3) for microarray signal coupling with the model (8) for PCR quantitation and explore the performance of different approaches to selecting the significant genes. In the example below, we select the top 5% of genes with the highest true differential expressions and apply three filtering procedures for recovering these genes from simulated data. TABLE 2 shows the sensitivities, that is, the fractions of truely differentially expressed genes that were successfully recovered from data. (We do not show the corresponding specificities because the vast majority of genes

TABLE 2. Sensitivities of different procedures for discovering differentially expressed genes

| | Number of replicates | | | |
Method	2	3	5	10
P values	0.099	0.144	0.274	0.403
q-PCR	0.208	0.263	0.323	0.712
Bio-weight	0.181	0.281	0.387	0.504

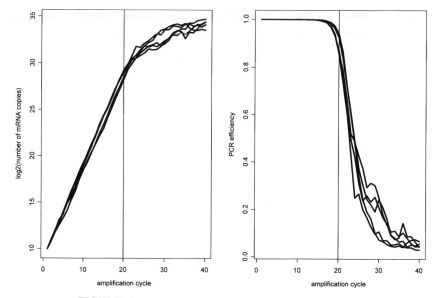

FIGURE 4. Examples of PCR amplification growth curves.

are not differentially expressed and are not declared to be differentially expressed; therefore, specificities are always trivially close to 100%.)

Examining TABLE 2, we may draw several conclusions. First, the method based on the t test P values is most unreliable for a small number of replicates (which is always the case in practice). Performance of the t test becomes reasonably close to that of the bio-weight only for sample size approaching 10, which is still a fairly small number for a reliable application of the t test, but already is a fairly large number from the cost/labor standpoint. Performance of the bio-weight is always substantially better than that of the t test. The advantages of the bio-weight over the t test diminish only for a comparatively large sample size. These results seem to be quite natural. Although replicated experiments are much more reliable than the single-slide experiments, nevertheless the use of a small number of replicates is not sufficient to experience a full advantage of the inference based on the t test over the "brute force" method based on the direct utilization of log-ratios. For these cases, the

TABLE 3. Quantiles of bio-weight for removing insignificant genes

	Number of replicates			
λ	2	3	5	10
0.1	0.96	0.93	0.90	0.82
0.35	0.82	0.76	0.67	0.52
0.5	0.71	0.62	0.53	0.41

method of bio-weight is a natural intermediate scheme taking advantage (or, better yet, compensating for weaknesses) of both extreme approaches. As seen from TABLE 2, for sample size up to 5, the bio-weight produces results reasonably close to those inferred from PCR quantitation, thus reflecting the fact that the genes selected using the bio-weight have a better chance to be confirmed by quantitative PCR.

There are some other useful properties of the bio-weight. A natural preliminary step in hunting for significant genes is first removing the genes that are the most unlikely to be significant. The bio-weight provides a convenient framework for this kind of data reduction. Because the reproducibility, λ, of a cDNA experiment is a positive value (in DADS data, it is about 0.35), there always exists such a quantile of bio-weight below which the cumulative reproducibility is zero. TABLE 3 shows these quantiles obtained by Monte Carlo simulation using the above formulated computational model. The numbers in this table are to be interpreted as follows. If we have a poorly reproducible experiment with a small number of replicates (top left corner of TABLE 3, $\lambda = 0.1$, 2 replicates), then as many as 96% of all the genes with the lowest bio-weight can be safely removed from further consideration as not containing anything except random noise. In the opposite case of a reasonably high reproducibility and a large number of replicates (right bottom corner of the table, $\lambda = 0.5$, 10 replicates), the data are much more reliable and hence only 41% of them can be removed as having no value. In the DADS data ($\lambda = 0.35$, 3 replicates), all the genes below the 76% percentile of bio-weight may be safely removed. After this kind of housecleaning, the dimensionality of the problem becomes much smaller and the cost of any computationally intensive procedure is greatly reduced.

DETERMINATION OF PLAUSIBLE THRESHOLDS FOR OVER/UNDEREXPRESSION

Having at our disposal the computational model, we can foresee, to a certain extent, how the outcome of our experiment would look if the number of replicates increases beyond that actually available. Let us imagine a hypothetical microarray experiment with no signal, that is, with absence of differentially expressed genes. In reality, this kind of experiment could be performed by competitive hybridization of two identical cell samples. In simulation, this assumption corresponds to a negligibly small variance of the $\eta_{i,j}$ term in the above described simulation model. FIGURE 5 shows a series of volcano plots that would be obtained as a result of 2, 3, 5, and 10 replications of the experiment. The thick vertical lines correspond to the threshold of over/underexpression 1.5. If we declare significant all the genes outside the

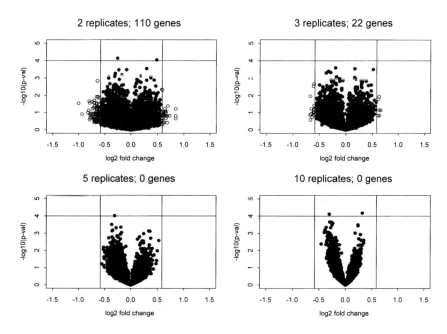

FIGURE 5. Simulation of replicated experiment under the assumption of absence of differentially expressed genes.

interval $(-1.5, 1.5)$, then the number of such genes will be 110 and 22 in the duplicated and triplicated experiments, respectively. These genes represent nothing more than false discoveries due to the assumption of absence of differentially expressed genes used in simulation. As seen from FIGURE 5, we need at least 5 replicates to avoid false discoveries. This intuitive consideration suggests the idea of how we should select plausible cutoff values for the over/underexpression. We will declare significant all the genes that are found outside the interval formed by the average extreme values of no-signal distributions. In the samples with size about 10,000, the probability of finding a random value outside the interval bounded by average extremes is about 0.00006 and may be safely ignored. If in a particular experiment we still find genes outside this interval, then we conjecture that these genes could not be attributed to the random noise only and consider these genes as plausible candidates to be declared significant. TABLE 4 shows expectations of extreme values for fold change versus number of replicates obtained by Monte Carlo simulation. This table should be interpreted as follows: in the duplicated experiment, we can safely call "overexpressed" only the genes with fold change above 1.89. Quite possibly, the log-ratios below these levels arise from random noise. With 3 replicates, our requirements become less stringent and the reasonable threshold for the fold change decreases to 1.68. A comfortable level 1.51 may be reached with 5 replicates. It is worth noting that, even if we increase the number of replicates up to 10, the gain would be comparatively modest: the threshold fold change would only reduce to

TABLE 4. Expectations of extreme fold changes in case of absence (*clear cells*) and presence (*shaded cells*) of genomic signal

	Number of replicates							
	2		3		5		10	
Maximum fold change	1.89	2.35	1.68	2.21	1.51	2.05	1.35	1.94
Maximum −log 10 (*P* value)	3.87	4.29	3.97	4.31	4.06	5.34	4.40	6.62
Maximum bio-weight	1.97	2.82	1.78	3.16	1.75	3.69	1.68	5.33

1.35. This conclusion can be used as an argument that 5 is a reasonable number of replicates for the type of cDNA chips similar to those used in the DADS experiment. It may be noted, however, that even these modest requirements may turn to be impracticable due to cost considerations.

The extreme value considerations may be also applied to the distribution of the *t* test *P* values. In the case of absence of differentially expressed genes, simulation shows that the average minimum of the *P* value does not change substantially with increasing number of replicates and remains in the vicinity of 10^{-4}. Presence of even a weak signal draws the *P* values toward much smaller values (i.e., toward the top of the volcano plot). There has been an extensive discussion in the statistical literature about the natural threshold of significance based on *P* values. This problem, known as the problem of multiple hypothesis testing, is fairly complex and a number of sophisticated methods have been devised to solve it.[14] Unfortunately, so far none of the existing methods has been recognized as completely satisfactory and adopted as a standard in the microarray community. A comprehensive critical review of these methods may be found in the report by Ge *et al.*[19] A multitude of approaches to multiple testing do not help much in practical analysis because the initial problem of selecting significant genes is replaced by a much more complicated problem, both logically and computationally. We believe that the extreme value considerations suggested in this paper introduce a simple method for selecting the natural threshold for the *P* values. Although this method suggests a fairly stringent criterion, note that it is still much milder than that imposed by the Bonferroni adjustment.

RESULTS

The above formulated method has been applied to the DADS data. Each triplicate of cDNA slides corresponding to different experimental conditions has been analyzed separately and all the genes were ranked by their total bio-weight computed as a sum of bio-weights in all the triplicates. Such ranking means that the selected genes demonstrate the most noticeable differential expressions under at least one of the experimental conditions, thus representing the best possible candidates for the follow-up study. TABLE 5 shows the top 10 genes resulting from our study. PCR validation of these genes as well as the biological interpretation of findings are intended to be future steps in our research.

TABLE 5. Top 10 genes ranked by their total bio-weight

Symbol	Gene name	Location	Bio-weight
SFRP5	Secreted frizzled related protein 5	15 pter-qter	7.95
TCOF1	Treacher Collins-Franceschetti syndrome	5q31.3-q33.3	7.27
NFIC	Nuclear factor I/C (CCAAT-binding transcription factor)	19p13.3	6.96
STMN1	Stathmin 1/oncoprotein 18	1p35-36.1	4.25
YAF2	YY1-associated factor 2	12q12	4.07
ICAM3	Intercellular adhesion molecule	19p13.3-p13.2	4.03
PPIG	Peptidyl-propyl isomerase G (cyclophilin G)	N/A	3.99
TUBGCP2	Tubulin, gamma complex–associated protein 2	10q26.3	3.91
CDSN	Corneodesmosin	6p21.3	3.59
SLC4A1	Solute carrier family 4, anion exchanger, member 1	17q12-q21	3.32

SUMMARY

As a result of our simulation study, we suggest two amendments to the commonly used algorithms for cDNA microarray data analysis. First, we suggest to take into consideration the actual probabilistic structure of log-intensities, thus avoiding restrictive assumptions of normality. Better knowledge of this structure allows one to make reasonable predictions of genomic signal and reduce the influence of random noise. The second modification consists in introducing the concept of bio-weight as a key parameter for identification of the genes deserving a follow-up validation. This criterion seems to be a reasonable measure of significance for a small number of replicates when the power of the t test is fairly low. It is shown that application of the bio-weight provides a much better true-positive rate than the criterion based only on P values.

REFERENCES

1. BROWN, P. & D. BOLSTEIN. 1999. Exploring the new world of the genome with DNA microarrays. Nat. Genet. Suppl. **21:** 33–37.
2. JAGOTA, A. 2001. Microarray data analysis and visualization. Department of Computer Engineering, University of California, Santa Cruz.
3. EISEN, M.B., P.T. SPELLMAN, P.O. BROWN & D. BOLSTEIN. 1998. Cluster analysis and display of genome-wide expression patterns. Proc. Natl. Acad. Sci. USA **95:** 14863–14866.
4. TAMAYO, P., D. SLONIM, J. MESIROV et al. 1999. Interpreting patterns of gene expression with self-organizing maps: methods and application to hematopoietic differentiation. Proc. Natl. Acad. Sci. USA **96:** 2907–2912.
5. EFRON, B., R. TIBSHIRANI, J. STOREY & V. TUSHER. 2001. Empirical Bayes analysis of microarray experiment. JASA **96**(456): 1151–1160.
6. KERR, K.. & G. CHURCHILL. 2001. Experimental design for gene expression microarrays. Biostatistics **2:** 183–201.

7. DONOHO, D.L. 2000. High-dimensional data analysis: the curses and blessings of dimensionality. Aide-Memoire. Department of Statistics, Stanford University.
8. KERR, M., M. MARTIN & G. CHURCHHILL. 2000. Analysis of variance for gene expression microarray data. J. Comput. Biol. **7**(6): 819–837.
9. HASTIE, T., R. TIBSHIRANI, D. BOLSTEIN & P. BROWN. 2001. Supervised harvesting of expression trees. Genome Biol. **2**(1): 1–12.
10. WOLFINGER, R., G. GIBSON, E. WOLFINGER *et al.* 2001. Assessing gene significance from cDNA microarray expression data via mixed models. J. Comput. Biol. **8**: 625–637.
11. YANG, Y., S. DUDOIT, P. LUU *et al.* 2002. Normalization for cDNA microarray data: a robust composite method addressing single and multiple slide systematic variation. Nucleic Acids Res. **30**(4): 15.
12. JUHLIN, K. 2003. Assessing and managing experimental noise from small-sample microarray experiments. *In* Proceedings of the Cambridge Healthcare Third Annual Meeting on Microarray Data Analysis, September 21–23, 2003, Baltimore.
13. PINHEIRO, J. & D. BATES. 2000. Mixed-Effects Models in S and S-PLUS. Springer-Verlag. New York/Berlin.
14. DUDOIT, S., J. SHAFFER & J. BOLDRICK. 2002. Multiple hypothesis testing in microarray experiments. Technical Paper 110. U. C. Berkeley Division of Biostatistics Working Paper Series.
15. RAJEEVAN, M., D. RANAMUKHAARACHCHI, S. VERNON & E.R. UNGER. 2001 Use of real-time quantitative PCR to validate the results of cDNA array and differential display PCR technologies. Methods **25**: 443–451.
16. TICHOPAD, A., M. DILGER, G. SCHWARZ & M. PFAFFI. 2003. Standardized determination of real-time PCR efficiency from a single reaction set-up. Nucleic Acids Res. **31**(20): 122.
17. MEIJERINK, J., C. MANDIGERS, L. VAN DE LOCHT *et al.* 2001. A novel method to compensate for different amplification efficiencies between patient DNA samples in quantitative real-time PCR. J. Mol. Diagn. **3**(2): 55–61.
18. AL TAHER, A., A. BASHEIN, T. NOLAN *et al.* 2000. Global cDNA amplification combined with real-time RT-PCR: accurate quantification of multiple human potassium channel genes at the single cell level. Yeast **17**: 201–210.
19. GE, Y., S. DUDOIT & T. SPEED. 2003. Resampling-based multiple testing for microarray data analysis. Test **12**(1): 1–77.

Automated Interpretation of Protein Subcellular Location Patterns

Implications for Early Cancer Detection and Assessment

ROBERT F. MURPHY

Departments of Biological Sciences and Biomedical Engineering, and Center for Automated Learning and Discovery, Carnegie Mellon University, Pittsburgh, Pennsylvania 15213, USA

ABSTRACT: Fluorescence microscopy is a powerful tool for analyzing the subcellular distributions of proteins, but that power has not been fully utilized because most analysis of those distributions has been done by visual examination. This limitation can be overcome using automated pattern recognition methods widely used in other fields. This article summarizes work demonstrating that automated systems can recognize the patterns of major organelles in both two- and three-dimensional images of cultured cells, and that these systems can distinguish similar patterns better than visual examination. The basis for these systems are sets of Subcellular Location Features that capture the essence of subcellular patterns without being sensitive to the extensive variation that occurs in the size, shape, and orientation of cells in microscope images. These features can also be used to make sensitive, statistical comparisons of the distribution of a protein between two conditions, such as in the presence and absence of a drug. The possible use of automated pattern analysis methods for improving detection of abnormal cells in cancerous or precancerous tissues is also discussed.

KEYWORDS: Subcellular Location Features; protein localization; fluorescence microscopy; pattern recognition; location proteomics; image similarity; protein distribution comparison

LOCATION PROTEOMICS

Basic research in biology has been revolutionized by the advent of *genomics*, defined as the study of entire genomes rather than individual genes. As the sequences of complete genomes (and lists of suspected genes making up those genomes) have become available, the focus of much biological research has shifted from *genomics* to *proteomics* in order to understand the behavior and function of all proteins and the roles they play in development and disease. Most proteomics efforts to date have

Address for correspondence: Robert F. Murphy, Departments of Biological Sciences and Biomedical Engineering, and Center for Automated Learning and Discovery, Carnegie Mellon University, 4400 Fifth Avenue, Pittsburgh, PA 15213. Voice: 412-268-3480; fax: 412-268-6571. murphy@cmu.edu

Ann. N.Y. Acad. Sci. 1020: 124–131 (2004). © 2004 New York Academy of Sciences. doi: 10.1196/annals.1310.013

focused on methods for determining protein *sequence, structure, abundance,* and *interactions.* Far less attention has been paid to determining and understanding the *locations* of protein within cells, although knowledge of the subcellular location of a protein is critical to understanding how it functions. The primary method by which information has been obtained about the organelles and other subcellular structures that contain a specific protein is by labeling that protein with a fluorescence probe (e.g., using a monoclonal antibody) and collecting images of cells using a fluorescence microscope. The main reason for the absence of prior systematic, large-scale efforts to determine subcellular location for all proteins has been the difficulty of automatically and quantitatively describing subcellular location in cells with varying sizes and shapes.

A major goal in my group in the past few years has therefore been to perform *automated interpretation of fluorescence microscope images* depicting the subcellular distribution of proteins.[1–7] While the primary motivation behind this work has been to enable the new field of *location proteomics*, the work also has potential applications in cancer detection, assessment, and treatment.

This chapter will therefore review previous work demonstrating that changes in the subcellular distributions of proteins and organelles can be recognized in fluorescence microscope images in a fully automated manner.

DEVELOPMENT OF SUBCELLULAR LOCATION FEATURES AND CLASSIFICATION OF SUBCELLULAR PATTERNS

The most critical component of our work to date has been the development of sets of numerical features that capture the essence of subcellular distributions without being overly sensitive to the position or rotation of a cell within an image.[1,3,6] We have used these features to create automated *classifiers* that can recognize the patterns of all major subcellular structures in 2D images.[3,6]

The input was a collection of images of HeLa cells that were labeled with antibodies against protein markers for various organelles. Examples of the images used in these studies are shown in FIGURE 1. We specifically included markers whose distributions are quite similar: the proteins giantin and GPP130 are both found primarily in the Golgi apparatus, and the patterns of LAMP2 (primarily lysosomal) and transferrin receptor (TfR, primarily endosomal) are difficult to distinguish visually.

The general pattern recognition problem is to learn the patterns present in two or more *classes* of image, where each class is known to differ from the others by at least one descriptor external to the image (called a *label*), such that the class of new images not used in the learning can be predicted correctly. The accuracy of prediction for new images is usually assessed by dividing any available *labeled* images into a *training* set used to train the classifier and a *test* set used to evaluate performance by comparing the class predicted by the classifier to the known class. There are two basic approaches to recognizing patterns in images. The first involves learning a model of the distribution of the pixels in each class so that the model can be compared to the pixel values in new images. The second involves describing the images using numerical features and learning rules to associate the feature values to the classes.

For recognizing protein patterns, the variability of cell size, shape, and orientation within the microscope field, and the variability in the number, position, and

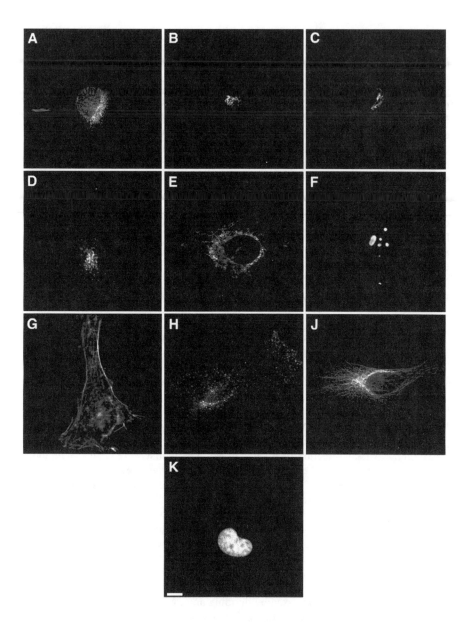

FIGURE 1. Representative images from the 2D HeLa cell data set described in the text. These images have had background fluorescence subtracted and have had all pixels below an automatically chosen threshold set to 0. Images are shown for HeLa cells labeled with antibodies against an ER protein (**A**), the Golgi protein giantin (**B**), the Golgi protein GPP130 (**C**), the lysosomal protein LAMP2 (**D**), a mitochondrial protein (**E**), the nucleolar protein nucleolin (**F**), transferrin receptor (**H**), and the cytoskeletal protein tubulin (**J**). Images are also shown for filamentous actin labeled with rhodamine-phalloidin (**G**) and DNA labeled with DAPI (**K**). Scale bar: 10 μm. (Reprinted from ref. 3.)

orientation of organelles within each cell, make it difficult to use model-based approaches. We have therefore evaluated a number of types of numerical features for describing the patterns in cell images. These have been described in detail previously[3,7] and are briefly summarized here. Zernike moment features describe the overall pattern in a cell by measuring the degree to which the pattern matches a set of radially symmetric functions (the Zernike polynomials). Haralick texture features describe the frequency with which particular pixel values are found adjacent to other pixel values. Morphological features describe the properties of objects derived from thresholding the image (e.g., average object size). Edge features describe the distribution of edges (regions of sharply varying intensity) in an image (e.g., the fraction of fluorescence found along an edge). Last, hull features describe the pattern relative to the convex hull of the image, which connects the outermost set of above-threshold pixels.

We have used these features in various combinations to analyze cell images. To facilitate referring to a specific feature or combination of features, we have described a nomenclature for these Subcellular Location Features, or SLF. Sets of SLF are referred to by a set name (e.g., SLF3), and individual features are referred to by a set name and the number of the feature within that set (e.g., SLF3.7).

Obviously, the quality of classification results depends critically on the quality of the features used. For many classification approaches, the presence of uninformative features (features that have similar values for all classes) or the presence of redundant features (features whose values are correlated with those of other features) can complicate the learning task sufficiently so that poorer results are obtained than would have been obtained with a smaller set of informative, nonredundant features. One approach to creating such a set is to only describe images using features known to meet this criterion, which is often very difficult. A second approach is to describe each image using many features (some of which may be redundant or noninformative) and then use a method that automatically identifies which features best distinguish the classes being analyzed. There are many such methods and we have evaluated a number of them in the context of subcellular pattern analysis.[8] The best results were obtained with Stepwise Discriminant Analysis (SDA) and we have defined some SLF sets as the results of applying SDA to a larger SLF set. A description of each feature and set can be found at http://murphylab.web.cmu.edu/services/SLF/.

Results for one of our automated classification systems are shown in TABLE 1 in the form of a *confusion matrix* that tabulates how often images of a known class (shown in the row headings) are placed by the classifier in each predicted class (shown in the column headings). As can be seen, the classifier can distinguish all classes (including the two Golgi proteins) with an accuracy over 70%.

An important finding of our initial work on the HeLa data set[3] was that an automated system could recognize subtle differences in protein patterns that are not readily distinguishable by visual examination. To confirm that these patterns were indeed difficult to distinguish visually, we tested the ability of a human observer to learn this task.[7] The results are shown in TABLE 2. While our automated classifiers can distinguish the Golgi proteins giantin and GPP130 with an average accuracy of 75% (TABLE 1), a human observer, even after training until no further improvement occurred, had an average accuracy of only 50% (which is what is expected for random guessing). Both the automated system and visual examination had a similar overall accuracy when the two proteins were combined and considered as a single Golgi class.

TABLE 1. Confusion matrix for classification of images from the 2D HeLa data set combined with a parallel DNA image

True class	Output of the classifier									
	DNA	ER	Gia	GPP	LAM	Mit	Nuc	Act	TfR	Tub
DNA	**99**	1	0	0	0	0	0	0	0	0
ER	0	**89**	0	0	4	4	0	0	1	2
Giantin	0	0	**76**	20	0	1	1	0	1	0
GPP130	0	0	23	**73**	0	1	2	0	1	0
LAMP2	0	2	0	0	**83**	1	0	0	13	0
Mitochon.	0	5	0	0	2	**90**	0	0	1	2
Nucleolin	0	0	0	0	0	0	**98**	0	0	0
Actin	0	0	0	0	0	0	0	**99**	0	1
TfR	0	3	0	0	16	3	0	1	**75**	2
Tubulin	0	2	0	0	0	2	0	0	3	**93**

NOTE: The SLF13 feature set was used with a BPNN with a single layer of 20 hidden units over 10 cross-validation trials. The number of images in each predicted class is shown as a percentage of the number of test images for each known class (averaged across the 10 cross-validation trials). The average correct classification rate was 88% (91% when the two Golgi proteins, giantin and GPP130, are considered as a single class). Data from ref. 7.

TABLE 2. Confusion matrix for visual classification of images from the 2D HeLa data set

True class	Output of the classifier									
	DNA	ER	Gia	GPP	LAM	Mit	Nuc	Act	TfR	Tub
DNA	**100**	0	0	0	0	0	0	0	0	0
ER	0	**90**	0	0	3	6	0	0	0	0
Giantin	0	0	**56**	36	3	3	0	0	0	0
GPP130	0	0	53	**43**	0	0	0	0	3	0
LAMP2	0	0	6	0	**73**	0	0	0	20	0
Mitochon.	0	3	0	0	0	**96**	0	0	0	0
Nucleolin	0	0	0	0	0	0	**100**	0	0	0
Actin	0	0	0	0	0	0	0	**100**	0	0
TfR	0	13	0	0	3	0	0	0	**83**	0
Tubulin	0	3	0	0	0	0	0	3	0	**93**

NOTE: The number of images in each predicted class is shown as a percentage of the number of images for each known class (the results are from the last round of testing, after the classification accuracy had reached a maximum). The average correct classification rate was 83% (92% when the two Golgi proteins, giantin and GPP130, are considered as a single class). Data from ref. 7.

The above results are for classifying single cells, but even better performance can be obtained if we assume that all of the cells on a given slide show the same pattern. With this assumption, we can form small sets of cells from the same set, classify each individually, and then choose as the prediction for the whole set whichever class had the most cells. We have shown that such a "plurality voting" scheme can use a classifier with an average accuracy of 83% to classify sets of ten cells with an average accuracy greater than 98%.[3]

The improvement over visual examination demonstrated above for our automated systems on 2D images might be expected to be even greater for the analysis of 3D images, given the difficulty of visualizing and remembering complex patterns in more than two dimensions. To test this hypothesis, we collected a data set of 3D HeLa images covering the same patterns in the 2D data set.[5] Using only morphological features, these images could be classified with an average accuracy of 91%. This was about 5% better than that obtained for 2D classification using just the central slice from each 3D image.[5]

COMPARISON OF CELL POPULATIONS

The work described above addresses the assignment of cell images to defined classes, such as organelles. An equally important problem frequently addressed by fluorescence microscopy is determining whether the pattern of a protein changes in response to some treatment (such as the addition of a drug). More generally, this problem can be described as determining whether two sets of images represent statistically different patterns. Since the SLF contain sufficient information about subcellular patterns to allow those patterns to be accurately classified, it is reasonable to expect that they can be used to measure changes in those patterns as well. We have thus developed a system (called SImEC for Statistical Imaging Experiment Comparator) that performs rigorous statistical comparison of image sets.[4]

SImEC begins by converting image sets into a matrix in which each row represents a cell image and the columns contain the values of the chosen SLF set. The statistical question is then whether it is likely, at a given confidence level, that the matrices for the two sets could have resulted from images drawn from the same set. This hypothesis can be tested using the Hotelling T^2 test, which yields an F statistic with two degrees of freedom: the number of features and the combined number of images in the two sets minus the number of features. If the F statistic for two sets is greater than the critical F value for those degrees of freedom at the chosen confidence level, the hypothesis that the sets are drawn from the same population can be rejected. TABLE 3 shows the F statistics for all pairwise comparisons between the ten classes in the 2D HeLa cell data set. Not unexpectedly given that all of these classes can be distinguished by a classifier, the results indicate that all ten classes are statistically different at the 95% confidence level. To test that the test does not falsely identify all sets as different, random subsets drawn from the same class were compared at the same confidence level. Over repeated trials, approximately 95% of the randomly drawn subsets were considered to be the same (as expected). The conclusion is that the SLF can be used to create a statically sound method for comparing subcellular protein distributions.

TABLE 3. Pairwise comparison of classes from the 2D HeLa data set using SImEC

Class	No. of images	DNA	ER	Gia	GPP	LAM	Mit	Nuc	Phal	TfR
DNA	87									
ER	86	90.6								
Giantin	87	138.9	49.9							
GPP130	85	154.1	51.3	2.6						
LAMP2	84	92.3	22.6	11.7	11.6					
Mitochon.	73	179.2	11.0	56.1	61.6	17.4				
Nucleolin	73	91.3	60.3	18.7	17.1	20.0	67.0			
Actin	98	523.5	58.1	374.2	358.2	127.4	17.0	274.2		
TfR	91	101.3	8.6	19.1	17.5	3.1	9.0	30.3	26.4	
Tubulin	91	185.5	12.5	97.3	102.4	31.3	8.0	100.5	21.4	6.5

NOTE: The values shown are F values from the T^2 test for the comparison of each class with each other class. Larger F values indicate that the two classes are more dissimilar. To determine whether two classes differ at a particular confidence level, the F value is compared to the critical F value for that confidence level. The critical values of the F distribution for a 95% confidence level range from 1.42 to 1.45 for the comparisons shown here (the critical value depends on the total number of images in the comparison and the number of features being used). Since all F values shown in the table are greater than this, all classes can be considered to be distinguishable from each other with 95% confidence. Note that the lowest F values were observed for the comparisons of giantin with GPP130 and of transferrin receptor with LAMP2. The highest F values were seen for pairs that are very different, such as for the DNA distribution compared with any of the others. Data from ref. 4.

IMPLICATIONS FOR IMPROVED DETECTION OF CANCEROUS AND PRECANCEROUS TISSUE

It is becoming increasingly clear that what may be largely normal-appearing tissue in the vicinity of skin (and other) cancers may be precancerous to a sufficient degree that recurrence at that site is likely. For nonmelanoma skin cancers, the most common current approach to surgery is to remove tissue until pathology indicates that the margins of the removed tissue are clear. For melanoma, additional tissue is removed until a 1- to 3-cm margin beyond the tumor is created. A difficulty with these approaches is that current methods cannot always determine whether the margins are indeed fully normal tissue.

Fluorescent probe staining has the potential to provide a dramatic increase in sensitivity and accuracy over traditional pathology stains. Probes that may be useful include antibodies against proteins known to localize in specific organelles, antibodies against proteins implicated in oncogenesis, or dyes that stain specific organelles or biochemical processes. However, a significant current limitation in the use of fluorescence microscopy for pathology is that fluorescence microscope images are difficult to interpret because the structural context visible with traditional stains is absent. One possible solution to this problem is the use of automated image analysis methods such as those described here. The prior work has been carried out on model systems consisting of cultured cells grown on coverslips, and thus one task to be accomplished is to extend them to images of cells in intact tissues. The next step is to identify proteins whose subcellular patterns change at various stages during the development of malignancies in a particular tissue (if they exist). This knowledge can potentially be used to screen for abnormalities (e.g., in biopsies) and to assess the stage or risk for a given abnormality.

ACKNOWLEDGMENTS

I thank John Kirkwood for helpful discussions on potential applications of our work to skin cancer detection. The original research described above was supported in part by Research Grant No. RPG-95-099-03-MGO from the American Cancer Society; Grant No. 99-295 from the Rockefeller Brothers Fund Charles E. Culpeper Biomedical Pilot Initiative; NSF Grant Nos. BIR-9217091, MCB-8920118, and BIR-9256343; NIH Grant Nos. T32 GM08208 and R33 CA83219; and a research grant from the Commonwealth of Pennsylvania Tobacco Settlement Fund.

REFERENCES

1. BOLAND, M.V., M.K. MARKEY & R.F. MURPHY. 1998. Automated recognition of patterns characteristic of subcellular structures in fluorescence microscopy images. Cytometry **33:** 366–375.
2. MURPHY, R.F., M.V. BOLAND & M. VELLISTE. 2000. Towards a systematics for protein subcellular location: quantitative description of protein localization patterns and automated analysis of fluorescence microscope images. Proc. Int. Conf. Intell. Syst. Mol. Biol. **8:** 251–259.
3. BOLAND, M.V. & R.F. MURPHY. 2001. A neural network classifier capable of recognizing the patterns of all major subcellular structures in fluorescence microscope images of HeLa cells. Bioinformatics **17:** 1213–1223.
4. ROQUES, E.J.S. & R.F. MURPHY. 2002. Objective evaluation of differences in protein subcellular distribution. Traffic **3:** 61–65.
5. VELLISTE, M. & R.F. MURPHY. 2002. Automated determination of protein subcellular locations from 3D fluorescence microscope images. *In* 2002 IEEE International Symposium on Biomedical Imaging (ISBI-2002), pp. 867–870.
6. MURPHY, R.F., M. VELLISTE & G. PORRECA. 2002. Robust classification of subcellular location patterns in fluorescence microscope images. *In* 2002 IEEE International Workshop on Neural Networks for Signal Processing (NNSP 12), pp. 67–76.
7. MURPHY, R.F., M. VELLISTE & G. PORRECA. 2003. Robust numerical features for description and classification of subcellular location patterns in fluorescence microscope images. J. VLSI Sig. Proc. **35:** 311–321.
8. HUANG, K., M. VELLISTE & R.F. MURPHY. 2003. Feature reduction for improved recognition of subcellular location patterns in fluorescence microscope images. Proc. SPIE **4962:** 307–318.

Data-Driven Computer Simulation of Human Cancer Cell

R. CHRISTOPHER,[a] A. DHIMAN,[a] J. FOX,[a] R. GENDELMAN,[a] T. HABERITCHER,[a] D. KAGLE,[a] G. SPIZZ,[a] I. G. KHALIL, AND C. HILL

Gene Network Sciences, Ithaca, New York 14850, USA

ABSTRACT: Using the Diagrammatic Cell Language™, Gene Network Sciences (GNS) has created a network model of interconnected signal transduction pathways and gene expression networks that control human cell proliferation and apoptosis. It includes receptor activation and mitogenic signaling, initiation of cell cycle, and passage of checkpoints and apoptosis. Time-course experiments measuring mRNA abundance and protein activity are conducted on Caco-2 and HCT 116 colon cell lines. These data were used to constrain unknown regulatory interactions and kinetic parameters via sensitivity analysis and parameter optimization methods contained in the DigitalCell™ computer simulation platform. FACS, RNA knockdown, cell growth, and apoptosis data are also used to constrain the model and to identify unknown pathways, and cross talk between known pathways will also be discussed. Using the cell simulation, GNS tested the efficacy of various drug targets and performed validation experiments to test computer simulation predictions. The simulation is a powerful tool that can in principle incorporate patient-specific data on the DNA, RNA, and protein levels for assessing efficacy of therapeutics in specific patient populations and can greatly impact success of a given therapeutic strategy.

KEYWORDS: Gene Network Sciences (GNS); Diagrammatic Cell Language (DCL); DigitalCell; cancer; cell; computer; data; drug; model; simulation

INTRODUCTION

The last few decades have seen a tremendous growth in the knowledge of the underlying molecular mechanisms of cancer. Many genes and pathways that control cell growth and proliferation and underlie cancer have been discovered and the mechanisms by which mutations in these genes and pathways lead to uncontrolled cellular proliferation have been elucidated.[1] There have even been a handful of new therapies that have been developed on the basis of this knowledge: Herceptin for breast cancer, Gleevac for chronic myeloid leukemia, and Velcade and Avastin for other cancers. However, the apparent progress that has been made in understanding and treating cancer has also revealed many layers of complexity that thwart our abilities to rationally diagnose, treat, and understand the disease. The majority (~80%)

Address for correspondence: C. Hill, Gene Network Sciences, 31 Dutch Mill Road, Ithaca, NY 14850. Fax: 607-257-5428.

colin@gnsbiotech.com

[a]These authors contributed equally to this work.

Ann. N.Y. Acad. Sci. 1020: 132–153 (2004). © 2004 New York Academy of Sciences.
doi: 10.1196/annals.1310.014

of cancers do not appear to be dependent on the presence of a single predisposing mutant allele, such as the BRCA1 or BRCA2 gene for breast cancers.[2] Rather, a number of subtle mutations may act synergistically, resulting in the initiation of the cancerous phenotype.[3,4] The collective actions of mutations that lead to tumorigenesis arise in the context of highly regulated gene expression networks and signal transduction pathways. These complex biochemical circuits often give rise to nonintuitive cellular phenotypic outcomes because of feedback loops and cross talk between pathways. This complexity makes the process of connecting molecular interactions and events to cellular and tissue level outcomes very difficult, errorprone, and information-intensive. Even in the cancer drug development success stories of Gleevac and Herceptin, where the drug mechanism of action is believed to be well understood, this understanding has been later revealed to be much murkier than once thought. The stark reality is that the growth in the knowledge of the underlying molecular mechanisms of cancer has not allowed for a more fully predictive and reliable process for matching the correct existing drugs with the particular patient (diagnostics), and discovering and developing new drugs with significantly greater efficacy (therapeutics).

The completion of the Human Genome Project and the discovery of many cancer-related genes from the application of genomics, DNA microarray, and proteomics technologies have offered the opportunity to create a more complete picture of the underlying molecular biology of cancer. Much insight has been gained into the underlying genetic pathogenesis of cancers via high-throughput microarray analysis of gene expression in tumor samples.[5–12] However, the current reality is that this recent explosion of data has exacerbated a problem that was already beyond the control of cancer researchers: *how to integrate all of the relevant knowledge in a systematic way that can provide the best strategy for halting the uncontrolled growth of cancer cells and tumors*. Current bioinformatics methods have focused on (1) the creation of efficient databases for the storage and retrieval of genomic data and (2) the creation of algorithms for identifying patterns of biological significance (i.e., binding motifs in DNA sequence and correlations or clusters of similarly behaving genes or similarly behaving biological samples in DNA microarray data). While these approaches are a very powerful way of housing and querying large data sets, these methods will always lack the *context dependence* and *dynamic interconnectedness* that is at the core of biological function. An example of the importance of context dependence is the *p53* protein, which will lead to cell cycle arrest only under certain conditions, but will perform a different function or no function at all under other conditions. Dynamic interconnectedness is evident as the change in the "effective" circuitry of a cell (a function of its physiological state) that dictates which genes are expressed and which are not expressed, and therefore which pathways are active. Most importantly, these methods do not allow for *extrapolation* and *generalization* from existing biological data to new biological data, nor do they allow for the ability to iteratively perturb and adjust system variables. With these methods, knowing the concentration of a key protein marker and the phenotype of a cancer cell under different concentrations of a growth factor receptor does not allow rapid extrapolation to a prediction of the effect of varying the growth factor receptor concentration to one of millions of different values. In other words, the full power of inductive logic and massive computational capacity is not being fully exploited to find new biological implications from what we already know.

How would medicine improve if we were able to systematically deal with the complexity of cancer biology to make accurate predictions of drug response in cell lines, animals, and human patients? We would be able to ask complicated questions of our data, such as "What is the predicted effect of applying a particular chemotherapy with this new targeted cancer drug to a cell line with a particular genetic background?"; or more subtle questions could be posed, such as "What is the optimal dose or binding rate of a drug that is necessary to achieve a maximal apoptotic effect?". Being able to answer these types of questions would allow the creation of therapeutic and diagnostic strategies that effectively treat different forms of cancer and are tailored to specific groups of patients.

Achieving such a predictive understanding of cancer cells and their response to drugs requires a platform that can relate underlying molecular circuitry to the time-varying molecular expression profiles that determine cellular phenotypes. This would involve the integration of pathway data from the literature and the ability to predict from a particular pathway structure the resulting molecular concentration profiles, both under varying conditions and as a function of time. These molecular concentration profiles correspond to various phenotypic states of the cell, such as proliferation, cell cycle arrest, and apoptosis, so that predicting molecular concentration profiles from a particular pathway structure allows one to predict phenotype changes that result from perturbations to this circuitry. For such predictions to be accurate, quantitative, and time-dependent, dynamic mathematical equations are needed. The platform that can provide a predictive understanding of cancer cells and their response to drugs is a data-driven computer simulation that solves the mathematical equations describing the underlying molecular circuitry of a cell.

This ultimate goal of predicting how perturbations to the "molecular wiring diagram" change the molecular profile and cellular phenotype is extremely challenging because (1) only 5–10% of the circuitry of a human cell is known[13] and (2) high-throughput measurements of molecular concentration profiles have great variability. These challenges necessitate a two-pronged approach. The first is the forward predictive modeling of known curated signal transduction pathways. This provides the foundation that describes the basic cellular functions, such as response to mitogenic signals, cell proliferation, and apoptosis. This core model can generate predictions of phenotypes resulting from genetic knockouts/knockdowns or applying drugs, as well as characterizations of the mechanism of action of a drug. This core model also provides a framework to rationally place genes and proteins with little known function into a cell model and enables a more complete prediction of the function of such a gene or protein. The second approach combines inferential data mining (which extracts patterns and correlations from genomic and proteomic data) with the forward predictive model of known pathways. This is called dynamical network inference and it provides a more complete and more data-driven characterization of cell circuitry. Network inference enables the discovery of new pathways, the discovery of the function of uncharacterized genes and novel targets, and the automatic inference of the mechanism of action of a drug.

Using the tools described below, GNS has created a data-driven model of an HCT 116 colon cancer cell. The model describes the cross talk between the major cellular pathways and the interactions involved in determining the phenotypic fate of a cell. The GNS graphical colon cancer model contains over 1000 genes and proteins (several hundred of which are contained in the simulation model) that comprise the major signal transduction pathways and gene expression networks that control human cell growth and cell homeostasis. The GNS cancer model integrates a wide variety of data types into a predictive platform for testing hypotheses in an iterative manner. This model has the ability to explore the subtle questions posed earlier. The model in its current form has been successful in conducting "virtual" knockdown experiments that have been experimentally validated with siRNA methods.

The number of literature references that define pathway circuitry is approximately 3560. The circuitry data are typically extracted from cell systems other than HCT 116 and sometimes species other than human. Data collected specifically on HCT 116 cells are crucial in further specifying the circuitry. One thousand mRNA expression (DNA microarray, SAGE) data points were used to determine if a pathway component is present, and 274 knockdown/knockout data points were also used. Time-course measurements on approximately 15 proteins expressed in the HCT 116 cells were used to quantitatively refine the model by applying the parameter estimation methods described in the MODELING METHODOLOGY section. FACS data were also collected and used to constrain the cell cycle phase durations in the model. The molecular and cell biology contained in the cancer cell model covers the G1-S-G2-M components of the cell cycle, including pathways such as Ras, Wnt/β-catenin, p53, and apoptosis. An example pathway of apoptosis is shown in FIGURE 1.

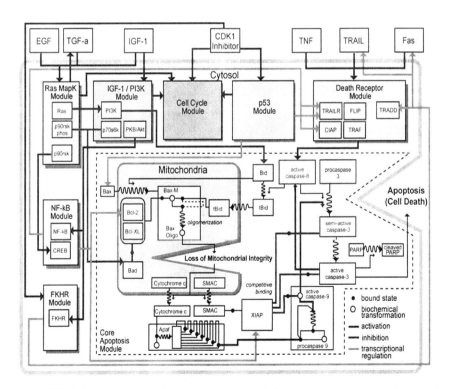

FIGURE 1. Apoptosis model: Schematic description of key apoptotic and survival pathways and their interplay in the determination of phenotypic end point.

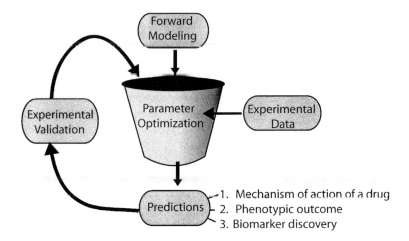

FIGURE 2a. Schematic of GNS methodology used to construct data-driven model.

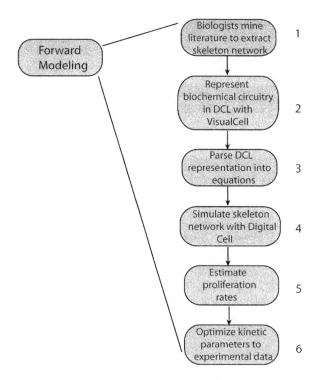

FIGURE 2b. Elements of forward predictive modeling listed sequentially.

In this paper, we will describe the methodology and tools used to construct large-scale, data-driven cell simulations, the application of this model to predicting cellular phenotypes and growth assay results from gene knockdowns, and additional and future applications of our technology.

MODELING METHODOLOGY

The methodology that has been used to create the GNS colon cancer cell model includes the following steps: (i) mining the literature and public databases for possible interactions and kinetic data; (ii) representing the interactions in the Diagrammatic Cell Language (DCL)[14] using the VisualCell™ platform; (iii) parsing DCL representations into reactions and equations; (iv) simulating the system via the DigitalCell engine; (v) extracting estimates of proliferation rates from the single cell model; (vi) using experimental data to estimate unknown parameters in the model. Once the model has been developed, it can generate specific predictions that can be tested experimentally. Experimental validation is used to iteratively refine the model and generate new predictions. This methodology is diagrammed in FIGURES 2a and 2b.

Mining the Literature and Public Databases for Possible Interactions and Kinetic Data

In this step, either a pathway or a group of genes and corresponding proteins is identified for inclusion in the computer model. Systematic searches are then conducted in multiple databases to establish gene function, protein-protein interactions, mRNA and protein expression in the tissue/cell of interest, and presence of splice variants and isoforms. LocusLink and OMIM are used as a starting point. Then, Pub-Gene, Science STKE, and KEGG are used for delineation of the skeleton networks. The search is expanded to Entrez-PubMed for supporting data from primary literature for protein-protein interactions and further network expansion. A minimum of three articles per interaction must be extracted for inclusion of that interaction into the curated forward model. The experimental data obtained from primary literature is further classified on the basis of experimental methods used to identify the interactions. For example, experiments done *in vivo* with endogenous proteins are given more weight than those utilizing stable transfections. In addition, the cell line or tissue used in the experiment is recorded to determine the relevance of the interaction in an epithelial cell line. The individual molecular components, interactions between them, and experimental papers used to determine the interactions are annotated and entered into the GNS database for future querying and updating.

Representing the Interactions in the DCL Modeling Language Using the VisualCell Platform

Once the components of the biological system to be modeled have been defined and the interactions between them elucidated from the body of biological knowledge

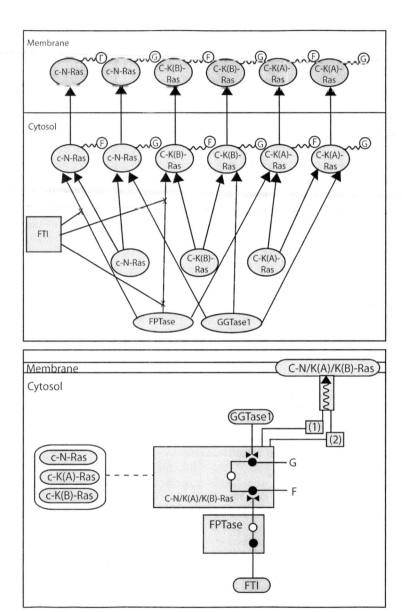

FIGURE 3. Comparison of a conventional diagram of a network with the same network drawn in the DCL. The boxed structures representing C-N/K(A)/K(B)-Ras and FTPase are linkboxes. The open circles within each linkbox represent different states for each protein, while the filled circles represent binding nodes. Relevant states are resolved by resolution boxes [□ with (1) or (2)]. The double-headed arrows (►◄) translate into "enables binding". The smooth-edged rectangle is a likebox that represents proteins with similar function (in this case, the different isoforms of Ras).

(literature, databases, or even direct experimental measurements), one needs to assemble this knowledge in a manner that represents the connectivity between the components: a circuit diagram of the genes and proteins underlying the cell or biological system. This requires a representation that is rich enough to represent the complex context-dependent functions of biomolecules, and algorithmically precise enough to be translated into a mathematical framework and a set of computer instructions. This also requires a representation that can be scaled to an arbitrary size and complexity so that one can use it to represent the complete wiring diagram of the cell. GNS has developed the DCL to address these needs.

The interactions between the genes, proteins, metabolites, and other cellular constituents are represented in DCL. DCL is designed to allow biologists and modelers to express a complete, precise, and functional diagram of the cell that is readable by both humans and computers. The language is designed to be compact and scalable; the current graphical model of the colon cancer cell contains over 1000 genes/proteins, 3000 components (a gene or protein in a particular state), and their interactions. The key elements that make DCL powerful are linkboxes and likeboxes.

Linkboxes are a physical combination of different molecular species, which can be anything from binding sites on a protein to regulatory regions of DNA. Likeboxes, on the other hand, represent chemicals, binding sites, or even reactions that act alike. FIGURE 3 illustrates a portion of the Ras Map Kinase pathway drawn in a traditional representation side by side with the DCL representation. In the traditional representation, there are two major limitations. The first limitation is scalability. This unstructured representation will not allow the creation of networks of hundreds of components or more. The second limitation is the ambiguity of the functions of the components. The context-dependent functions of the components cannot be described in a mathematical model, necessitating the need for a written description. Conversely, the DCL representation concisely represents the 22 protein states present in the model (e.g., C-N-RAS Geranylated, C-N-RAS Farnesylated, C-N-RAS Geranylated and in the membrane, etc.) without the need for the written caption. It concisely represents the following biological interactions:

- Farnesyl protein transferase (FPTase) catalyzes the addition of a farnesyl group onto C-N-Ras, C-K(A)-Ras, and C-K(B)-Ras. Farnesyl transferase inhibitor (FTI) blocks this reaction. Geranyl-geranyl transferase 1 (GGTase1) catalyzes the addition of a geranyl-geranyl moiety onto the same group of Ras molecules. After lipid modification, each Ras molecule translocates from the cytosol to the membrane.

The DCL is computationally complete. The language contains complex objects that may inherit properties from their constituents. This type of inheritance is inspired by object-oriented languages, but it is different in one crucial way: the objects do not lie in a hierarchy. Whenever a number of objects produce a new object by any process, the resulting object inherits all the properties of all the objects, except for those specifically excluded. DCL is also extensible; for example, if additional modifications should arise, the linkbox representing Ras can be expanded to include those modifications and the enzyme that modifies it. The functions of the components are what the language seeks to represent, not their sequence or structure. Whatever its structure, the function of a protein determines the same DCL biochemical network topology or graph. To be more precise, it determines one of a number of equivalent graphs.

Parsing DCL into Reactions and Equations

GNS has developed the VisualCell, a software tool to facilitate the use of DCL. VisualCell is a graphical application that provides visual editing of cellular signaling networks and other biochemical networks. VisualCell is currently used to create, annotate, and communicate the network. The networks are typically constructed by biologists specializing in a particular pathway or system, and then passed digitally to a mathematical modeler who uses the detailed diagram and the annotations to create a simulation model that simplifies the complexity of the graphical model so that a simulation of the network is computationally tractable. Next, VisualCell automatically generates lists of reactions, chemicals, and parameters that serve as input into the DigitalCell (see next subsection). Since the simulation of even a simple network can require transcribing thousands of reactions, this step is particularly important. The environment also enables the seamless communication between a graphical application that typically runs on a personal computer and a numerical application that typically runs on a computer cluster.

The environment is designed and built to enable high performance and large capacity. File load speeds, smooth graphical manipulation, direct interaction with the model and the model parameters, and rapid expansion of the concise graphical representation into data structures suitable for the generation of equations all affect the operators' ability to rapidly set up and perform *in silico* experiments. In addition, the ability of the system to handle networks of thousands of components is essential to effective simulation of the systems under study. The current environment is meeting these performance requirements for current networks and is projected to be able to efficiently handle networks with tens of thousands of components. For example, a network of 3600 components loads from disk into memory and is displayed on-screen in less than 3 s on a P4 2.2-GHz laptop computer. Benchmarks indicate that load times scale linearly, so we can expect to load a 100,000-component network in under 90 s. The 3600-component network requires only 650 kbytes of disk storage and has an in-memory footprint of roughly 25 MB. Expansion of states is very time-efficient as well. While state expansion time is very dependent on the topology of the network, current benchmarks (again on a P4 2.2-GHz laptop) show a single molecular representation expanding to 11,200 states in under 4 s, and a more topologically challenging set of molecules (with a high degree of interconnection) expanding to over 28,000 states in under 19 s. It is important to note that the expansion cost is incurred only once for each network unless the network topology changes, and then only for the parts of the network connected to the changed region. Multiple simulation runs, even after changes in chemical or reaction parameters, do not require reexpansion of the states.

Simulating the System via the DigitalCell Engine

Once the biochemical network has been parsed into reactions, the reactions are then translated into a system of ordinary differential equations (ODEs) or stochastic reaction probabilities by the DigitalCell. This set of ODEs is then solved numerically.

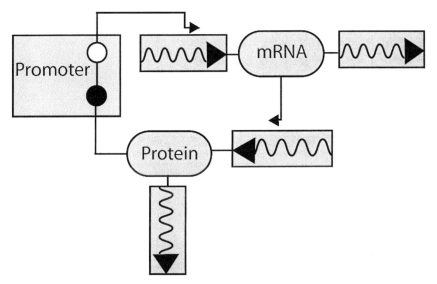

FIGURE 4. DCL representation of a single gene circuit in which mRNA is transcribed and translated when promoter is unbound. The gene product binds the promoter, preventing transcription.

The DigitalCell is a dynamical simulation engine developed by GNS that supports integration of ODEs and stochastic systems, as well as parameter estimation if experimental data are available. It is currently being used to study extremely large-scale (several hundred state variables and parameters) models of signal transduction and gene expression in colon cancer cells. DigitalCell takes as input chemical species, parameters, experimental data, and a set of reactions describing a biochemical network. It is written in C++ and makes use of object-oriented programming techniques such as polymorphism; hence, it is highly extensible. This structure makes adding new reactions to the code very simple. A simple one-gene network can be used to illustrate how the DigitalCell works. In this example, the presence of a free promoter ($[fP]$) induces transcription of mRNA, which is then translated into a protein. This protein then binds the promoter to form a complex ($[bP]$), preventing further transcription (FIG. 4).

   The network and the time variation of the concentration of network components can be described mathematically by the following set of equations:

$$d[fP]/dt = -k_b[fP][protein] + k_u[bP],$$

$$d[bP]/dt = k_b[fP][protein] - k_u[bP],$$

$$d[protein]/dt = k_b[fP][protein] + k_u[bP] + k_t[mRNA] - k_d[protein],$$

$$d[mRNA]/dt = k_{tm}[fP] - k_{dm}[mRNA].$$

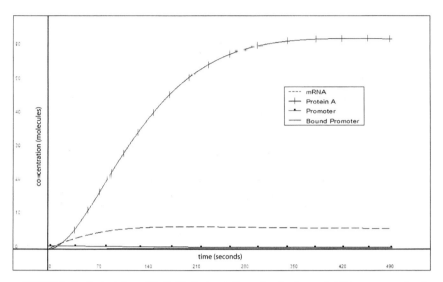

FIGURE 5. Output from DigitalCell simulation of a single autoinhibitory gene circuit. The mRNA and protein concentrations approach equilibrium values. For this plot and other simulation plots in this paper, units are arbitrary.

For a particular set of parameter values and initial concentrations ($k_b = 0.001$, $k_u = 0.1$, $k_{tm} = 0.1$, $k_{dm} = 0.01$, $k_t = 0.1$, $k_d = 0.01$; at time = 0, $[fP] = 1$, $[bP] = 0$, $[mRNA] = 0$, $[protein] = 0$; where $k_b \equiv$ rate of protein binding to promoter, $k_u \equiv$ rate of protein unbinding from promoter, $k_{tm} \equiv$ transcription rate, $k_{dm} \equiv$ mRNA degradation rate, $k_t \equiv$ protein translation rate, $k_d \equiv$ protein degradation rate), the network was simulated and the resulting time course is displayed in FIGURE 5.

The DigitalCell takes four pieces of information as input. First, the initial conditions for the network are defined and algebraic constraints in the network are identified. For example, the concentrations of bound and free promoter always add up to a constant in this one-gene model. Second, the parameters are defined. Parameters can be defined as fixed or free. Free parameters can be estimated using optimization routines. If bounds are known for some free parameters, they are explicitly defined as well. Third, the reactions are defined by listing the type of reactions that occur in the network. Each reaction contains as input the chemicals and parameters that are involved. For each reaction in the list, DigitalCell adds a term to the right-hand side of the appropriate equations. For example, the binding reaction of the protein to the free promoter is responsible for the first term in the rate equations for $[fP]$, $[bP]$, and $[protein]$. The DigitalCell includes at least 20 different reaction types as well as the ability to include user-defined reactions. Fourth, the experimental data, if available, are utilized in the parameter estimation routine (see later subsection).

The DigitalCell can include compartmentalization of molecular components as well as transport between compartments. For example, the colon cancer simulation is divided into a nuclear compartment, cytosolic compartment, endosomal compartment, mitochondrial compartment (on the membrane and inside the membrane), plasma membrane, and extracellular compartment. General switches, time delays, and other functions can be used to model processes and interactions if not enough is known about the detailed biology.

Finally, often the equilibrium solution for a simulation is unknown. The equilibrium solution must first be found before perturbing the system to observe its behavior forward in time. Before solving the systems of equations underlying the circuitry of the cell to produce simulation output, initial values for parameters in the model must be estimated. These parameter values describe the kinetic rates for various biological processes, such as for transcriptional activation, translation of proteins, binding between proteins, binding between upstream regions of the gene and proteins, and translocation of components between various cellular compartments, as well as other quantities such as initial concentrations of molecules in the cell. Initial parameter values can be estimated in three ways: (i) from the biological literature and databases, (ii) via experimental measurements, and (iii) from known values of genes and proteins with similar function. For example, one can use the initial value of a particular ligand binding to a particular receptor that is representative of other ligand receptor binding rates. For mammalian cells, one finds binding rates that range from 10^{-5} to 10^{-2} (molecules min/cell)$^{-1}$. Similarly for concentration levels, one finds that receptor levels range from a few thousand molecules per cell to tens of thousands.

Extracting Proliferation Rates

The DigitalCell simulation predicts the time course of the chemical concentrations of a single cell as it progresses through the cell cycle. However, many experimental growth assays only measure the total number of cells in a population at a few time points to estimate growth rates. We have devised the following approach that allows the output from the single cell simulation to be used to estimate population growth. First, a particular experimental condition (e.g., knockdown of cyclin D) is simulated using four different initial conditions corresponding to the four phases of the cell cycle (G1, S, G2, and M). Then, the number of cell cycle divisions that occur during the simulated experiment is recorded, and a population average number of cycles is obtained by weighting the results of the four simulations. The weights are assigned to each simulation based on the fraction of cells in each phase, as determined by FACS assays. Finally, the population average number of cycles can be converted into an estimate of the total number of cells in an experimental preparation after the completion of the experiment. This number can then be directly compared to experimental results. Mathematically, the approach is as follows:

- Assume a homogeneous population of cells (all cells divide at same rate), except

   (i) a fraction α of the cells are unaffected by the experimental condition;
   (ii) a fraction β of the cells die during each division ($\beta_0 \equiv$ fraction of cells that die in control).

After n_0 divisions (where N_0 is the initial population size), the number of cells N_c in the control sample is

$$N_c = N_0[2(1 - \beta_0)]^{n_0}$$

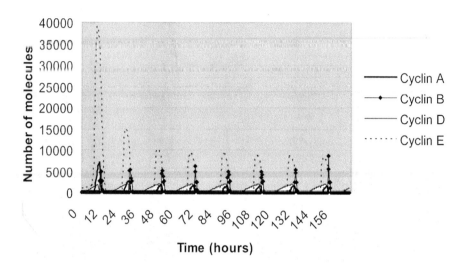

FIGURE 6. Unperturbed HCT 116 cell. Simulation results showing the levels of active cyclin D, cyclin E, cyclin A, and cyclin B oscillating over a 7-day period. Transient is due to initial stimulation of cells by serum.

and the number of cells in the experimental sample is

$$N_e = \alpha N_0[2(1 - \beta_0)]^{n0} + (1 - \alpha)N_0[2(1 - \beta)]^n.$$

Dividing the two yields,

$$r = N_e/N_c = \alpha + (\{(1 - \alpha)[2(1 - \beta)]^n\}/[2(1 - \beta_0)]^{n0}).$$

FIGURE 6 shows simulation results of key cell cycle proteins in an unperturbed HCT 116 cell. For each round of the cell cycle, the figure shows a sequential increase of active cyclin D (which is complexed with cdk4/6), followed by increases in the levels of cyclin A. Subsequent increases in cyclin B levels indicate entry into mitosis, followed by cell division. Note that the cell goes through 8 cell divisions in approximately 7 days.

Estimating Parameters

Each simulation depends on a set of M parameters that includes the initial concentrations of mRNA and protein components, and the kinetic rate constants. Experimental data on each cell line are used to optimize the cell simulation. For example, experimental time-course data of specific proteins are collected in response to various stimuli. These data are generated by the stimulation of cultured mammalian cells with growth factors. Cells are collected at varying times after stimulation and then protein levels are assayed using Western blot analysis. Western blot analysis also allows the phosphorylation state and cleavage of a protein, both of which may indi-

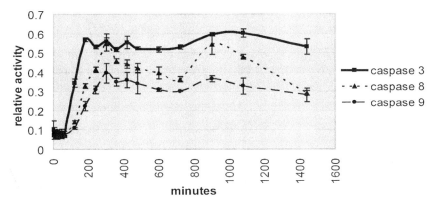

FIGURE 7. Experimental time-course data of caspases 3, 8, and 9 generated from HCT 116 cell lines during induction of apoptosis. HCT 116 cells were treated with 2 ng/mL TRAIL. For each time point, cells were washed with PBS, scraped from their dish, spun down, and then resuspended in lysis buffer. Protein concentration in each sample was measured and adjusted to 1 mg/mL. Then, 100 μg of each sample was assayed for caspase 3, 8, and 9 activity using colorimetric assay kit from R&D Systems (Minneapolis, MN).

cate activation or inactivation, to be assayed. In this way, a single experiment can provide information about the dynamics of protein levels and activity over relatively short (hours) or relatively long (days) time periods. FIGURE 7 illustrates an example of time-dependent caspase activity in response to Trail stimulation. In addition to this time-course data, other data types such as FACS data and growth assay data are useful in constraining the model.

The DigitalCell simulation engine contains a variety of optimization algorithms that use experimental data to improve estimates of parameters. These routines include local and global minimizers. Local minimizers (which are usually gradient-based) start from an initial vector in parameter space and attempt to make "downhill" moves towards the nearest local minimum. In contrast to local methods, global minimizers search the entire parameter space in an attempt to find the lowest possible cost. All of these methods have been parallelized.

Each optimization routine uses a global cost function that is a quantitative measure of the "distance" between simulation results and experimental data. For example, a common choice for the cost function $CF(M)$ is

$$CF(M) = \Sigma_{i,j}(Exp\_data^i_j - Sim\_data^i_j)^2/\sigma^i_j{}^2$$

where $Exp\_data^i_j$, $Sim\_data^i_j$, and σ^i_j are the experimental data point, simulation data point, and error on each data point for the i-th chemical, respectively. The sum over j is taken over all time points collected for each experimentally measured chemical. The cost function can also be generalized to include fitting to multiple conditions. The more conditions entered, the more constrained and accurate the model becomes.

The cost function can also take on other forms such as those that would incorporate error in the time dimension or data structures with various statistical distributions. It can also incorporate data in the form of fold change in molecular concentrations or phenotypic measurements. The cost function merely needs to be of a mathematical form that penalizes the simulation output for deviating from the experimental data. Ideally, experimental data are available under multiple conditions. These conditions may include the cell or biological system under different growth and/or cytokine media, with the addition of a chemical compound or drug, a knockout of a particular gene, or knockdown of the RNA level using siRNA or antisense methods. If such data are available, one minimizes the global cost function over all possible experimental conditions k given by

$$CF(p) = \Sigma_k CF^k(p).$$

The goal is to find the parameter values that minimize the overall global cost function $CF(M)$. To minimize the global cost function, one perturbs the parameters away from the starting values, the simulation is repeated, and the cost recalculated. If the cost is lower, the optimizer takes the new set of parameters that gave the lower "cost" and a better fit to the data. The optimizer iterates the process of changing the parameters, simulating the network, and evaluating the change in the "cost" until the simulation nearly matches the data. For example, the Levenberg-Marquardt optimization algorithm minimizes the cost function by searching through parameter space using information on the slope (first derivative of the global cost function with respect to parameters) and curvature (second derivative of the global cost function with respect to parameters) in M-dimensional parameter space. A general strategy for optimization used by GNS modelers is to identify modules that are activated as a result of a given condition (such as stimulating the cell with a particular growth factor) and then optimize parameters contained in those modules, while leaving other model parameters fixed. This strategy reduces the number of parameters to optimize at a given time.

Experimental Validation

After the model parameters have been optimized using available data, *in silico* experiments can be conducted to predict the effect of a variety of perturbations. These predictions can then be tested to either validate or invalidate the model and to suggest further refinements to the model. For example, if the model predicts potential cancer drug targets within a specific cell type, knockdown experiments with siRNA or antisense technology are conducted to verify the accuracy of the prediction. Cancer cells consistent with the cell line on which the model is based are grown in a monolayer and transfected with siRNA. The cells are then assayed for the phenotypic effect of this knockdown by trypan blue exclusion, alamar blue, or MTT assays. These assays generate a quantitative output that is proportional to the number of living cells and that can be directly compared to estimates from experiments.

DRUG DISCOVERY APPLICATIONS OF DATA-DRIVEN CELL MODEL

Target Validation and Phenotype Prediction

After the model has been constructed and trained against experimental data via the parameter estimation process described in the MODELING METHODOLOGY section, the model is able to generate a variety of predictions. One important application is phenotype prediction and target validation. For example, *in silico* "knockdown" experiments consist of lowering the translation rate or increasing the degradation rate of a component in the model, such as AKT2. The model is then simulated with the knockdown perturbation. Depending on the resulting molecular concentration profiles, a particular phenotype will be indicated (i.e., an increase of caspase 3 levels indicates apoptosis). FIGURE 8 lists representative example phenotype predictions after target knockdown. The great advantage that this *in silico* knockdown method has over other target validation methods is that the molecular mechanism of action can be explored in great detail. This advantage is illustrated by the simulation results for a control (unperturbed) HCT 116 cell and for two *in silico* knockdown experiments described below.

Target	G1-S	S	G2-M	M	Multi-nucleation	apoptosis	sensitivity to apoptosis	no effect
Bcl2							X	
Bcl-xl							X	
AKT2						X		
ERK	X						X	
MEK	X						X	
CDK1			X				X	
CTNNB1	X					X		
NFkB							X	
Bax						X		
h-MDM2	X		X				X	

FIGURE 8. Phenotype prediction and target validation. Use of the cancer cell model to predict resulting phenotype after knockdown of gene product by siRNA.

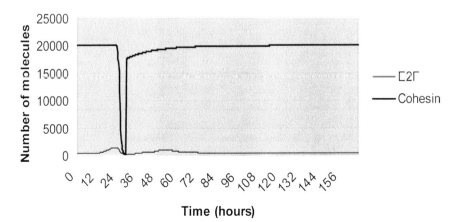

FIGURE 9. Cyclin D knockdown. Unperturbed HCT 116 cell as in FIGURE 6. Simulation results showing the levels of active E2F and cohesin.

FIGURES 6 and 9 show simulation results for an unperturbed HCT 116 cell during a total simulation time of 166 h (7 days) in the presence of serum. As shown in FIGURE 6, a sequential increase in levels of active cyclin D (early G1 phase), then cyclin E (late G1 phase), followed by cyclin A (S phase), and finally cyclin B (M phase), occurs in each cell cycle, in agreement with progression through G1-S-G2-M. FIGURE 9 shows cycling of active E2F (G1/S transition) and cohesin (metaphase to anaphase transition) levels for each cell cycle. Degradation of cohesin indicates separation of sister chromatids, followed by cell division.

Next, a cyclin D knockdown experiment was simulated. FIGURES 10a and 10b show simulation results that indicate that the cyclin D knockdown cell goes through

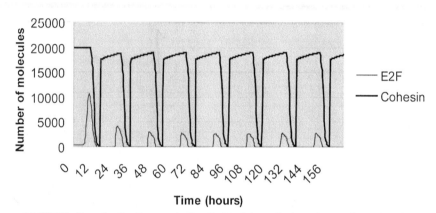

FIGURE 10a. Cyclin D perturbed cell. Model predictions for cyclin D knockdown HCT 116 cell showing levels of active cyclin D, cyclin E, cyclin A, and cyclin B. Note that the cell arrests after the first cell cycle.

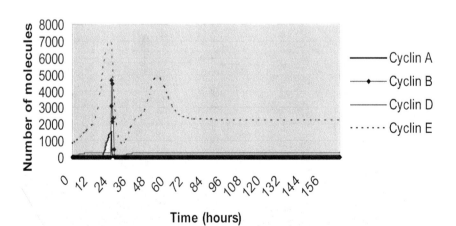

FIGURE 10b. Cyclin D perturbed cell. Model predictions for cyclin D knockdown HCT 116 cell showing levels of active E2F and cohesin for each cell cycle. Note that the cell arrests after the first cell cycle.

only one cell division followed by cell cycle arrest. This result is consistent with the important role played by cyclin D in progression through G1 and validates evidence present in the literature on the effects of knocking down cyclin D in cancer cells.[15-18]

Another example that demonstrates the capabilities of the GNS model focuses on the effects of inhibiting the kinase Akt/PKB. Under normal conditions, Akt mediates growth-factor-induced survival by inactivating pro-apoptotic proteins such as Bad. In addition, Akt activation leads to increases in active levels of the anti-apoptotic protein NFkB. Active NFkB upregulates transcription of survival proteins such as XIAP, Bcl2, and Bcl-xl. FIGURE 11a shows simulation results for levels of active NFkB in the presence of active Akt. Note that there is no detectable active (nuclear) Forkhead protein (FKHR). The oscillations in the levels of NFkB are due to a negative feedback loop included in the model that regulates NFkB levels via IkB.

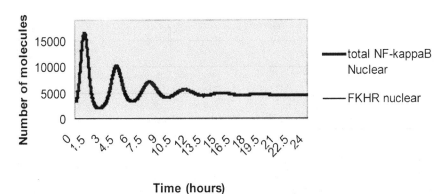

Time (hours)

FIGURE 11a. Effect of knocking down Akt in an HCT 116 cell. Simulation results showing levels of NFkB and FKHR proteins in an unperturbed (AKT2 on) HCT 116 cell.

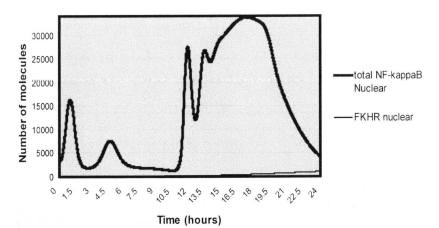

Time (hours)

FIGURE 11b. Effect of knocking down Akt in an HCT 116 cell. Simulation results showing levels of NFkB and FKHR proteins in an Akt knockdown HCT 116 cell.

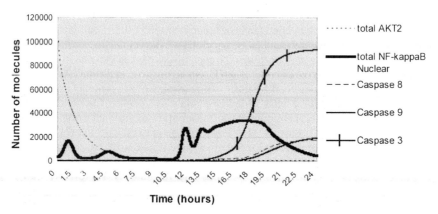

FIGURE 11c. Effect of knocking down Akt in an HCT 116 cell. Increases in levels of the caspase proteins (AKT2 knockdown) indicate that cells go through apoptosis following knockdown of Akt.

Upon inhibition of Akt (FIG. 11b), NFkB levels initially decrease for the first 11 h of the simulation. At the same time (~12 h), levels of active FKHR protein increase in the nucleus, leading to the production of the pro-apoptotic TNF-related apoptosis-inducing ligand (Trail). Newly synthesized Trail has two effects: (1) it drives the cell toward apoptosis; (2) as a stress response, it leads to increases in levels of NFkB. As a result, NFkB levels rise again starting at 12 h. However, as shown in FIGURE 11c, despite the rise in NFkB levels, the cell cannot override the initiation of apoptosis. This is indicated by the increase in the levels of caspases 3, 8, and 9 starting at ~15 h.

Biomarker Discovery and Elucidating Mechanism of Drug Action

In addition to mechanistic target validation and phenotype prediction, the data-driven cell model has other important applications. As a result of the concentration profile that is generated for every molecule in the model, concentration changes in particular molecules that correlate with a particular change in biological state can be identified as biomarkers. Also, the model can be useful in better determining the mechanism of action for a drug. Since the molecular mechanism for most drugs is unclear, the detailed molecular information produced by the simulation is likely to be quite valuable.

CONCLUSIONS AND FUTURE DIRECTIONS

In this paper, we have described methods of model creation, the cancer cell model, and pharmaceutical applications of the data-driven cell model. This modeling methodology allows for the iterative integration of experimental biological and chemical data of many different kinds. The range and accuracy of model predictions depend crucially on this integration of data. Once the experimental data, software tools, and algorithms have been brought together to create this model, predictions of

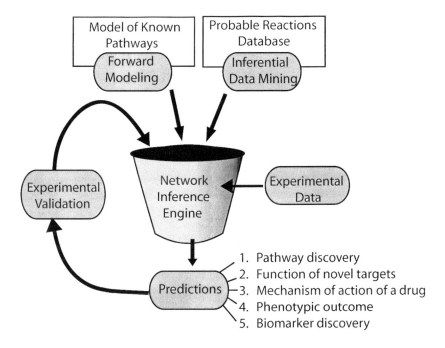

FIGURE 12. Methodology for integrating genomics data into the network inference method used to determine unknown pathway structure.

gene knockdown/knockout, drug response, and combination drug response can be made. The robustness of predictions can be calculated to estimate a confidence level in a particular model prediction. In the future, we hope to extend the capability of this methodology using a technique known as network inference.

Network inference is a potentially powerful combination of forward modeling and data mining. This methodology uses the forward predictive model of known pathways as a foundation (or core model) on which to attach genes and proteins of little or unknown function. The potential interactions between genes, proteins, and pathways outside of the core model are generated from the application of bioinformatics and data mining tools to sequence data and DNA microarray and proteomic data. FIGURE 12 displays this methodology. This pool of potential biochemical interactions, the Probable Links Database, admittedly contains many false positives and false negatives. However, when these speculative interactions serve as input into the Network Inference Engine that compares hypothetical network structure to quantitative experimental data, true interactions can be found. Network inference allows new genes with unknown function and unknown connection to known pathways to be placed into the model and into pathways of biological function. This provides a more complete target validation process and produces a sophisticated and accurate methodology for inferring the mechanism of action of a drug.

While an accurate data-driven computer model of a human cell has obvious applications to drug discovery and development such as the ones outlined above (i.e., target validation and phenotype prediction, better determining of mechanism of action of a drug), there is still a major gap between the effectiveness of a drug in a petri dish and the effectiveness of a drug in a human body. Recent studies that have examined the correlation between drug efficacy in cell lines and animal models versus clinical trials have pointed to little correlation in certain tissues and cancers.[19] Therefore, there is a need for the incorporation of historical and current clinical and animal data and for the extension of single cell models to a better approximation of the *in vivo* microenvironment of a human tissue or organ.

The pharmaceutical industry is at a crossroads. With an aging demographic, the market for life-saving and life-extending drugs continues to grow. However, the ability of the pharmaceutical industry to turn tens of billions of dollars of annual research and development investment into new safe and effective medicines is at an all-time low. Drug discovery and development technologies such as combinatorial chemistry, rational drug design, and high-throughput screening have been exploited without the hoped-for productivity increases. It currently takes upwards of $800 million and 12 years to bring a drug from discovery to market.[20] Success rates from discovery to FDA approval are approximately 1 in 10,000, and from the entry of human clinical trials to FDA approval is 1 in 10.[20] One reasonable hypothesis for this lack of drug development productivity is the simple fact that our current understanding of human biology is not sufficient to allow for rational creation of a drug to change a disease state. The Human Genome Project, DNA microarray technologies, and proteomic technologies have generated huge quantities of data and many new possible drug targets. This is an important and necessary first step in developing a deeper understanding of human biology that will make drug discovery and development more predictable and successful. The next steps that will make this dream of predictive medicine a reality include the systems biology approach of data-driven computer models. The successful integration of massive quantities of biological and chemical data into computer models will eventually improve the industry's ability to forecast clinical trial outcomes and improve drug development success rates. The description of the data-driven cancer cell model presented here is an important step in that direction.

ACKNOWLEDGMENTS

We would like to thank Robert Miller, David Byrne, Basudev Chaudhuri, Larry Felser, Rama Hoetzlein, and Ron Maimon for their contributions to this project. This work was performed under the support of the U.S. Department of Commerce, National Institute of Standards and Technology, Advanced Technology Program, Cooperative Agreement Number 70NANB2H3060.

REFERENCES

1. LUNDBERG, A.S. & R.A. WEINBERG. 1999. Control of the cell cycle and apoptosis. Eur. J. Cancer **35**(4): 531–539.
2. BALMAIN, A., J. GRAY & B. PONDER. 2003. The genetics and genomics of cancer. Nat. Genet. **33**(suppl.): 238–244.

3. ANTONIOU, A.C., P.D. PHAROAH, G. MCMULLAN *et al.* 2001. Evidence for further breast cancer susceptibility genes in addition to BRCA1 and BRCA2 in a population-based study. Genet. Epidemiol. **21:** 1–18.

4. ANTONIOU, A.C., P.D. PHAROAH, G. MCMULLAN *et al.* 2002. A comprehensive model for familial breast cancer incorporating BRCA1, BRCA2, and other genes. Br. J. Cancer **86:** 76–83.

5. HEDENFALK, I., D. DUGGAN, Y. CHEN *et al.* 2001. Gene expression profiles in hereditary breast cancer. N. Engl. J. Med. **344:** 539–548.

6. GRUVBERGER, S., M. RINGNER, Y. CHEN *et al.* 2001. Estrogen receptor status in breast cancer is associated with remarkably distinct gene expression patterns. Cancer Res. **61:** 5979–5984.

7. HEDENFALK, I., M. RINGNER, A. BEN-DOR *et al.* 2003. Molecular classification of familial non-BRCA1/BRCA2 breast cancer. Proc. Natl. Acad. Sci. USA **100:** 2532–2537.

8. PEROU, C.M., T. SORLIE, M.B. EISEN *et al.* 2000. Molecular portraits of human breast tumours. Nature **406:** 747–752.

9. SORLIE, T., C.M. PEROU, R. TIBSHIRANI *et al.* 2001. Gene expression patterns of breast carcinomas distinguish tumor sub-classes with clinical implications. Proc. Natl. Acad. Sci. USA **98:** 10869–10874.

10. VAN'T VEER, L.J., H. DAI, M.J. VAN DE VIJVER *et al.* 2002. Gene expression profiling predicts clinical outcome of breast cancer. Nature **415:** 530–536.

11. VAN DE VIJVER, M.J., Y.D. HE, L.J. VAN'T VEER *et al.* 2002. A gene-expression signature as a predictor of survival in breast cancer. N. Engl. J. Med. **347:** 1999–2009.

12. WEST, M., C. BLANCHETTE, H. DRESSMAN *et al.* 2001. Predicting the clinical status of human breast cancer by using gene expression profiles. Proc. Natl. Acad. Sci. USA **98:** 11462–11467.

13. PERI, S., J.D. NAVARRO, R. AMANCHY *et al.* 2003. Development of human protein reference database as an initial platform for approaching systems biology in humans. Genome Res. **13:** 2363–2371.

14. MAIMON, R. & S. BROWNING. 2001. Diagrammatic notation and computational grammar for gene networks. International Conference on Systems Biology.

15. ARBER, N., Y. DOKI, E.K-H. HAN *et al.* 1997. Antisense to cyclin D1 inhibits the growth and tumorigenicity of human colon cancer cells. Cancer Res. **57:** 1569–1574.

16. SAUTER, E.R., M. NESBIT, S. LITWIN *et al.* 1999. Antisense cyclin D1 induces apoptosis and tumor shrinkage in human squamous carcinomas. Cancer Res. **59:** 4876–4881.

17. SAUTER, E.R., M. HERLYN, S.C. LIU *et al.* 2000. Prolonged response to antisense cyclin D1 in a human squamous cancer xenograft model. Clin. Cancer Res. **6:** 654–660.

18. ZHOU, P., W. JIANG, Y-J. ZHANG *et al.* 1995. Antisense to cyclin D1 inhibits growth and reverses the transformed phenotype of human esophageal cancer cells. Oncogene **11:** 571–580.

19. JOHNSON, J., S. DECKER, D. ZAHAREVITZ *et al.* 2001. Relationships between drug activity in NCI preclinical *in vitro* and *in vivo* models and early clinical trials. Br. J. Cancer **84**(10): 1424–1431.

20. LEHMAN BROTHERS/MCKINSEY & CO. 2001. Report: The Fruits of Genomics. Lehman Brothers/McKinsey & Co.

Application of the Random Forest Classification Algorithm to a SELDI-TOF Proteomics Study in the Setting of a Cancer Prevention Trial

GRANT IZMIRLIAN

Biometry Research Group, Division of Cancer Prevention, National Cancer Institute, Bethesda, Maryland, USA

ABSTRACT: A thorough discussion of the random forest (RF) algorithm as it relates to a SELDI-TOF proteomics study is presented, with special emphasis on its application for cancer prevention: specifically, what makes it an efficient, yet reliable classifier, and what makes it optimal among the many available approaches. The main body of the paper treats the particulars of how to successfully apply the RF algorithm in a proteomics profiling study to construct a classifier and discover peak intensities most likely responsible for the separation between the classes.

KEYWORDS: random forest (RF) algorithm; SELDI-TOF; cancer; classifier; classification tree (CT); detection; prevention; MDM; statistic

INTRODUCTION

Overview

One of the most promising developments in the field of biomarkers and early detection has been the advent of genomic expression profiling using microarray technology as it has provided the ability to profile the expression of an entire genome on a single chip. Thus, researchers can determine the expression level of thousands of genes simultaneously and thereby "hunt" for differentially expressed genes across a variety of mRNA samples. For example, an experiment designed to study a potential cancer prevention agent could be designed by treating several samples of LNCaP cells with the agent, while designating another set of samples of LNCaP cells as controls. Then, mRNA collected from each cell population is hybridized to a gene microarray in order to search for differentially expressed genes among them. However, microarray technology has inherent limitations because the actual biological effectors are usually the resulting protein molecules. Thus, any study of the genomic expression levels is blind to posttranslational modifications and, because of this, levels

Address for correspondence: Grant Izmirlian, Biometry Research Group, Division of Cancer Prevention, NCI, DHHS, Executive Plaza North, Suite 3131, 6130 Executive Boulevard, MSC 7354, Bethesda, MD 20852. Voice: 301-496-7519; fax: 301-402-0816.
izmirlian@nih.gov

Ann. N.Y. Acad. Sci. 1020: 154–174 (2004). © 2004 New York Academy of Sciences.
doi: 10.1196/annals.1310.015

of mRNA expression often correlate poorly with the actual *in vivo* protein concentration due to differential rates of mRNA translation and varying protein half-lives.[1]

For several decades, the identification of serum proteins and peptides has been conducted using mass spectrometry and electrophoresis gels. The limitations of these techniques are similar to those that existed in genomics before the advent of microarray technology. Until recently, only a relatively small number of proteins could be studied simultaneously. Now, however, as in genomics, recent high-throughput technology coupled with the analytic tools of bioinformatics have accelerated the rate of discovery within the realm of serum protein chemistry, giving birth to the field of proteomics.

Specifically, the first widely used such mass spectrometric technique is known as surface enhanced laser desorption ionization (SELDI) coupled with time of flight (TOF) mass spectrometric detection.[2] The principle behind this is that, in the presence of an energy-absorbing matrix such as sinapinic acid (SPH), large molecules such as peptides ionize instead of decomposing when subjected to a nitrogen UV laser. Thus, partially purified serum is crystallized with an SPH matrix and placed on a metal slide. Depending upon the range of masses the investigator wishes to study, there are a variety of possible slide surfaces. For example, among hydrophilic exchange media, one choice is the strong anion exchange (SAX) surface, which has a range from 2 to 50 kDa. This can be used for a "first pass", while the weak cation exchange (WCX) surface has greater precision over a more narrow range (2 to 20 kDa). The peptides are ionized by the pulsed laser beam and then traverse a magnetic field–containing column. Masses are separated according to their times of flight as the latter are proportional to the square of the mass-to-charge (m/z) ratio. Since nearly all of the resulting ions have unit charge, the mass-to-charge ratio is in most cases a mass. Therefore, the terms "m/z ratio" and "mass" will be used interchangeably in the following. The *spectrum* (intensity level as a function of mass) is actually recorded digitally, so the resulting data obtained on each serum sample (hereafter, *subject*) are a series of intensity levels at each mass value on a common grid of masses (hereafter, *peaks*, *peak intensities*, or *features*). A typical machine has a digitized spectrum of length in the tens of thousands, with masses ranging from 2 to 50 kDa. Notice, at this level of resolution, that which is conceptualized as "a protein" translates into at least several consecutive peaks. For instance, it is known there are variations in isotopic ratios from person to person so that, at the level of resolution attainable by SELDI-TOF, the identity of a given protein in an aggregate of human subjects is most likely a range of similar masses differing by a fraction of a dalton.

The organization of the remainder of this paper is as follows. First, it is pointed out that, from the point of view of classical statistical methodology, most (if not all) data sets arising in a proteomics profiling study are underspecified problems so that no unique classification rule can be assigned to a given data set using any of these methods of classical statistics. Consequently, the analyst must turn to machine learning for answers. This will open a short synopsis of some of the available machine learning tools that have enjoyed popular use, especially in the substantive literature (such as a single classification tree, neural network, or genetic algorithm). The following discussion will attempt to give one appreciation for the reasons why many of these algorithms tend to overfit the training data, giving results that are not reproducible. Following will be a thorough discussion of the random forest (RF) algorithm:[3,4] specifically, what makes it an efficient, yet reliable classifier, and what makes it optimal among the many available approaches. The main body of the paper treats the particulars of how to successfully apply the RF algorithm in a proteomics profiling study to construct a classifier and discover peak intensities most likely responsible for the separation between the classes. Towards that end, a nominal t statistic for the important peak discovery component of analysis is investigated This has recently become available in the current release of the software.[4] This discussion is illustrated via a Monte Carlo study using "realistic" simulated data generated from characteristics of a proteomics study from the author's previous work. The case of null relationship between spectra and outcome and the case of a specific relationship of a given magnitude between spectra and outcome will be considered at a range of sample sizes. The newest RF (version 5) was posted in 2003 and is available as FORTRAN.[4] There are versions in R and in S-plus[5] and these are most closely related to version 3 of the original author.

The Preprocessing Step

Since it is arguably one of the most crucial steps and because it offers the chance to introduce concepts required in the rest of the paper, we next make brief mention of the preprocessing step. However, as it is not the focus of this research, only the approach that is recommended by the spectrometer manufacturer is briefly outlined here. First is the issue of normalization. A typical approach is to standardize the *total charge*, that is, the area under the curve, to a reference value. Without normalization, the comparison of peak intensities among different spectra is impossible. Next, the alignment step is required to eliminate slight horizontal axis shifts that exist among the spectra. There are differing opinions regarding the final phase of preprocessing, which is peak detection. As discussed below, because of the underspecified statistical nature of most profiling studies, analysis tools are required that can operate even when the number of features exceeds the sample size, even by orders of magnitude. For this reason, some will argue that this final phase of preprocessing, that of *peak detection*, is not necessary at all, but that the raw normalized and aligned spectra should be the target of analysis instead. This argument, however, is easily put into perspective by considering that the purpose of the investigation is not just classification, but most primarily peak and ultimately biomarker identification. As mentioned above, that which is conceptualized as a protein may translate into a large number of consecutive peaks in the raw spectrum. For this reason, a raw spectrum is unsuitable and so data reduction in the form of peak detection is necessary, not because the analysis tool depends upon it, but because we desire the target of analysis to be an equivalence class of proteins of similar mass. Once again, the manufacturer's supplied algorithm, while ad hoc in nature, seems to perform quite well and works as follows. Subject to three tuning parameters (the signal-to-noise ratio, θ; the window width, w; and the threshold proportion, r), the algorithm uses the entire pooled sample of spectra beginning with the lowest recorded m/z value and proceeds as follows. The first m/z value (denote its value m_1), corresponding to a local maximum intensity within a given spectrum at which the signal exceeds the background noise by a factor of more than θ, is considered a candidate *mass cluster*. Next, all spectra in the sample pool are scanned within the window centered at m_1 of half-width $w \times m_1$. If a total of at least $r \times n$ out of n (including the first) spectra are identified that share an intensity level exceeding the background noise by a factor of more than θ, then the candidate, m_1, is determined to be a *mass cluster* in the data set (hereafter, peak or feature). The algorithm continues in this manner to identify all such *mass clusters* present in the pooled sample of spectra. The study in which I was involved used $\theta =$ 3 and $r = 0.05$, values typical in the literature. The value of w depends upon the machine resolution. In the case that I encountered, $w = 0.003$. This means that a local maximum value of intensity in a given sample spectrum is considered to be a candidate peak for the data set if its signal exceeds the background by a factor of 3 or more, and that candidacy of that peak is confirmed whenever candidate peaks are detected in at least 5% of the pooled sample spectra, within a window of half-width that is three-tenths of a percent of the candidate mass value. Depending on the sensitivity range of the surface being used, this final step produces on the order of 100 or so *mass cluster*/intensity level pairs. For example, one such study used both SAX and WCX surfaces. The above-mentioned peak detection step produced 138 and 72 peak intensities in the m/z ranges of 2–50 kDa and 2–20 kDa, respectively. It is important to realize that, after this peak detection has been carried out, the data contained in each spectrum are now a series of intensity levels at each mass cluster value in a common grid of mass clusters. We will continue to refer to each of these intensity level/mass cluster pairs as peaks, peak intensities, or features.

Since it allows the high-throughput mass spectrometry of partially purified serum, use of SELDI-TOF and the field of proteomics have attracted tremendous interest and show promise for the fields of early cancer detection, drug discovery, and cancer prevention. A typical application in cancer research is to analyze serum collected from two or more clinically distinct populations. For example, in the area of cancer detection, these populations could be "normal" versus "ovarian cancer"; likewise, in the area of cancer prevention, these populations could be "responded to preventive therapy" versus "did not respond to preventive therapy".

Classifiers: An Overview

The goal of a proteomics profiling study is to try to relate these proteomics profiles to the clinical population of origin (hereafter, *class membership* or *class*). In general, this relationship could involve an arbitrary degree of complexity. Since a variety of methods for elucidating this relationship will be discussed, they will in general be referred to as *classifiers*. A classifier is an algorithm that uses *training data*, containing both the proteomics profile and the class membership on each element in a sample of a reasonable size, and uses it to define a classification algorithm whereby all future proteomics profiles with unknown class membership can be assigned a predicted class. After the training step, a validation step is necessary in order to estimate the generalization error in the trained classifier, and a variety of strategies exist for accomplishing this task. The one point in common among such strategies is that all require a validation set made up of samples not in the training set. The overall generalization error rate is one minus the fraction of predictions concordant with the truth. In two-class problems ("1" = "affected" or "responds", "0" = "healthy" or "doesn't respond"), the *sensitivity* and *specificity* are defined as the fraction of predictions that are concordant with the truth among those in the "1" and "0" classes, respectively. Below, we will briefly outline some of the alternate strategies for the validation step. At that point, we will see that the way in which the RF algorithm does this is optimal among all such strategies in the literature.[3,4] An important point can be made here. Suppose that a choice of classifier has been made and imagine an idealized situation in which such an abundance of data exist that, for each unique proteomics spectrum, there is a reasonable sample size sharing, nearly identically, that proteomics spectrum. Given a particular spectrum, X, and then among the sample sharing the spectrum X, the average proportion of predictions for each class, j, obtained in the validation phase, is an estimate of the true underlying conditional probability: $P\{Y=j \mid \text{spectrum is } X\}$, where Y denotes the class membership of a randomly drawn subject from the universe of individuals having spectrum X. In the remainder, we refer to this as the *science* underlying the problem since the presence or absence of true dependence of the outcome upon the spectrum is the target of any such investigation. Furthermore, one should keep in mind that the complement of the true underlying conditional probability given above provides a lower limit to the *expected* error rate attainable by any classifier (the Bayes risk). Another important point to be made is that the credibility of the estimated error rate (including estimated sensitivity and specificity) depends entirely upon the robustness of the classifier to slight perturbations in the training data and the manner in which it is validated.

Generalization Error: Some Caveats

Perhaps the first notable work in the cancer detection area was a case-control study of sera collected from ovarian cancer patients and controls, which used proteomics (SELDI-TOF) spectra to train a classification algorithm to distinguish sera of ovarian cancer patients from those of controls.[6] Interestingly, that study very quickly drew a lot of attention as sensitivity, specificity, and positive predictive value (PPV) were reported to be 100%, 96%, and 94%, respectively. However, since the appearance of that work, it has been the topic of much controversy. First, the 94% PPV is misleading as it is based upon the nearly 50% prevalence of ovarian cancer in the case-control study. When based instead upon the fraction of a percent prevalence that is known to exist in the population at large, this translates to a PPV of roughly 9%.[7,8] Second, it has been observed that the use of these findings to screen a healthy population would require a much higher specificity.[9] Finally, the difficulty in reproducing these results has called into question the validity of the findings.[10]

Underspecified Statistical Problems

In order to better appreciate the origin of the above-mentioned caveats, an intuitive discussion of an *underspecified statistical problem* in classical statistics is now presented. In other words, why isn't linear or quadratic discriminant analysis (LDA, QDA) or even (polytomous) logistic regression appropriate for most proteomics profiling studies? The reason is that there is too much data on too few subjects. This has been called the "curse of dimensionality" by some authors.[11] Consider that a typical proteomics spectrum, even after peak detection, has on the order of 100 peaks, while typical sample sizes are less than 100. To compound the problem, since it is believed that the true mechanism at the level of the proteome that distinguishes one class from another is highly complex, all possible interactions among the peaks must be considered. In the case of the two-class problem and logistic regression, one is faced with 2^{100} regression coefficients with a sample size of less than 100. To say that the system does not have a unique solution is putting it mildly. Consider that one can assign arbitrary values to an arbitrary choice of *all but 100* of the 2^{100} regression coefficients, and still there will exist a solution for the remaining 100. Consequently, nothing can be said about the values of any of the regression coefficients with any degree of certainty at all, so it is impossible to construct a classifier based upon maximum likelihood. This includes LDA and QDA and classification using categorical regression, unless one is willing to a priori throw away a large portion of the available features. As an aside, we remark that penalized maximum likelihood is a viable alternative and, in fact, support vector machines, one of the popular methods for analyzing proteomics profiling studies, is equivalent to ridge stabilized maximum likelihood.[12] The disadvantage of this family of approaches is the large degree of tuning required as well as its vulnerability to the curse of dimensionality.[11]

Classification Trees

For these reasons, machine learning techniques must be used instead of the tools of classical statistical inference in proteomics profiling studies. One of the simplest machine learning classifiers is the classification tree (CT).[13] It functions by using features from the spectra to successively split the training set into two portions or *nodes* until all subjects belonging to the same node share the same class. The training phase begins with all subjects in the *root node*. The root node is split into two child nodes by selecting the m/z value that separates the sample pool according to a threshold intensity level so that the split results in the greatest decrease in node class heterogeneity between parent and child nodes. Heterogeneity is measured in the CT using the Gini index, which is one minus the sum of squared class proportions. The decrease in heterogeneity is measured as the difference between the Gini index at the parent node and the weighted average Gini indices at the child nodes. In this manner, all resulting nodes are split until either the within-node class purity is 100% or further splitting is impossible due to identical feature profiles (not likely to occur in proteomics studies). Such nodes are called *terminal nodes*. Notice that the 100% node purity requirement sometimes results in a node containing a single subject. Thus, the algorithm just described is a complete decision rule and class membership prediction is done for spectra of unknown origin by placing it into the *trained* tree and assigning the class label corresponding to the terminal node into which it falls.

Bias and Variance

Because the "best variable" selection is repeated each time a node is split until the training set is fit perfectly, it is easy to see why a single CT represents an extreme case of overfit in the training data. Recall the language of the introductory paragraphs above, that is, at the validation step and within a group of similar spectrum profiles, the average proportion of predictions for a given class, j, is an estimate of the true underlying conditional probability: $P\{Y=j \mid \text{spectrum is } X\}$, where X and Y denote the spectrum of peak intensities and class membership of a randomly drawn subject from our source population. Classifiers such as a single CT, which fit the training data perfectly, can be shown to have high variance, but low bias.[14] This is to say that, in an idealized series of individual studies, attempts to replicate the same

TABLE 1. Bias/variance characteristics of several base classifiers

	Low variance	High variance
Low bias		CT, NN, GA
High bias	kNN, LDA, QDA, BDA	

NOTE: BDA, Bayesian discriminant analysis; CT, classification trees; GA, genetic algorithms; kNN, k-nearest neighbors; LDA, linear discriminant analysis; NN, neural nets; QDA, quadratic discriminant analysis.

conclusions, using separate (but equally distributed) data sets, will result in highly variable error rates obtained in the validation step of each study. However, if the classifier contains enough potential for complexity, that is, a suitably rich span of possible associations between spectrum and class membership (hereafter, *complexity span* of the classifier), as does the CT, then the average estimate among those individual studies would be an accurate estimate of the true underlying conditional probability of misclassification. TABLE 1 lists various *base* classifiers by the magnitude of bias and according to the magnitude of variance. The term "base classifier" is used here to distinguish a classifier that is a single instance of itself from *aggregate classifiers*, discussed shortly, that are constructed by aggregating over the predictions made by multiple instances of a base classifier. Notice first, in TABLE 1, that a single CT, genetic algorithms (GA), and artificial neural nets (ANN) are all algorithms that have low bias, but high variance. Recall that LDA and QDA are unsuitable for proteomics studies because they require sample size to be larger than the number of features plus interactions. It is still worth mentioning that LDA and QDA have low variance, but their complexity span is limited by the fact that they function by partitioning the space of spectrum intensities into regions of homogeneous predicted class and these regions are constrained to have linear (or quadratic) boundaries. This can result in bias. While Bayesian discriminant analysis can handle underspecified problems and has a richer range of boundary types, the investigator is required to choose a particular type of richness at the outset, and the algorithm is highly sensitive to this choice in underspecified problems, so this too results in bias. The k-nearest neighbors (kNN) classifier is low in variance because it does not necessarily fit the training data perfectly. However, its ability to detect trend between a few peaks and class membership deteriorates as the spectrum size increases, and thus has potentially a high bias as dimensionality increases and a strong signal among just a few peaks becomes overwhelmed by noise. Incidentally, support vector machines share this caveat—that is, become overwhelmed by noise.[11] Clearly, an ideal classifier belongs to the low variance/low bias cell, which is empty in the diagram. However, construction of an aggregate classifier from a base classifier such as the CT, ANN, or GA having low bias, but high variance, has the effect of variance reduction, producing a classifier of low bias *and* low variance.

Bootstrap Aggregation or Bagging

This can be explained as follows. Ideally, if every proteomics study could be replicated under identical circumstances, each producing data sets statistically independent from one another, but drawn from the same underlying distribution, then a separate classifier could be trained on data from each study. Next, given a spectrum, x, the ensemble could be used to predict class membership corresponding to x by giving each of the classifiers a vote, counting votes for each of the classes, and assigning, as the predicted class, the one with most votes. If the number of independent studies is B and the variance of any given statistic derived on a single base classifier in a single study is v, then the same statistic derived on the aggregate classifier has variance v/B. The summary statistic(s) could be, for example, the generalization error and a list of peak importances, as done in the Monte Carlo study that follows. Realistically, however, one never has a series of independent and identically distributed (i.i.d.) studies, just the outcome of a single study. However, a series of bootstrap replicates of the data set can be formed by drawing (with replacement) a sample of the same size. Note that drawing with replacement allows the possibility that a single element in the original sample is multiply represented in the bootstrap sample. It is well known that drawing a sample of size n with replacement from an original sample of the same size tends to include roughly two-thirds of the original sample, with duplication in the remaining third. These bootstrap replicates approximate a series of i.i.d. studies.[15] In this manner, a low bias/high variance base classifier such as CT can be aggregated, resulting in a classifier having both low bias and variance. In the machine learning literature, this is called *bagging* (an acronym for *b*ootstrap *agg*regat*ing*) the base classifier.[16] To reiterate, the training phase proceeds by training multiple base classifiers on each of a series of bootstrap replicates of the training set. This produces an ensemble of trained classifiers, each returning a predicted class when presented with a new spectrum. The aggregate classifier assigns predicted classes using majority vote. Another advantage of aggregate classifiers is that they offer a validation scheme whereby all of the available data can be used for training and for validation, while maintaining separation between training and validation, ensuring reliable estimates of error rates and related statistics. This validation scheme works as follows. Consider a data set consisting of a sample of size n. Each base classifier in the ensemble is trained on a bootstrap replicate from the entirety of available data. However, each of these bootstrap replicates (being samples of size n drawn with replacement from the original sample of size n) tends to leave out roughly one-third of the sample. Thus, each classifier in the ensemble is trained on roughly two-thirds of the original data. Consequently, each element in the sample of size n trains roughly $(2/3)B$ of all classifiers in the ensemble so that it can be used to validate the remaining $B/3$ classifiers. The use of bagging and the related out-of-bag cross-validation method has been called "632 cross-validation" by some authors[17] because the "roughly 2/3" above is in actuality $1 - 1/e$, which is ~0.632. Notice how this differs from "leave one (or more) out cross-validation". In the latter validation scheme, the training set size is $n - 1$ (or less) instead of n and, more importantly, due to the high degree of overlap among the ensemble of resulting data sets, these data sets do not approximate an i.i.d. series of studies, so there is neither reduction in variance nor increase in accuracy of the error rate estimate. Next, it is easy to see why 632 cross-validation is superior to split-sample cross-validation because in the latter method one is forced to train on only a portion (half, two-thirds, etc.) of the data. Finally, none of these other schemes has the effect of increasing the reliability of the error rate estimates as does the combination of bagging and 632 cross-validation.

THE RF ALGORITHM

RF Is Bagging Coupled with Random Feature Selection

The RF algorithm is conducted by bagging a CT, with 632 cross-validation, with an additional modification. Random feature selection in the construction of each tree and at each node is done in order to enhance the degree of independence among trees in the ensemble. This means that, during the training phase, within each CT, at each time a node needs to be split, the search for the best feature to split on is limited to

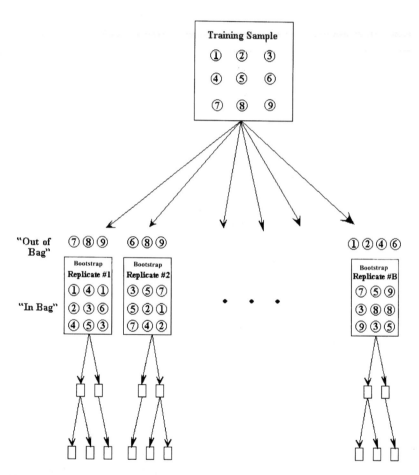

FIGURE 1. Schematic of "bagging" or bootstrap aggregation using the classification tree as the base classifier. Note that out-of-bag samples are used to validate all trees for which they are "out-of-bag". In ordinary bagged classification trees, splitting is done at every node in every tree by selecting the best feature to split on, resulting in purest nodes. In the RF algorithm, the search for best feature is limited to a randomly drawn subset of size around the square root of the total number of features. Random subsets are drawn repeatedly every time a node is split. Each trained classification tree gets one vote in the ensemble.

a subset of all features, and that subset is randomly drawn from the entirety of features. This random draw is made separately for all nodes in each tree in the ensemble and is of fixed size, m, a parameter set by the analyst. The default value of m is the square root of the total number of features, but results are fairly insensitive to this choice. Note that the subset selection process will tend to include each of the available features roughly at an equal number of nodes among all trees in the ensemble. Second, random feature selection still results in a low bias/high variance base classifier since each CT is "grown" (continues splitting) until 100% node purity is reached. Consequently, random feature selection has the effect of reducing correlation between individual classifiers in the ensemble, while maintaining *strength* of the aggregate, that is, its sensitivity to the true structure underlying our data.[3] To summarize, bagging always outperforms the base classifier both from the standpoint of reliability and from the standpoint of strength. The level of reliability and strength attained by bagging is enhanced by random feature subset selection (see FIG. 1).

Important Peak Discovery: The MDM Measure

The next topic of discussion is the manner by which the RF algorithm detects important peaks once the classifier has been trained. The principle behind the quantification of the importance of a given peak to the classification algorithm is intuitively clear. The investigator is interested in identifying peaks that differentiate the classes from one another. Thus, if a particular peak lends discriminatory ability to the classification algorithm, then replacing its values by noise should attenuate the discriminatory ability of the algorithm as a whole. This attenuation is measured via the *mean decrease in margin* (MDM) measure, which is computed at each peak, j, as follows. First, during the out-of-bag (o.o.b.) validation stage, each subject's amenability to classification is quantitated by the *margin*, which (in the two-class situation) is the amount by which o.o.b. votes for the correct class exceed those for the incorrect class. Once the margin for each subject is computed, each margin is recomputed using the same spectrum, only with intensity values at the peak j "noised" by selecting at random from the intensity values at peak j from among the other spectra in the data set. If the peak j is important to the classifier, then the margin should have decreased. The MDM measure is the average over subjects of this decrease in margin at the subject level (true margin minus margin of noised spectra), and larger values of MDM are indicative of greater importance. The newly released version 5 of RF (available as FORTRAN) computes an estimated variance in the MDM importance measure corresponding to each peak in the spectrum, and resulting Z scores and corresponding P values are returned.[4] Thus, it is possible to do important peak selection within the realm of statistical inference.

Adjustments for Multiple Testing: The Benjamini-Hochberg FDR

As is the case in the analysis of gene expression microarrays, multiple hypothesis testing is an issue here as well. We recommend use of the Benjamini-Hochberg (BH) step-down procedure to control the false discovery rate (FDR).[18] This can be described as follows. If one does nothing about multiple hypothesis testing and applies the naive "nominal P value is less than 0.05" filter to a list of more than 100 hypotheses, that is, the per comparison error rate (PCER) procedure, then it is expected that roughly 5 peaks having purely happenstance relationship with the outcome will be determined to be significant. This may be alright if the resulting list is much longer than 5; however, if the important list is of length 5 or so, then decisions based upon this analysis will probably end up wasting someone's time and money in the lab. The strictest way to adjust for multiple testing is the Bonferroni procedure. It works by comparing nominal P values corresponding to each test to 0.05 divided by the total number of hypothesis tests (peaks in this case). This controls the global type I error, which means that the chance of falsely identifying *at most* one or more peaks is <0.05. While this is appropriate in the analysis of multi-arm clinical trials, in which a single false-positive finding is clearly undesirable, it is clearly too conservative for filtering a list of candidate peaks. The BH step-down procedure is somewhere in between the Bonferroni and PCER procedures, and works by controlling the false discovery rate, which is more in keeping with the philosophy of this type of biologic investigation. The BH procedure controls the proportion of falsely identified peaks among the number of peaks identified as significant. While Bonferroni controls the chance of falsely identifying one or more, BH controls any expected proportion falsely identified among those identified. To illustrate the BH step-down procedure, consider the analysis of a hypothetical proteomics profiling study, here using simulated data. The manner in which this hypothetical data set was simulated is described below. Imagine that the peak detection phase of the preprocessing step produced 138 peaks. TABLE 2 lists the top 25 peaks, sorted by nominal P values based upon the MDM importance measure and nominal t statistics. Column 1 lists the "mass name"; column 2, the MDM measure (difference in percent of o.o.b. votes × 100); column 3, the nominal t statistics; column 4, nominal P values; column 5, true P values; and column 6, the BH step-down values (so called because the direction is from higher to lower P values, even though one starts at the end of the list and works upward). The latter are calculated as the peak rank (row number) times the desired FDR, in this case 0.10, divided by the total number of hypothesis tests, in this case 138. The procedure works by starting at the bottom of the list and comparing nominal P with BH step-down value. As we move from row 138 upward, the *first* row in which the nominal P is *less than* the corresponding BH step-down value becomes the dividing line—all rows including this one are considered to be "discoveries". Assuming that the hypothesis tests in question are statistically independent, this procedure controls the expected FDR.[18] Thus, of the discoveries made according to this procedure, the expected proportion that occurred purely by chance is guaranteed to be less than or equal to the stipulated FDR value if the total number of discoveries is "large". Under violations to the independence assumption, the procedure is supposed to be conservative. Notice that, in TABLE 2, the first 5 lines are considered to be discoveries. If, in reality, #22 is the only true discovery, then the observed proportion of false discoveries would be 80%. However, in the above-described procedure, replacing the nominal P values with the true P values (discussed below) results in no peaks identified as significant, that is, observed FDR of 0%. To summarize, the results of RF analysis consist of the overall o.o.b. error rate, sensitivity, and specificity, and additionally a list of peak importances. Here, we use the MDM importance measures sorted by P values combined with the BH step-down procedure.

TABLE 2. The top 25 MDM importance measure nominal t values sorted by P value

Mass no.	MDM	t stat	Nominal P	True P	BH
M.062	1.930	4.200	$1.33e{-}05$	0.004	0.000725
M.022	7.520	4.040	$2.67e{-}05$	0.005	0.001450
M.037	1.290	3.090	$9.89e{-}04$	0.011	0.002170
M.026	1.260	3.060	0.001	0.012	0.002900
M.060	1.270	2.780	0.003	0.015	0.003620
M.044	1.020	2.480	0.006	0.021	0.004350
M.055	0.295	2.200	0.014	0.029	0.005070
M.029	0.291	2.080	0.019	0.033	0.005800
M.036	0.665	1.470	0.070	0.073	0.006520
M.009	0.603	1.470	0.071	0.074	0.007250
M.002	0.226	1.430	0.076	0.078	0.007970
M.020	0.539	1.170	0.121	0.114	0.008700
M.004	0.484	1.150	0.124	0.117	0.009420
M.068	0.495	1.130	0.129	0.121	0.010100
M.069	0.455	1.120	0.132	0.123	0.010900
M.042	0.154	1.100	0.136	0.127	0.011600
M.067	0.474	1.090	0.138	0.129	0.012300
M.053	0.149	1.070	0.143	0.133	0.013000
M.085	0.136	1.040	0.149	0.139	0.013800
M.045	0.396	0.964	0.168	0.156	0.014500
M.028	0.317	0.786	0.216	0.204	0.015200
M.064	0.304	0.771	0.220	0.209	0.015900
M.135	0.320	0.770	0.221	0.209	0.016700
M.019	0.316	0.768	0.221	0.210	0.017400
M.131	0.111	0.703	0.241	0.231	0.018100

NOTE: Data simulated under the "alternative".

MONTE CARLO SIMULATION STUDY

Simulation of "Realistic Spectra"

Next, we turn the discussion to benchmarking the algorithm via Monte Carlo study. This is done using simulated data. An attempt was made to simulate "realistic looking" proteomics spectra by using moments derived from a proteomics study in which the author was involved. These profiles will be generated first according to the peak intensity distribution described below. Second, the "outcome" variable, class membership, will be simulated conditional upon each spectrum. The next subsection describes results of a Monte Carlo investigation in which there is no association between spectra and class membership (i.e., under the global null hypothesis), while the subsequent subsection describes results of a second Monte Carlo investigation using data simulated under a specific type of "alternative hypothesis".

Specifically, each data set consisted of a sample of 100 spectra, while each spectrum contained 138 peaks. Each spectrum was generated according to a 138-dimensional correlated log-normal distribution (i.e., logged values are multivariate normal) with mean vector and marginal variances taken from the author's previous work. There was an indication of a high degree of correlation in the proteomics study, but the sample size available was not sufficient for a stable estimate. However, correlations over 0.9 were considered as high, while others were considered low. Thus, the correlation matrix used in the simulation consisted of values of 0 and 0.9 off the diagonal, with 78 of the 138 peak intensities belonging to a correlation pair of 0.9. This type of correlation produces realistic-looking spectra sharing many gross visual features with the real proteomics study from the author's previous work and is in accordance with biological intuition, which states that practically all of what one sees in a human serum spectrum are the proteins of normal cellular processes. For example, consider a group of proteins that are involved with a specific process part of normal metabolism. If that process is running faster in a given subject, then one expects concentrations of all proteins in that group to be affected.

Data under the "Global Null"

Having a reasonable mechanism in place for simulating spectra, the next topic of discussion is the conditional distribution of class membership given the spectrum distribution. Of interest is the behavior of the RF classification algorithm and, more specifically, its criteria for selecting important peaks and also for quantifying the level of confidence in this selection. Moreover, of particular interest is this behavior both in the presence of true effect and in the absence of any effect. In order to do this systematically, the properties of the algorithm are first investigated via Monte Carlo (MC) study using a series of 1000 replicated i.i.d. data sets under the global null hypothesis (no association between spectra and outcome). Each of these data sets was given a sample size of 100 and an overall prevalence of 50%. The RF algorithm was fit to each MC replicate data set using 1000 trees. The median, 5th, and 95th MC percentiles for the sensitivity (Se) and specificity (Sp) were 48.1% (11.4%, 81.7%) and 49.0% (12.2%, 82.1%), respectively. While it appears that high values of each had nonnegligible probability of occurring, it is important to note that such high values never occurred together as the Youdin index,[19] $(Se + Sp - 1)$, and overall error rate had median, 5th, and 95th MC percentiles of -3.8% (-23.5%, 15.9%) and 50% (40%, 62%), respectively. Notice that the latter of these, the overall o.o.b. error rate, and its 95% MC confidence interval are precisely that expected from 100 flips of a fair coin, the mechanism that generated the outcomes. Next, MC variance estimates for the per-peak MDM importance measures were derived and compared with the variance estimate used in the FORTRAN version 5. It was discovered that the latter are up to 10-fold larger than those estimated via MC. Next, nominal t statistics based upon the correct standard error were obtained by dividing each MDM measure by its MC standard error estimate. A kernel density estimate was formed from the pooled sample of nominal t statistics across peaks and MC replicates. This is displayed in FIGURE 2. Quite puzzling is the fact that it appears to be skewed and largely kurtotic,

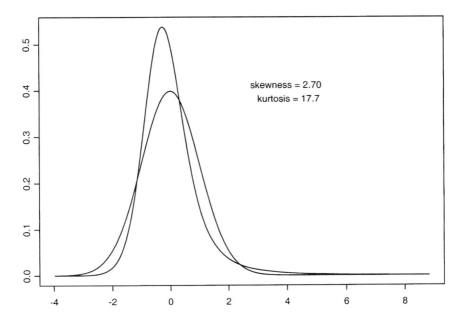

FIGURE 2. (*Upper*) Kernel density plot for *t* statistics from a Monte Carlo study (no. of reps: 1000) generated from the global null, pooled across 138 peaks with skewness and kurtosis shown. (*Lower*) Standard normal.

with values of 2.72 and 18.0, respectively. In passing, we remark that the individual peakwise distributions of these nominal *t* statistics behaved similarly to the distribution of the aggregate mentioned here. The areas to the right of the point of intersection, 2.29, under the true distribution and under the standard normal distribution are 0.023 and 0.0085, respectively. In the following, important peak discovery was conducted using nominal *t* statistics based upon MDM importance measures divided by MC estimates of standard error. To get a feel for the chance of committing "type I" errors at the peak discovery phase, the BH procedure was applied to sorted lists in each of the 1000 MC data sets generated under the global null. The BH criterion for selecting important peaks at FDR of 10% was applied in two ways: by referring *t* statistics to the standard normal curve and by referring them to a kernel density estimate of their true (nonnormal) underlying distribution. The latter was obtained via MC simulation. When referring to the nominal (but incorrect) null distribution, the empirical FDR (proportion of the MC reps in which any peak was identified using the BH criteria) was 79%. This is quite inflated relative to the nominal FDR of 10%. However, when referring to the true null distribution, the empirical FDR was 9.5%, which is very close to and below the stipulated upper bound of 10%. To summarize, the MC study of data simulated under the "null hypothesis" has demonstrated that RF has a very low chance of committing "type I" errors from the standpoint of the estimated error rate. However, at the stage of important feature selection using MDM nominal t statistics, it has been demonstrated that, in order to maintain control over the expected FDR, P values should be derived using the true underlying null distribution, which is nonnormal. The ramifications for the study of a given data set when the true null distribution is unknown are to use resampling by random allotment of class membership in order to determine percentiles under the null for use in a peak selection procedure such as the BH-FDR procedure.

Data under the "Alternative"

Having studied the application of the RF algorithm to data under the global null via MC simulation, a similar study using data generated under "the alternative" is now presented. The data set will contain a signal that will hopefully be detected using the RF classifier and peak importance MDM measure. Before describing the manner in which these "data under the alternative" were generated, some clarification is in order. If the analytic tools are well understood in terms of formal statistical inference and an approximation exists for the power function, then (given a parameter value and sample size) one can derive the approximate power to detect it. The accuracy of the above-mentioned approximation can be tested by simulating data according to parameters specified and simply measuring the proportion of times the null was rejected (simple enough). That being said, the reader now can appreciate the caveats faced in the present situation. There is no approximate power function. The APPENDIX (found at the end of this paper) provides a variance formula for the MDM importance measure, but the null distribution is of unknown form. Consequently, one cannot have any feel for the magnitude in signal that is detectable at a particular sample size. Instead, a particular choice of signal is made. This will be followed up with a statement about efficiency, and a heuristic argument that can be used to give a rough estimate for sample size will be given. Towards this end, three peaks, #22, #88, and #96, were chosen more or less arbitrarily to be designated as "truly important". This choice was made arbitrarily, but in accordance with reality the selection was made from among the peaks present at smaller concentrations. Next, these intensity levels were categorized at their respective medians. Next, 8 categories were constructed from all of the possible combinations among the 3 intensities being above or below their respective medians. The conditional probabilities for class "1" membership that were assigned to each of the 8 cells are listed in TABLE 3. Note that, in each of the columns corresponding to one of the 3 "important" masses, #22, #88, and #96, a "1" indicates that the particular intensity at that mass is greater than its corresponding median value. The last column lists the probability of membership in the "1" class that was assigned to each cell. Thus, the generation of the data set is accomplished by first simulation of spectra as described in the above and then, to each complete spectrum, generating the appropriate $\{0, 1\}$-valued variable having success probability from column 4 in TABLE 3, corresponding to the particular cell among the 8 listed in TABLE 3 to which the spectrum belongs. Note that the "classification space" is the nonnegative octant of 3D space, there are 8 regions within this space of homogeneous class membership distribution, and these 8 cells are divided by 3 planes, one through each axis at a median. This fairly simplistic situation has linear boundaries and, as such, does not test the might of RF to detect oddly shaped boundaries. However, the intended purpose is to demonstrate

TABLE 3. Class "1" membership probabilities

#22	#88	#96	$\mathbb{P}\{Y = 1 \mid X\}$
0	0	0	0.05
1	0	0	0.15
0	1	0	0.70
1	1	0	0.70
0	0	1	0.10
1	0	1	0.30
0	1	1	0.10
1	1	1	0.99

NOTE: Class "1" membership probabilities assigned to each of the 8 cells defined by categorizing 3 arbitrarily chosen peak intensities at their respective medians. In each of the first 3 columns, a "1" indicates that it "is greater than its corresponding median value".

the ability of RF to identify truly important peaks having a sufficient level of strength for classification, even in the presence of an abundance of peaks completely unassociated with class membership. Notice as well that, while the cell shapes are simplistic, the model is not linear on the logit scale in the intensity levels categorized at the medians. The above generation of data sets was carried out within a Monte Carlo study, using 1000 such generated data sets, each having sample size $n = 100$. Each of these data sets was analyzed using the RF algorithm, again using 1000 trees. The median, 5th, and 95th MC percentiles corresponding to the overall o.o.b. error rate, sensitivity, and specificity were 32% (24.9%, 40%), 76.9% (64.4%, 87.1%), and 63.8% (54.2%, 73.4%). Once again, the BH step-down procedure was applied in two ways to the sorted lists of MDM importance measure t statistics that resulted from analyses of each of the 1000 simulated data sets—by referring t statistics to the nominal (but incorrect) standard normal curve and by referring instead to their true underlying distribution under the global null as described above. Of the three peaks, #22, #88, and #96, the strongest of these, mass #22, with a mean value of 4.4, was detected in 39% of the MC data sets when referring to the standard normal curve using the BH step-down procedure with an FDR of 10%, but the 39% power dropped to only 1.5% when referring to the true null distribution. Thus, an empirical estimate of the power to detect an important peak having MDM = 4.4 at a sample size of 100 under an FDR of 10% is only 1.5%. Notice that inference on the MDMs is in reality based only on a sample size of ne^{-1} since the asymptotic variance is of order equal to the size of the average o.o.b. sample size. For sake of comparison, consider a power calculation for the two-by-two table for association between class membership and the intensity at mass #22, categorized at its median. The overall prevalence and true logged relative odds are given by

$$\sum_{j=0}^{7} \pi_j \, p_j = 0.34$$

and

$$\text{logit}(\sum_{j \text{ odd}} \pi_j p_j) - \text{logit}(\sum_{j \text{ even}} \pi_j p_j) = 2.23$$

where the π values are the probabilities listed in the rightmost column of TABLE 3, that is, the conditional probability for class "1" given the spectrum, and the p values are the population fractions in each of the cells. The 8 cell proportions were estimated from a data set of size 10,000. Next, note that, given an overall prevalence of 0.34, the sample size required for a power of 90% to detect a logged odds ratio of 2.23 in a simple one-way association under type I error of 10% is $n = 70$. Since, as remarked above, inference on the MDM measures in the RF algorithm is based upon the average o.o.b. sample, then an o.o.b. sample of 70 corresponds to a total sample of size $n = e \times 70 = 190$. A second MC study based upon data generated under the "alternative hypothesis" mentioned above, having sample size $n = 190$, was conducted. This resulted in median, 5th, and 95th MC percentiles for the overall o.o.b. error rate, sensitivity, and specificity of 31.1% (25.3%, 36.3%), 79.1% (70.1%, 86.4%), and 64.0% (57.0%, 71.2%), respectively. This time, the MDM corresponding to mass #22, with a mean value of 7.0, was detected using the BH procedure with an FDR of 10% with an empirical power of 93% when referring to the nominal (but incorrect) standard normal curve, but only 2.5% when referring to the true null distribution. The first result, based upon assumed normality of the null distribution, suggests, at least under the current set of circumstances, that peak discovery using RF is no less efficient in the use of data in discovering a single peak of a given strength among 137 other nonsignificant peaks than knowing the correct peak and the correct split in advance and using the two-by-two table test for association, except for the factor of e. This is not to imply that RF's ability to sort through noise does not result in loss of efficiency as it was shown above that referral to the wrong null distribution is not fixed at the same type I error (in this case, FDR). In truth, the power to detect the above effect at a sample size of 190, when referring to the true underlying null distribution, is only 2.5%.

DISCUSSION

The topic of aggregating base classifiers has been one of intense and fruitful activity in the area of machine learning. Nonetheless, even among the most current substantive work in medical bioinformatics, the analysis tools of popular choice are base classifiers.[20]

It cannot be stressed enough that, from the standpoint of reproducibility and validity, no other tool can be expected to match the performance of a bagged classifier. The reason for this is that the bagged classifier gives the closest and most reliable approximation to the *true* relationship between the spectra and the outcome. Furthermore, 632 cross-validation is made possible and this is clearly the most efficient use of available data. The reason for this is that bootstrapped replicates are sent to train each classifier so that each element in the sample will have been left out of roughly one-third of the training sets of all of the classifiers in the ensemble; hence, validation is done by sending each element in the sample to classifiers that it did not train. This is nearly as good as having an independent validation sample in addition to a bagged classifier, depending upon the degree of overlap (statistical dependence) of the classifiers in the ensemble. Bootstrapping ensures a degree of independence, depending upon how large a series of bootstrapped replicates and how large the sample size. The RF algorithm reduces the level of correlation even further by using random feature selection every time a node is split.

The performance of the RF algorithm was investigated via MC simulation. This was done both under the assumption that no relationship exists between the spectra and outcome (the global null) and under a stipulated "effect" of a given magnitude at two different sample sizes. The first MC investigation using data under the global null demonstrated a nonnormal asymptotic distribution for the mean decrease in margin (MDM) t statistics, having a larger tail to the right of the moderate-to-extreme value, 2.48. It was noted that this has a profound effect on important peak selection using multiple testing selection criteria such as the BH FDR. Peaks selected using MDM t statistics filtered using the BH criteria controlled at FDR = 10% resulted in an empirical FDR of 79% when referring to the incorrect (standard normal) null distribution. When referred to the correct null distribution, the empirical FDR was 9.5%. In addition, the relative efficiency of peak selection using importance measures returned by RF filtered using BH at FDR = 10% relative to logistic regression *endowed with the knowledge of the correct peak and the correct split* was hinted at, but not resolved. Further work needs to be done to understand the nature of the true null distribution and, in the mean time, an additional series of simulation studies may shed light upon the efficiency of RF relative to logistic regression in the hands of a deity. For now, it can be said that the upper bound is e^{-1} and, most likely, the correct answer is substantially smaller. The implications of this are profound. If an investigator is putting together a proteomics profiling study from scratch (as opposed to adding onto a completed clinical trial), the question posed is as follows: "what kind of reasonable effect is expected of the strongest single predictor split at the most informative threshold?" From this, one can easily obtain the required sample size from a binomial test of proportions. The required sample to sift through all of the extraneous information (i.e., to do data mining) is going to be substantially larger than three times the above.

In conclusion, the most striking advantages of the RF algorithm are its robustness to noise, its simplicity, its lack of dependence upon tuning parameters, and its speed in computation. As an additional note, we mention that an entirely new set of visual diagnostic tools has been made available.[4] Two such new diagnostic tools are the person-peak specific MDM measure (to assess the influence at the person by peak level) and predicted prototypes (to create meaningful summary displays of a trained classifier). A thorough investigation of these is recommended.

Finally, there has recently appeared a plethora of publications promising a comparison of various statistical techniques in the analysis of proteomics profiling data. Usually, these apply a range of techniques to one or more data sets taken from profiling studies.[1] Presumably, the use of clinically obtained data is intended to attach a greater level of credibility within the audience of bench scientists and medical researchers. However, several clinically obtained data sets cannot begin to illuminate the statistical properties of an analytic tool in the way that can be done using "realistic-looking data" generated in a Monte Carlo study. For example, "how does the method fare when there really is no relationship between the spectra and the outcome variable" and "how does the method fare when there really is a relationship between the spectrum and the outcome variable of a given strength" are questions that can only be answered via a thorough simulation study. This paper only begins to provide a thorough study and, as one does not yet exist, this can be taken as an invitation to the reader to write one. One important issue would be to pay better attention than time has permitted here to the generation of even more realistic looking spectra. By "realistic", it is meant that the goal is to create data that share a reasonable amount of statistical characteristics with proteomics spectra of human serum. For this purpose, spectra from several studies could be combined to provide stable estimates of the required cross-moments, and substantive experts would be required to weigh in on the level of "reality" having been attained. The most thorough kind of "methods benchmarking" work should contain "real data" as well as a thorough MC study. While this paper has not quite made the cut stipulated by the above razor, it is hoped that a convincing case has been made.

REFERENCES

1. Wu, B., T. Abbott, D. Fishman et al. 2003. Comparison of statistical methods for classification of ovarian cancer using mass spectrometry data. Bioinformatics 19: 1636–1643.
2. Yip, T-T. & L. Lomas. 2002. SELDI ProteinChip array in oncoproteomic research. Technol. Cancer Res. Treat. 1: 273–280.
3. Breiman, L. 2001. Random forests. Mach. Learn. 45: 5–32.
4. Breiman, L. & A. Cutler. 2003. The random forest package, version 5, in FORTRAN [http://www.math.usu.edu/~adele/forests/index.htm/].
5. Liaw, A. & M. Weiner. 2003. The random forest package, version 3.91 in R [http://cran.us.r-project.org/].
6. Petricoin, E.F., A.M. Ardkani, B.A. Hitt et al. 2002. Use of proteomic patterns in serum to identify ovarian cancer. Lancet 359: 572–577.
7. Elwood, M. 2002. Correspondence: proteomic patterns in serum and identification of ovarian cancer. Lancet 360: 170.
8. Rockhill, B. 2002. Correspondence: proteomic patterns in serum and identification of ovarian cancer. Lancet 360: 169.
9. Diamandis, E.P. 2002. Correspondence: proteomic patterns in serum and identification of ovarian cancer. Lancet 360: 170.
10. Pollack, A. 2004. New cancer test stirs hope and concern. N.Y. Times. Section F, p. 1.
11. Hastie, T., R. Tibshirani & J.H. Friedman. 2001. The Elements of Statistical Learning. Springer Pub. New York.
12. Svetnik, V. & A. Liaw. 2003. Personal communication.
13. Breiman, L., J.H. Friedman, R.A. Olshen et al. 1984. Classification and Regression Trees. Chapman & Hall. London/New York.
14. Breiman, L. 1998. Arcing classifiers. Ann. Stat. 26: 801–823.
15. Efron, B. 1979. Bootstrap methods: another look at the jackknife. Ann. Stat. 7: 1–26.
16. Breiman, L. 1996. Bagging predictors. Mach. Learn. 26: 123–140.
17. Efron, B. & R. Tibshirani. 1995. Cross-validation and the bootstrap: estimating the error rate of a prediction rule. Technical Report.
18. Benjamini, Y. & Y. Hochberg. 1995. Controlling the false discovery rate—a practical and powerful approach to multiple testing. J. R. Stat. Soc. B57: 289–300.
19. Youden, W.J. 1950. Index for rating diagnostic tests. Cancer 3: 32–35.
20. Yanagisawa, K., Y. Shyr, B.J. Xu et al. 2003. Proteomic patterns of tumour subsets in non-small-cell lung cancer. Lancet 362: 433–439.
21. Durrett, R. 1991. Probability: Theory and Examples. Wadsworth & Brooks/Cole. Belmont, CA.

APPENDIX

Derivation of the MDM Variance

Denote the data by $T_n = \{(X_i, Y_i): i = 1,\ldots,n\}$, where $X_i \in R_d$, a bounded subset of $\mathbb{R}^d$, has distribution $F(dx) = \mathbb{P}\{X_i \in dx\}$ and $\pi(x) = \mathbb{P}\{Y_i = 1 \mid X_i = x\}$. Attention is restricted here to the two-class situation for ease in exposition, but the ideas presented here generalize easily. Call T_n the training set. For $b = 1,\ldots,m$, let $T_n^{(b)} = \{(X_i, Y_i): i \in \mathcal{T}_{n,b}\}$ denote a bootstrap sample from T_n, which is to say that $\mathcal{T}_{n,b}$ is a random sample with replacement from $\{1,\ldots,n\}$. In the language of the text, $\mathcal{T}_{n,b}$ is the portion of the training sample that is "in-bag" for the b-th bootstrap set. Denote its complement as $\mathbb{O}_{n,b} = \mathcal{T}_{n,b}^c$, which is the portion of the training sample that is "out-of-bag" for the b-th bootstrap set. Next, let $C(\cdot, T_n^{(b)}, \xi_b)$ denote the b-th classifier in the ensemble, which has trained on $T_n^{(b)}$ and is considered a stochastic function from R_d to $\{0, 1\}$. Here, ξ_b is a random vector containing codings for all random feature subset selections at each node of the b-th tree in the ensemble. For a given subject i, a tree b, and a feature j, the raw margin[3] is defined as

$$\Delta_{n,i,b}^{(j)} = 2\{I[C(X_i, T_n^{(b)}, \xi_b) = Y_i] - I[C(X_i^{(j)}, T_n^{(b)}, \xi_b) = Y_i]\}$$

where $X_i^{(j)}$ is equal to X_i at all components, except at the j-th, which is replaced with a random draw from the j-th components of the rest of the sample, that is,

$$X_{i,\ell}^{(j)} = \begin{cases} X_{\eta(i),j} & \text{for } \ell = j \\ X_{i,\ell} & \text{otherwise,} \end{cases}$$

and η is a uniform random permutation on $\{1,\ldots,n\}$. Let $N_{n,b} = |\mathbb{O}_{n,b}|$. The MDM importance measure can now be defined as

$$\overline{\Delta}_{m,n,j} = \frac{1}{m} \sum_{b=1}^{m} \frac{1}{N_{n,b}} \sum_{i \in \mathbb{O}_{n,b}} \Delta_{n,i,b}^{(j)}.$$

By the subadditive ergodic theorem,[21] for fixed n, this converges almost surely as $m \to \infty$ to a finite sample approximation of

$$2 \int_{R_d} \max_{y \in \{0, 1\}} \mathbb{P}\{Y_i = y \mid X_i = x\} - \max_{y \in \{0, 1\}} \mathbb{P}\{Y_i = y \mid X_i = \xi\} F(dx) F^{(j)}(d\xi)$$

where $F^{(j)}$ is the distribution of $X_i^{(j)}$, that is, the product of the joint distribution of all components except the j-th times the marginal of the j-th. Next, the dependence of the variance upon n and m is investigated. One obtains

$$\text{var}[\Delta_{m,n,j}] = \mathbb{E}[\text{var}[\Delta_{m,n,j} | \{N_{n,b} : 1 \leq b \leq m\}]]$$

$$= m^{-1}\mathbb{E}[N_{n,b}^{-1}]\text{var}[\Delta_{n,1,1}^{(j)}] + m^{-1}\mathbb{E}\left[\frac{N_{n,b}-1}{N_{n,b}}\right]\text{cov}[\Delta_{n,1,1}^{(j)}, \Delta_{n,2,1}^{(j)}]$$

$$+ \frac{m-1}{m}\mathbb{E}[N_{n,b}^{-1}]\text{cov}[\Delta_{n,1,1}^{(j)}, \Delta_{n,1,2}^{(j)}]$$

$$\approx \frac{e}{mn}\text{var}[\Delta_{n,1,1}^{(j)}] + \frac{n-1}{mn}\text{cov}[\Delta_{n,1,1}^{(j)}, \Delta_{n,2,1}^{(j)}] + \frac{e(m-1)}{mn}\text{cov}[\Delta_{n,1,1}^{(j)}, \Delta_{n,1,2}^{(j)}].$$

Note that the second term, the variance of the conditional expectation, is absent because the conditional expectation has zero variance, being independent of $N_{n,b}$. The rest is just the variance of a correlated sum of identically distributed terms with identical pairwise correlations. Given that one always has control over m, it can be assumed that m is much larger than n. Consequently, the dominating term, which is of order n^{-1}, arises from the covariance between the raw margins corresponding to a single subject in two different trees. Thus, an expression for the asymptotic variance of the MDM importance measure, $\Delta_{m,n,j}$, hinges upon obtaining either an exact or approximate value of

$$\lim_{n \to \infty} \text{cov}[\Delta_{n,1,1}^{(j)}, \Delta_{n,1,2}^{(j)}].$$

Improved Small Volume Lung Cancer Detection with Computer-Aided Detection: Database Characteristics and Imaging of Response to Breast Cancer Risk Reduction Strategies

MATTHEW FREEDMAN

*Department of Oncology, Division of Cancer Genetics and Epidemiology,
Division of Advanced Cancer Imaging, ISIS Imaging Science and Information Systems
Research Center, Georgetown University Medical Center,
Washington, District of Columbia 20057, USA*

ABSTRACT: Computer-aided detection (CAD) and diagnosis (CADx) of *in vivo* imaging studies are important tools based on bioinformatics. Currently, there are two diseases for which the United States Food and Drug Administration (FDA) has given premarket approval (PMA): the detection of signs consistent with lung cancer on chest radiographs and breast cancer on mammograms. There are systems for other diseases and other types of images under development; however, this process depends on the availability of an accurate database. The author helped in the development of the databases for such systems and management of the clinical trial that resulted in the FDA-PMA of the system that detects findings consistent with lung cancer. The characteristics of the database used will be described. Further, a woman's risk of developing breast cancer differs from those of other women. Risk can be high, average, or low. There are now pharmaceuticals that decrease the risk that women, as a group, will develop breast cancer and it has been suggested that dietary changes could have similar effects. The pharmaceutical agents, though, have some associated side effects, and it is clinically important to determine whether these agents have decreased an individual woman's risk of breast cancer. *In vivo* imaging biomarkers of risk and successful risk reduction are therefore sought, but the information on possible *in vivo* imaging biomarkers is less mature than activities in CAD. Bioinformatics will be an important contributor to this *in vivo* imaging biomarker development.

KEYWORDS: computer-aided detection; cancer; database; breast risk reduction; imaging biomarkers

Address for correspondence: Matthew Freedman, M.D., M.B.A., Associate Professor of Oncology, Division of Cancer Genetics and Epidemiology, Director of Division of Advanced Cancer Imaging, ISIS Imaging Science and Information Systems Research Center, Georgetown University Medical Center, Box 20057-1465, Washington, D.C. 20057-1465.
freedmmt@georgetown.edu

Ann. N.Y. Acad. Sci. 1020: 175–189 (2004). © 2004 New York Academy of Sciences.
doi: 10.1196/annals.1310.016

IMPROVED SMALL LUNG CANCER DETECTION
WITH COMPUTER-AIDED DETECTION:
DATABASE CHARACTERISTICS

Lung cancer is the most frequent cause of cancer deaths in the United States for both men and women. In fact, more people die from lung cancer than from breast, colon, and prostate cancer combined. For many years, a nihilistic view of lung cancer screening has persisted in the United States, but there is now increasing optimism that early detection could decrease mortality, and a prospective randomized study is now under way in the United States, the National Lung Screening Trial (NLST). The NLST is randomizing subjects to receive either a chest radiograph or a chest computer tomogram.

Currently, the most common method for the initial detection of lung cancer is the chest radiograph. The chest radiograph, however, is somewhat limited as a screening tool since small lung nodules are not always particularly conspicuous. It is well documented by the studies reported by Stitik[1,2] and Heelan[3] from the Hopkins and Memorial early lung cancer screening programs that 30–90% of lung cancers prospectively detected during screening with chest radiographs are visible on a prior chest radiograph obtained approximately one year earlier. This observation that many of the cancers were visible one year earlier encouraged several groups to work to develop computer tools that would provide prompts to radiologists so that the lung cancers might be detected earlier, resulting in an increased chance of effective therapy.

The author, along with scientists from the University of Chicago and Georgetown University, assisted Deus Technologies LLC (Rockville, MD) in their efforts to develop and test a commercial system for lung cancer detection.[a] Deus Technologies developed, tested, and received its premarket approval (PMA) from the United States Food and Drug Administration (FDA) and markets a commercial system for the detection of lung nodules on chest radiographs having characteristics of small lung cancers.

The data submitted to the FDA as the basis for the PMA indicated that radiologists using the RS-2000 computer-aided detection (CAD) system improved their detection of lung cancers 9–27 mm in diameter by 11%. The detection improvement was greatest for the cancers 9–14.5 mm (21%), intermediate for those 15–19.5 mm, and minimal for the larger nodules, mainly because the radiologists had already recognized almost all of the larger nodules without the assistance of the CAD prompts. In the setting of heightened awareness of small lung cancers, the radiologists with the RS-2000 detected 32% of the cancers that had been missed prospectively by two radiologists without the CAD and 44% with the aid of CAD. For the small sample size of 18 cases, this was not statistically significant.

The databases that had been assembled for developing, training, and testing the RS-2000 CAD system were sufficient to prove the system. The characteristics of these databases are described in the next sections of this chapter.

[a]The author of this chapter is a consultant to, Clinical Director of, and a stockholder in Deus Technologies LLC.

CHARACTERISTICS OF THE DATABASES USED TO DEVELOP, TRAIN, AND TEST THE RS-2000 SYSTEM

Two separate databases were developed for the development tasks for the Deus Technologies RS-2000. The first database was for development, training, and internal testing. The second database was separately developed and maintained for the clinical trial that was to be submitted to the FDA as part of the PMA application.

Fundamental Characteristics of the Database Needed to Develop, Train, and Internally Test a CAD System

One of the major impediments to the development of CAD and computer-aided diagnosis (CADx) systems is the lack of sufficient true cases of the disease. Cases (preferably several thousand) are required for development, training, and testing of the algorithm. Assembling such a large number of proven cases is both difficult and time-consuming. Because of the difficulty in obtaining a sufficient number of true confirmed cases, various other types of data can be used. Four types of data can be used during the process of CAD development and validation: (1) computer drawing can simulate images; (2) computers can synthesize images by combining portions of two images, either combining two real images or one real and one simulated; (3) images can be obtained in physical phantoms; and (4) images can be selected from true clinical data. The true clinical data can be of two types: images limited to the precise diagnosis under study or the image set can include images from diseases with similar patterns on images.

Typical types of synthesized images are either a combination of a real chest image with a simulated nodule or an extracted image of a true nodule superimposed on a real chest image that did not include a nodule. True clinical data can be limited to cases of lung cancer or can include cases of cancer that has metastasized to the lung. Optimally, validation should be done on the precise disease of interest—in this instance, cases of lung cancer.

The database for CAD development for the Deus Technologies RS-2000 consisted of several thousand normal and several thousand chest radiographs containing one or a limited number of lung nodules. Cases were gathered from multiple sites from multiple countries, and several different types of film were used for recording the chest images. Cases for training the algorithm were kept separate from the internal testing set. Training cases could have one or more nodules; the testing set consisted of cases containing only one nodule and nodule-free cases.

The database for the clinical trial was a completely separate set of cases. These were kept at Georgetown University and were kept completely separate from the cases used by Deus Technologies for development, training, and internal testing of the RS-2000. The film collection was from the Johns Hopkins Early Lung Cancer Program (JH-ELC). This program was a 5-year screening study of approximately 10,000 subjects, all of whom were screened with chest radiographs and sputum cytology. A text database indicating all subjects who had developed cancer during 5 or more years of follow-up was available along with the date of cancer diagnosis on the radiograph and final pathology diagnosis. The film set was a raw collection of films, substantially more than 100,000 films, from which the specific films demonstrating the cancers had to be extracted. All cancer cases had to be reviewed to find the best film and, from among the possible best films, a group of radiology experts selected the film to be used, confirmed the location of the cancer, and determined if the cancer had been present on a prior film.

A random selection of cases was made from those subjects who did not develop cancer. All cases to be used were screened for image quality. To create the active database for the research, three separate databases were assembled: a text description database in MS Excel, a film database maintained in film files, and a database containing the digitized version of each chest radiograph selected for possible inclusion in the final study. For the final study, randomization selection methods were used to select the cases for inclusion.

Inclusion Criteria for the FDA-PMA Study

Cancer Cases

All cases had to have a confirmed pathology diagnosis of primary lung cancer. The expert panel had to agree by consensus on the location of the cancer and that the film quality was within published current guidelines for quality.

Cancer-Free Cases

All cases had to have a minimum of 3 years of follow-up, during which time no cancer had developed. The quality of each film was confirmed to be within published current guidelines for quality. The cancer-free cases were not selected to be normal, but only cancer-free. If the CAD tool were to be effective, it would have to be effective in a population of suitable age and smoking history; it was recognized that the chest radiographs of such people would have focal scars from prior infections, areas of emphysema, and focal areas of fibrosis.

Selection of Cases

For each cancer case, the size of the cancer had been recorded. Cases were limited to those with cancer nodules 9–30 mm in size. The characteristics of the CAD algorithm defined the size limits for the nodules. Computer pseudorandom numbers were assigned to each case, the pseudorandom number was used to sort the cases, and then the first 80 cancer cases were selected for inclusion. A similar procedure was used for the cancer-free cases.

Method of Analysis

Receiver operating characteristic (ROC) analysis was used for this study. In ROC analysis, each observer radiologist is provided with the image and asked to provide a confidence rating on the likelihood that the case contains a cancer. For this study, the range of scores ranged from 1 to 100. Each radiologist was trained and encouraged to use the full range of scores available.

Characteristics of the Assembled Database

The ideal database for testing a CAD program is not agreed on. The principle that the Georgetown University group used was that the cases included must range in difficulty from easy to hard. If every radiologist could detect a specific case without the aid of the computer, the case would be too easy. If no radiologist could detect a specific cancer, working either without or with the CAD prompts, the case was too hard. There is, however, no way to know that this will be the result until the study is actually completed. Prospectively, we did not know which cases each radiologist and the computer would detect. The same is true for the normal cases. If the case appeared obviously normal to all radiologists, it was too easy. If the case was not considered cancer-free by at least one of the radiologists, it was too hard.

The following subsections describe some of the characteristics of the cases.

Size Distribution

The size of the cancer nodules measured on the radiograph ranged from 9.5 to 27 mm, with a mean and median of 15 mm (FIG. 1). Fifteen mm is approximately the mean size of missed cancers reported in previous studies.[3–5]

Measures of Difficulty of Cancer Cases

The cases for testing CAD systems should encompass a range of difficulties. The optimum would be a group of cases where only one radiologist would detect the hardest cases and where there would be only one case where all the radiologists were able to identify the cancer without the use of the CAD program. FIGURE 2 demonstrates the number of radiologists identifying each of the 80 cancer cases. There are only a few cases where no radiologist recognized the cancer without the use of CAD, but there are more cases where all the radiologists recognized the cancer without the use of CAD. The cases where all of the radiologists recognized the cancers without CAD are too easy. In running the trial, these cases will not be useful in demonstrating the effect of CAD and thus add cost without adding benefit. If this had been known in advance, these cases should, optimally, be removed from the trial.

Distribution of Scores

For each case, the radiologist has to provide a confidence rating on whether or not cancer is present. An indication of the difficulty of the cases is the range of scores that each case elicited from the radiologists. The wider the range of scores among the radiologists used for each case, the more appropriate the case is. FIGURE 3 demonstrates the range of scores used for each cancer case. The chart shows that, for most of the cancer cases, at least one radiologist considered the presence of cancer to be uncertain, while others were certain of the presence of cancer. This means that the cancer was visible on the radiograph and, therefore, the radiologist who initially missed it might be alerted to its presence by a computer prompt. The mean confidence rating shows that the difficulty of cases was reasonably linear.

Radiologists can vary in their level of skill and in their use of the confidence rating system. For this trial, radiologists were selected to be relatively equal in their

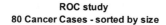

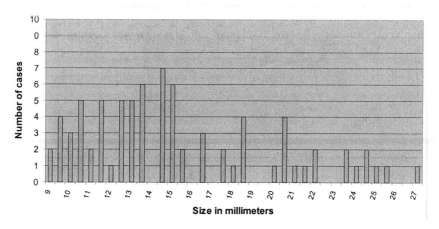

FIGURE 1. This chart demonstrates the size distribution of the cancers from the clinical trial. Note that it is weighted towards smaller cases.

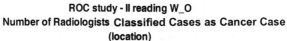

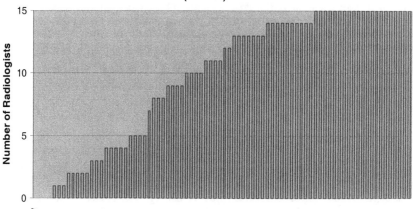

FIGURE 2. This chart demonstrates the number of radiologists who correctly identified each cancer case prior to using CAD. All of the radiologists recognized those cases to the right. For these, the CAD program analysis could provide no benefit since all of the radiologists have already made the correct diagnoses without it.

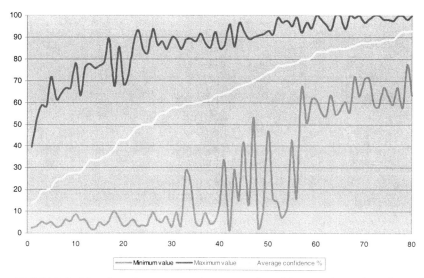

FIGURE 3. The chart demonstrates the range of confidence ratings given for each cancer case. The average line demonstrates that the cases were relatively linear in their mean confidence rating, showing a fairly even distribution from hard to easy.

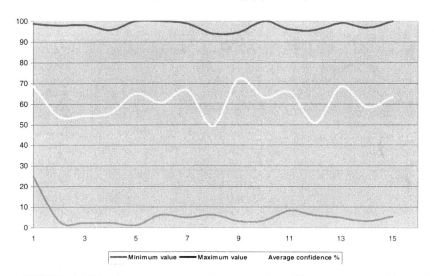

FIGURE 4. This chart demonstrates the range of confidence scores used by each radiologist for the cancer cases. The broad range of scores indicates that the radiologists found some cancer cases easy to detect and failed to detect at least some cases.

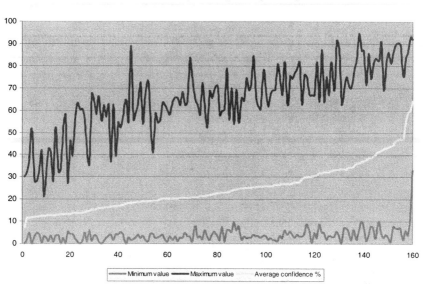

FIGURE 5. This chart demonstrates the range of confidence scores given for each cancer-free case by the 15 radiologists. The confidence levels are lower than for the cancer cases, but show a wide range of values. This indicates that, for approximately two-thirds of the cases, at least one radiologist considered the case suspicious for cancer and that, for almost all of the cases, at least one radiologist correctly identified it as cancer-free.

skill as they were recruited for the trial. FIGURE 4 demonstrates that each radiologist used nearly the full range of confidence scores available to them. Each radiologist detected some and missed some of the cancer cases.

Difficulty of Measurement of Cancer-Free Cases

In normal clinical practice, patients at risk for lung cancer often have scars from various other diseases. Thus, the cases selected to show the clinical benefits of CAD should reflect the population of people who would be studied by the technique. Hence, it is important that the "normal" cases not be completely normal, but rather reflect the types of nonindex diseases found in the population of interest. This means that some will have scars that look like cancer, but are not. In previously reported screening studies,[1,2] 9–25 people had findings (scars) that could be cancer for each cancer case found. The database of images for CAD work should contain such scars. The next few figures demonstrate some of the characteristics of the cancer-free cases used in the clinical trial. FIGURE 5 demonstrates the range of scores used by the 15 radiologists for each of the 160 cancer-free cases. FIGURE 6 demonstrates the range of scores used by each of the 15 radiologists for the normal cases. These indicate the range of difficulty of each case.

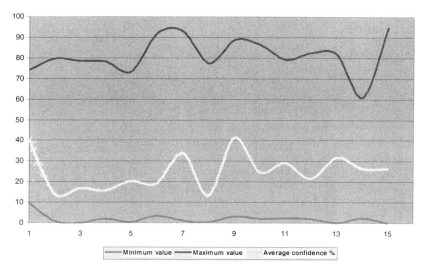

FIGURE 6. This chart demonstrates the range of scores used by each of the 15 radiologists for the cancer-free cases. It shows that each radiologist used a wide range of scores indicating that at least one of the cancer-free cases was considered to contain cancer. The average confidence score is lower for the cancer-free cases than for the cancer cases, indicating that the cancer-free cases were less suspicious than the cancer-containing cases.

SURROGATE END POINT BIOMARKERS OF CANCER PREVENTION

Surrogate end point biomarkers of cancer prevention strategies do not now exist, but are considered important. Clinical trials are complex, expensive, and time-consuming. In prevention trials, sample sizes must be substantially larger than in treatment trials because, in prevention trials, only a small percentage of participants will develop the disease under study. Thus, many subjects who would never develop cancer must be included so as to have a sufficient number of cases of cancer to document the probability of cancer prevention. Current accepted methods of breast cancer prevention, for example, are based on treatment with tamoxifen and there is evidence that treatment with raloxifene may also be effective. To prove that tamoxifen decreased the risk for breast cancer took many years of research and a large number of subjects. There are many potential agents that could reduce the risk of cancer, but providing proof of effectiveness is a difficult task. To avoid long clinical trials, it has been suggested that surrogate end point biomarkers could be used for the initial screening for prevention effectiveness. The Georgetown group has and continues to investigate *in vivo* imaging methods for use as potential bio-markers indicating risk reduction. Such markers, once validated, could be useful in the identification of new preventive strategies. In addition, such imaging biomarkers could indicate which individuals are not showing therapeutic advantage from the strategy. If no therapeutic advantage was present, then the strategies could be changed or discontinued. These pharmaceuticals cost more than $1000 per year. If the medicine is not effective for an individual, this is an unnecessary expenditure. Some women are reluctant to continue to take medicines that have some risk. If an imaging biomarker could show that the agent is helping that individual woman towards lower risk, she might be more willing to continue to follow the strategy.

At this point, we do not know if there are biomarkers that indicate that individual risk of cancer has been reduced. Thus, the task is to search for biomarkers. The problem can be approached potentially as follows: one can look at the effect of pharmaceuticals that decrease the risk of cancer (tamoxifen and raloxifene) and measure the types of changes that occur with their use. Such changes could potentially serve as biomarkers. This would enable one to look at new pharmaceuticals that have similar mechanisms of biological action and use these biomarkers to confirm that these biological actions occur with the newer agents. Even if the same effect is seen, one will not know that the change in biomarkers is related to the risk reduction since the change could be coincident, but not related. Final proof will require many cases collected and analyzed. Databases are essential for such analysis.

Our group is working to understand the changes that occur on *in vivo* images that could be used as imaging biomarkers of breast cancer chemoprevention and dietary prevention. We use both human subjects and animal models. An integral part of our work is the use of image guide biopsy to confirm the biological nature of the imaging changes seen. It is our assumption that careful selection of tissues and cells obtained using image-guided biopsies is important if genomic and proteomic analysis is not to be distorted by sampling error.

THE ROLE OF IMAGING IN CANCER RISK
ASSESSMENT AND PREVENTION TRIALS

There are three tasks involved in this work: (1) assessing the degree of risk, (2) identifying changes induced by risk reduction therapy, and (3) providing directed biopsy of regions likely to provide valid samples for gene array analysis. There are several accepted image-based measures of cancer risk. For lung cancer, the presence of obstructive airway disease and identification of nodules of atypical adenomatous hyperplasia are risk factors. For breast cancer, breast density is the imaging feature most associated with risk, although we propose that measures of breast metabolism are an additional feature.

Breast density is a known indicator of breast cancer risk with some subgroups having up to 8 times the risk of the age-matched population. Our group has reported on the changes in breast density induced by raloxifene.[6] We studied 168 women randomized to raloxifene at one of two doses, estrogen or placebo. The changes in breast density over a 2-year period of time were measured by computer-based interactive thresholding.

The study found the following results at 2 years: (1) breast density was significantly greater in the estrogen group compared to the others ($P < .01$); (2) placebo and raloxifene groups showed decreasing density ($P < .003$); and (3) placebo and raloxifene groups showed similar degrees of change.

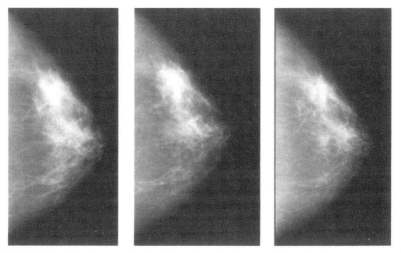

FIGURE 7. The decrease in glandular tissue in the breast identified by mammography in a woman receiving tamoxifen at baseline and after 3 and 6 months of medication.

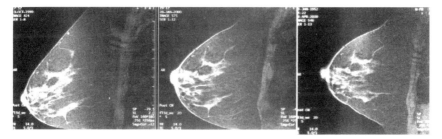

FIGURE 8. The decrease in breast glandular density shown by MRI at baseline and after receiving 3 and 6 months of medication.

We also performed a small pilot study where 27 women at high risk of developing breast cancer chose to take or not take tamoxifen. In the design, there were assessments of imaging and tissue biomarkers obtained at 0, 3, and 6 months. Each woman had the following: a mammogram, MRI without and with gadolinium enhancement, MR hydrogen (proton) spectroscopy of both the whole breast and of the site selected for image-guided biopsy, tissue and blood analysis for several biomarkers, RNA analysis, chromosome analysis, and gene array expression analysis. The results have not yet been reported.

The following analyses of the images are under way:

(1) mammogram breast density (FIG. 7);
(2) MRI breast glandular tissue volume (FIGS. 8 and 9);
(3) MRI degree of gadolinium enhancement (FIG. 10);[7,8]

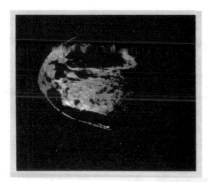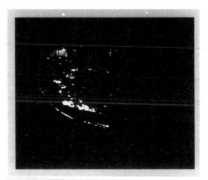

FIGURE 9. The locations of gadolinium enhancement in a woman in this research study. The *left image* shows the fibroglandular tissue, some of which shows contrast enhancement. The *right image* is a subtraction image of the preenhancement image subtracted from the postenhancement image, showing that the regions of gadolinium enhancement occur in only portions of the regions of fibroglandular tissue. Thus, different areas of the fibroglandular tissue have different degrees of vascularity.

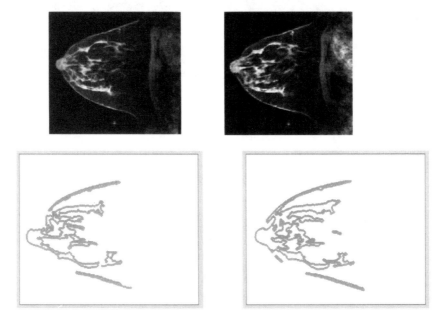

FIGURE 10. The segmentation of glandular tissue on serial MRI examinations performed 3 months apart: (*top*) the original MRI images; (*bottom*) the computer segmentation results outlining the glandular tissue.

(4) MR spectroscopy of measures of lipids:
 (i)   lipid-water ratio globally (FIG. 11),
 (ii) lipid-water ratio at site of repeated biopsy,
 (iii) saturated-unsaturated lipid ratio.

We are performing computer analysis of MR images in 3D and mammograms with the goal to detect changes in the amount of glandular tissue and the degree of breast

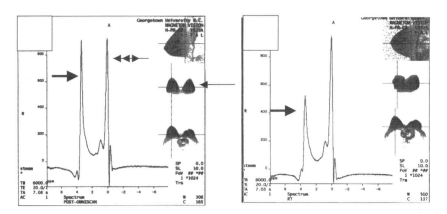

FIGURE 11. These two spectra demonstrate changes in the MR hydrogen (proton) spectroscopy of a woman on tamoxifen at baseline and at 6 months. The sequence shows a decrease in the height of the peak to the left, demonstrating a decrease in water content (*arrows*). This corresponds to a decrease in glandular tissue. The amplitude of the peak is proportional to molecular concentration.

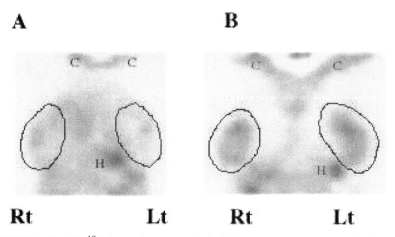

FIGURE 12. The ^{19}F-deoxyglucose uptake in the breasts of two women. There is more uptake in the breasts of the woman on the right. It is unknown if this increase in metabolic activity is related to breast cancer risk.

signal enhancement by gadolinium (vascularity), as well as MR spectroscopy to determine lipid-water ratio and lipid composition.

Metabolic Imaging and the Measurement of Breast Cancer Risk

Positron emission tomography (PET) with ^{19}F-deoxyglucose (FDG) demonstrates the degree of transport of glucose into cells. It is thus an imaging biomarker of cellular glucose metabolic activity. Women differ in their uptake of this agent into the breast tissue and this may or may not relate to the risk of subsequent breast cancer. It is an area of our current study (FIG. 12).

Animal Models

The complexity of the problems of understanding the assessment of risk of breast cancer by measurements of breast density, vascular flow, and breast tissue metabolism has led us to the use of animal models. We are using both ultrasound and MRI/S imaging of the rat breasts in this study as we investigate potential imaging biomarkers (FIGS. 13 and 14).

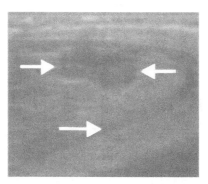

FIGURE 13. An ultrasound image of a normal rat breast in a living rat. The whiter strand-like densities (*white arrows*) represent the amount of stromal tissue in prepuberty by ultrasound imaging. This represents baseline data for studies now in progress.

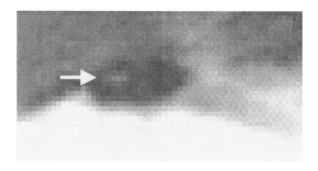

FIGURE 14. An MRI image of a normal rat breast obtained in a living rat. The few white strand-like densities (*white arrow*) represent the amount of stromal tissue in prepuberty by MRI.

SUMMARY OF IMAGING BIOMARKERS OF BREAST CANCER RISK

Our focus is on the interpretation and validation of biomarkers of breast cancer risk using several methods: mammographic density measurements, MRI and MRS measurements, FDG-PET, and animal models. Bioinformatics approaches to problems such as this will require databases able to contain multiple layers of information about spatial and temporal features of images where it is important to have each set of data related to the same small volume of tissue. The bioinformatics approach should be designed to allow combinations of the information obtained with imaging studies with multiple types of data. Data on biomarkers obtained from image-guided tissue biopsies are important so that such information as gene expression can be related not to the tissue in general, but to specified areas of interest. *In vivo* images can be used to guide biopsy for tissues likely to yield the best data. The interpretation of the importance of gene expression data should be location-specific to assure that the tissue studied is clinically correlated to the process under study and to minimize the effect of sampling error.

ACKNOWLEDGMENTS

The following people participated in various aspects of the findings summarized in this chapter: S-C. Benedict Lo, Teresa Osicka, Michael Yeh, Fleming Lure, Xin-Wei Xu, Jesse Lin, Ed Martello, Hui Zhao, Ron Zhang, Anita Sarcone, Ann Gallager, Chin Shoou Lin, Yue Joseph Wang, Jason Xuan, "Kathy" Kun Huang, "Andy" Rujirutana Srikanchana, Kelvin Woods, Lalitha Shankar, Leena Hilikivi-Clarke, Claudine Isaacs, Bassem Haddad, Baljit Singh, Minetta Liu, Robert Dickson, Jianchao Zeng, Marc Lippman, Daniel Hayes, Vered Stearns, Marie Pennanen, J. San Martin, J. O'Gorman, S. Eckert, and E. L. Walls.

REFERENCES

1. STITIK, F. & M. TOCKMAN. 1978. Radiographic screening in the early detection of lung cancer. Radiol. Clin. North Am. **16:** 347–366.
2. STITIK, F., M. TOCKMAN & N. KHOURI. 1985. Chest radiology. *In* Screening for Cancer, pp. 163–191. Academic Press. New York.
3. HEELAN, R.T., B.J. FLEHINGER, M.R. MELAMED *et al.* 1984. Non-small cell lung cancer: results of the New York Screening Program. Radiology 151: 289–293
4. AUSTIN, J.H.M., B.M. ROMNEY & L.S. GOLDSMITH. 1992. Missed bronchogenic carcinoma: radiographic findings in 27 patients with a potentially resectable lesion evident in retrospect. Radiology **182:** 115–122.
5. QUEKEL, L. *et al.* 1999. Miss rate of lung cancer on the chest radiograph in clinical practice. Chest **115:** 720–724.
6. FREEDMAN, M.T., J. SAN MARTIN, J. O'GORMAN *et al.* 2001. Digitized mammography in postmenopausal women receiving raloxifene or estrogen in a two-year placebo-controlled, randomized clinical trial. J. Natl. Cancer Inst. **93:** 51–56.
7. HUANG, K., J. XUAN, J. VARGA *et al.* 2002. MRI image-based tissue analysis and its clinical applications. Proc. SPIE Image Processing **4684:** 424–432.
8. SRIKANCHANA, R., J. XUAN, K. HUANG *et al.* 2002. Mixture of principal axes registration: a neural computation approach. Proc. SPIE Image Processing **4684:** 923–932.

Evolutionary Fuzzy Modeling Human Diagnostic Decisions

CARLOS ANDRÉS PEÑA-REYES

Swiss Federal Institute of Technology, EPFL, Lausanne, Switzerland

ABSTRACT: Fuzzy CoCo is a methodology, combining fuzzy logic and evolutionary computation, for constructing systems able to accurately predict the outcome of a human decision-making process, while providing an understandable explanation of the underlying reasoning. Fuzzy logic provides a formal framework for constructing systems exhibiting both good numeric performance (accuracy) and linguistic representation (interpretability). However, fuzzy modeling—meaning the construction of fuzzy systems—is an arduous task, demanding the identification of many parameters. To solve it, we use evolutionary computation techniques (specifically cooperative coevolution), which are widely used to search for adequate solutions in complex spaces. We have successfully applied the algorithm to model the decision processes involved in two breast cancer diagnostic problems, the WBCD problem and the Catalonia mammography interpretation problem, obtaining systems both of high performance and high interpretability. For the Catalonia problem, an evolved system was embedded within a Web-based tool—called COBRA—for aiding radiologists in mammography interpretation.

KEYWORDS: Fuzzy CoCo; fuzzy modeling; evolutionary computation; breast cancer

INTRODUCTION

A good computerized diagnostic tool should possess two characteristics, which are often in conflict. First, the tool must attain the highest possible diagnostic performance. Second, it would be highly beneficial for such a system to be human-interpretable. This means that the physician is not faced with a black box that simply spouts answers with no explanation; rather, we would like for the system to provide some insight as to *how* it derives its outputs. Any diagnostic tool bases its functioning on a model of the diagnostic decision, built upon available data and knowledge. Such a model is thus the main design goal when conceiving diagnostic tools.

White-box modeling approaches assume that everything about the system is known a priori, expressed either mathematically or verbally. In contrast, in *black-box modeling*, a model is constructed entirely from data using little additional a priori

Address for correspondence: Carlos Andrés Peña-Reyes, Swiss Federal Institute of Technology at Lausanne, EPFL, Logic Systems Laboratory, IN-Ecublens, CH-1015 Lausanne, Switzerland. Voice: +41-21-693-67-14; fax: +41-21-693-37-05.

carlos.pena@epfl.ch *or* c.penha@ieee.org

Ann. N.Y. Acad. Sci. 1020: 190–211 (2004). © 2004 New York Academy of Sciences.
doi: 10.1196/annals.1310.017

knowledge. For example, in artificial neural networks, a structure is chosen for the network and the parameters are tuned to fit the observed data as best as possible. Such parameters are not human-interpretable and do not offer any insight about the modeled system. A third, intermediate approach, called *gray-box modeling*,[1] takes into account certain prior knowledge of the modeled system to provide the black-box models with human-interpretable meaning.

Fuzzy modeling techniques can be viewed as gray-box modeling because they allow the modeler to extract and interpret the knowledge contained in the model, as well as to imbue it with a priori knowledge. The earliest fuzzy systems were constructed using knowledge provided by human experts and were thus linguistically correct. However, the difficulty of applying such an approach for ill-known or data-intensive models led to the coming of new data-driven fuzzy modeling techniques. These techniques initially concentrated on solving a parameter-optimization problem based on the numeric performance of the systems, paying little attention to linguistic aspects. Recently, as fuzzy modeling techniques have concentrated more on linguistic issues, the difficulty of improving system interpretability without losing performance has become evident. This accuracy-interpretability trade-off is currently one of the most active research lines in fuzzy modeling. However, the construction of fuzzy models of large and complex systems is a hard task demanding the identification of many parameters. One way to solve this problem is to use a nature-inspired method: evolution.

Evolutionary algorithms are based on two powerful principles of evolution: variability and selection. A population of individuals, each representing a possible solution to a given problem, evolves in the problem environment, reproducing among themselves according to their fitness. This constant competition drives the population toward individuals adapted to the problem environment, that is, toward good solutions.

We present Fuzzy CoCo, our evolutionary fuzzy modeling technique, which applies a recent evolutionary technique, cooperative coevolution, to the design of interpretable fuzzy systems. We demonstrate the efficacy of Fuzzy CoCo by applying it to two hard problems related with breast cancer diagnosis: mammography interpretation and biopsy-based diagnosis.

BACKGROUND

Fuzzy Modeling

Fuzzy logic is a computational paradigm that provides a mathematical tool for representing and manipulating information in a way that resembles human communication and reasoning processes.[2] It is based on the assumption that, in contrast to Boolean logic, a statement can be *partially* true (or false) and composed of imprecise concepts. A *fuzzy variable* (also called a *linguistic variable*; see FIG. 1) is characterized by its name tag, a set of *fuzzy values* (also known as *labels*), and the membership functions of these labels; these latter functions assign a membership value, $\mu_{label}(u)$, to a given real value, u, within some predefined range.

A *fuzzy inference system* is a rule-based system that uses fuzzy logic to reason about data.[2] Its basic structure consists of four main components, as depicted in FIGURE 2:

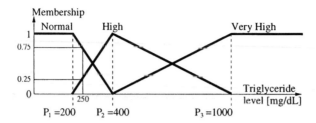

FIGURE 1. Example of a fuzzy (or linguistic) variable. Triglyceride level has three possible fuzzy values: *Normal*, *High*, and *Very High*, plotted as a degree of membership vs. input value. P_i values define the membership functions. The example input value of 250 mg/dL is assigned the membership values, $\mu_{Normal}(250) = 0.75$, $\mu_{High}(250) = 0.25$, and $\mu_{VeryHigh}(250) = 0$.

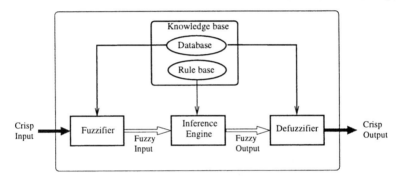

FIGURE 2. Basic structure of a fuzzy inference system.

(1) a fuzzifier, which translates crisp (real-valued) inputs into fuzzy values;
(2) an inference engine that applies a fuzzy reasoning mechanism to obtain a fuzzy output;
(3) a defuzzifier, which translates this latter output into a crisp value;
(4) a knowledge base, which contains both an ensemble of fuzzy rules, known as the rule base, and an ensemble of membership functions, known as the database.

The decision-making process is performed by the inference engine using the rules contained in the rule base. These fuzzy rules define the connection between input and output fuzzy variables. A fuzzy rule has the form,

if *antecedent* **then** *consequent*,

where *antecedent* is a fuzzy-logic expression composed of one or more simple fuzzy expressions connected by fuzzy operators and *consequent* is an expression that assigns fuzzy values to the output variables. The inference engine evaluates all the rules in the rule base and combines the weighted consequents of all relevant rules into a single output fuzzy set.

TABLE 1. Parameter classification of fuzzy inference systems

Class	Parameter
Logical	Reasoning mechanism
	Fuzzy operators
	Membership function types
	Defuzzification method
Structural	Relevant variables
	Number of membership functions
	Number of rules
Connective	Antecedents of rules
	Consequents of rules
	Rule weights
Operational	Membership function values

Fuzzy modeling is the task of identifying the values of the parameters of a fuzzy inference system so that a desired behavior is attained.[2] These parameters can be classified into four categories (TABLE 1):[3,4] logical, structural, connective, and operational.

Logical parameters are usually predefined by the designer based on experience and on problem characteristics. Structural, connective, and operational parameters may be predefined or obtained by synthesis or search methodologies. Generally, the search space, and thus the computational effort, grows exponentially with the number of parameters. Therefore, one can either invest more resources in the chosen search methodology or infuse more a priori, expert knowledge into the system (thereby effectively reducing the search space). The aforementioned trade-off between accuracy and interpretability is usually expressed as a set of constraints on the parameter values, thus complexifying the search process.

Evolutionary Computation

Evolutionary computation makes use of a metaphor of natural evolution, according to which a problem plays the role of an environment wherein lives a population of individuals, each representing a possible solution to the problem. The degree of adaptation of each individual to its environment is expressed by an adequacy measure known as the *fitness function*. The phenotype of each individual, that is, the candidate solution itself, is generally encoded in some manner into its *genome* (genotype). Evolutionary algorithms potentially produce progressively better solutions to the problem. This is possible thanks to the constant introduction of new "genetic" material into the population by applying so-called genetic operators, which are the computational equivalents of natural evolutionary mechanisms.

The archetypal evolutionary algorithm proceeds as follows (presented in pseudo-code format in FIGURE 3): An initial population of individuals, $P(0)$, is generated at random or heuristically. At every evolutionary step t, known as a *generation*, the

```
begin EA
  t:=0
  Initialise population P(t)
  while not done do
    Evaluate P(t)
    P'(t) := Select[P(t)]
    P''(t) := ApplyGeneticOperators[P'(t)]
    P(t + 1) := Introduce[P''(t),P(t)]
    t:=t+1
  end while
end EA
```

FIGURE 3. Pseudo-code of an evolutionary algorithm.

individuals in the current population, $P(t)$, are *decoded* and *evaluated* according to some predefined quality criterion, referred to as the fitness. Then, a subset of individuals, $P'(t)$—known as the *mating pool*—is selected to reproduce, according to their fitness. Thus, high-fitness ("good") individuals stand a better chance of "reproducing," while low-fitness ones are more likely to disappear.

Selection alone cannot introduce any new individuals into the population, that is, it cannot find new points in the search space. These points are generated by altering the selected population $P'(t)$ via the application of crossover and mutation, so as to produce a new population, $P''(t)$. Crossover tends to enable the evolutionary process to move toward "promising" regions of the search space. Mutation is introduced to prevent premature convergence to local optima by randomly sampling new points in the search space. Finally, the new individuals, $P''(t)$, are introduced into the next-generation population, $P(t+1)$; usually, $P''(t)$ simply becomes $P(t+1)$. The termination condition may be specified as some fixed, maximal number of generations or as the attainment of an acceptable fitness level.

As they combine elements of directed and stochastic search, evolutionary techniques exhibit a number of advantages over other search methods. First, they usually need a smaller amount of knowledge and fewer assumptions about the characteristics of the search space. Second, they are less prone to get stuck in local optima. Finally, they strike a good balance between *exploitation* of the best solutions and *exploration* of the search space.

The application of an evolutionary algorithm involves a number of important considerations. The first decision to make when applying such an algorithm is how to encode candidate solutions within the genome. The representation must allow for the encoding of all possible solutions, while being sufficiently simple to be searched in a reasonable amount of time. Next, an appropriate fitness function must be defined for evaluating the individuals. The (usually scalar) fitness value must reflect the criteria to be optimized and their relative importance.

Evolutionary Fuzzy Modeling

Fuzzy modeling can be considered as an optimization process where part or all of the parameters of a fuzzy system constitute the search space. Works investigating the application of evolutionary techniques in the domain of fuzzy modeling had first appeared about a decade ago,[5] focusing mainly on the tuning of fuzzy control systems. Evolutionary fuzzy modeling has since been applied to an ever-growing number of domains.[6]

Depending on several criteria—including the available a priori knowledge about the system, the size of the parameter set, and the availability and completeness of input/output data—artificial evolution can be applied in different stages of the fuzzy-parameter search. Three of the four categories of fuzzy parameters in TABLE 1 can be used to define targets for evolutionary fuzzy modeling: structural parameters, connective parameters, and operational parameters;[3] logical parameters are usually pre-defined by the designer based on experience.

Knowledge Tuning (Operational Parameters)

The evolutionary algorithm is used to tune the knowledge contained in the fuzzy system by finding membership function values.

Behavior Learning (Connective Parameters)

In this approach, one supposes that existing knowledge is sufficient in order to define the membership functions; this determines, in fact, the maximum number of rules. The genetic algorithm is used to find either the rule consequents or an adequate subset of rules to be included in the rule base.

Structure Learning (Structural Parameters)

In many cases, evolution has to deal with the simultaneous design of rules, membership functions, and structural parameters. In some methods that use a fixed-length genome encoding a fixed number of fuzzy rules along with the membership function values, the designer defines structural constraints according to the available knowledge of the problem characteristics. Other methods use variable-length genomes to allow evolution to discover the optimal size of the rule base.

Both behavior and structure learning can be viewed as rule-base learning processes with different levels of complexity. In the evolutionary-algorithm community, there are two major approaches for evolving such rule systems: the Michigan approach and the Pittsburgh approach.[7] Another method has been proposed specifically for fuzzy modeling: the iterative rule learning approach.[8] These three approaches are briefly described below.

The Michigan Approach. Each individual represents a *single* rule. The fuzzy inference system is represented by the *entire population*. Since several rules participate in the inference process, the rules are in constant competition for the best action to be proposed, and cooperate to form an efficient fuzzy system. Such a cooperative-competitive nature renders difficult the decision of which rules are ultimately responsible for good system behavior. It necessitates an effective credit assignment policy to ascribe fitness values to individual rules.

The Pittsburgh Approach. Here, the evolutionary algorithm maintains a population of candidate fuzzy systems. Selection and genetic operators are used to produce new generations of fuzzy systems. Since evaluation is applied to the entire system, the credit-assignment problem is eschewed. The main shortcoming of this approach is its computational cost since a population of fuzzy systems has to be evaluated for each generation.

The Iterative Rule Learning Approach. Each individual encodes a single rule. Evolution is used iteratively to discover single rules, sequentially, until an appropriate rule base is built. Even though this approach combines search speed with fitness-evaluation simplicity, it may lead to a nonoptimal partitioning of the antecedent space.

Interpretability Considerations

As mentioned before, the fuzzy modeling process has to deal with an important trade-off between *accuracy* and *interpretability.* The model is expected to provide high numeric accuracy, while incurring as little a loss of linguistic descriptive power as possible. Some works have attempted to define objective criteria to facilitate modeling interpretable fuzzy systems.[4,9,10]

Fuzzy systems (FIG. 2) process information in three stages: fuzzification, inference, and defuzzification. Fuzzification and defuzzification deal with linguistic variables and labels, defining the *semantics* of the system. Inference is performed using rules that define the connection between variables, that is, the *syntax* of the system. Fuzzy modelers must thus take into account both semantic and syntactic criteria to obtain interpretable systems.

Semantic Criteria

The notion of "linguistic variable" formally requires associating a meaning to each fuzzy label.[11] The following semantic criteria describe a set of properties that a fuzzy variable should possess in order to facilitate the task of assigning linguistic terms.[3,4] The focus is on the meaning of the ensemble of labels instead of the absolute meaning of each term in isolation.

Distinguishability. Each linguistic label should have semantic meaning and the fuzzy set should clearly define a range in the variable's universe.

Justifiable number of elements. The number of membership functions of a variable should correspond to the number of conceptual entities that humans can handle. It should not exceed the limit of 7 ± 2 distinct terms.

Coverage. The membership value of any element from the universe must be different from zero for at least one of the linguistic labels.

Normalization. For each label to have semantic meaning, at least one element of the universe should have a membership value equal to one.

Complementarity. For each element of the universe, the sum of all its membership values should be equal to one, guaranteeing uniform distribution of meaning among the elements.

Syntactic Criteria

A fuzzy rule relates one or more input-variable conditions, called antecedents, to their corresponding output fuzzy conclusions, called consequents. The linguistic adequacy of a fuzzy rule base lies on the interpretability of each rule as well as on that of the whole set of rules. The following syntactic criteria define some conditions that, if satisfied by the rule base, reinforce the interpretability of a fuzzy system.[4,10]

Completeness. For any possible input, at least one rule should be fired, or activated, to prevent the fuzzy system from getting blocked. (Note that a rule fires when the truth level of its antecedent is different from zero.)

Rule-base simplicity. The set of rules must be as small as possible. Otherwise, only a few rules must fire simultaneously for any input.

Single-rule readability. The number of conditions implied in the antecedent of a rule should be human-handleable (i.e., $\leq 7 \pm 2$).

Consistency. The consequents of two or more rules that fire simultaneously should not be contradictory, that is, they should be semantically close.

Strategies to Satisfy Semantic and Syntactic Criteria

The criteria presented above define a number of restrictions on the fuzzy parameters. Semantic criteria limit the choice of membership functions, while syntactic criteria bind the fuzzy rules. We present below some strategies to apply these restrictions.

Linguistic labels shared by all rules. All the labels defined for each variable are shared by all the rules,[4,10] resulting in a grid partition of the input space as illustrated in FIGURE 4. To satisfy the completeness criterion, a fully defined rule base is normally used, as that shown in FIGURE 5a.

Normal, orthogonal membership functions. The membership functions of two successive labels must be complementary in their overlapping region, whatever form they have. Moreover, in such regions, each label must ascend from zero to unity membership values (see FIG. 4).[4]

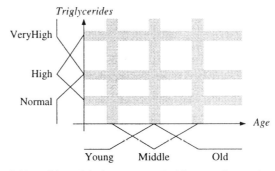

FIGURE 4. Grid partition of the input space. In this example, two input variables, each with three labels, divide the input space into a grid of nine regions.

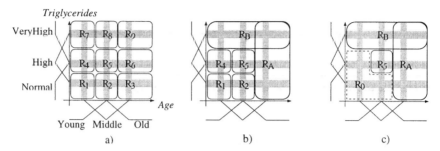

FIGURE 5. Strategies to define the rule base. **(a)** Fully defined rule base: the system contains all nine possible rules of the form **if** *Triglycerides* **is** *label* **and** *Age* **is** *label* **then** .... **(b)** *Don't-care* labels: two rules, R_A and R_B, containing *don't-care* labels cover almost half of the input space. In the figure, R_A is interpreted as **if** *Age* **is** *Old* **then** .... **(c)** Default rule, called here R_0, defines a default action to be performed as much as the so-called active rules—R_5, R_A, and R_B—do not apply.

Don't-care conditions. A fully defined rule base, as in FIGURE 5a, becomes impractical for systems with many inputs due to an exponential increase in the number of rules. Moreover, as each rule contains a condition for each variable, the rules might be too lengthy to be understandable and too specific to describe general circumstances. To tackle these two problems, one can allow variables, in a given rule, to be labeled as *"don't-care"*.[4,12] These variables are then considered as irrelevant (e.g., the rule R_A, in FIG. 5b, covers the space of three rules: R_3, R_6, and R_9). Thus, *don't-care* labels allow both reducing the rule base size and improving rule readability.

Default rule. In many cases, the behavior of a system exhibits only a few regions of interest, described by a small number of rules. To describe the rest of the input space, a default action provided by the default rule would suffice. The example in FIGURE 5c shows that the default rule, R_0, covers the space of rules R_1, R_2, and R_4. A fuzzy default rule is as true as all the others are false. Its activation degree is thus given by $\mu(R_0) = 1 - max[\mu(R_i)]$, where $\mu(R_i)$ is the activation degree of the *i*-th rule.

FUZZY CoCo: A COOPERATIVE COEVOLUTIONARY APPROACH TO FUZZY MODELING

Coevolution refers to the simultaneous evolution of two or more species with coupled fitness. Such coupled evolution favors the discovery of complex solutions whenever complex solutions are required.[13] Simplistically speaking, one can say that coevolving species can either compete (e.g., to obtain exclusivity on a limited resource) or cooperate (e.g., to gain access to some hard-to-attain resource). Cooperative coevolutionary algorithms involve a number of independently evolving species that together form complex structures, well suited to solve a problem. The fitness of an individual depends on its ability to collaborate with individuals from other species. In this way, the evolutionary pressure stemming from the difficulty of the problem favors the development of cooperative strategies and individuals.

Single-population evolutionary algorithms often perform poorly when confronted with problems presenting one or more of the following features:

(1) the sought-after solution is complex,
(2) the problem or its solution is clearly decomposable,
(3) the genome encodes different types of values,
(4) strong interdependencies are found among the components of the solution,
(5) component ordering drastically affects fitness.

Cooperative coevolution effectively addresses these issues, consequently widening the range of applications of evolutionary computation.[14]

The Coevolutionary Algorithm

A fuzzy modeling process usually deals with the simultaneous search for operational and connective parameters (TABLE 1), which provide an almost complete definition of the linguistic knowledge describing the behavior of a system, and the values mapping this description into a real-valued world. Fuzzy modeling can be thought of as two separate, but intertwined search processes: (1) the search for the membership functions that define the fuzzy variables and (2) the search for the rules used to perform the inference.

Fuzzy modeling presents several features discussed earlier that justify the application of a cooperative-coevolutionary approach: (1) the required fuzzy systems can be very complex since a few dozen variables may call for hundreds of parameters to be defined; (2) the proposed solution can be decomposed into two distinct components: rules and membership functions; (3) membership functions are continuous

```
begin Fuzzy CoCo
    g:=0
    for each species S
        Initialize populations P_S(0)
        Evaluate population P_S(0)
    end for
    while not done do
        for each species S
            g:=g+1
            E_S(g) = elite-select P_S(g − 1)
            P'_S(g) = select P_S(g − 1)
            P''_S(g) = crossover P'_S(g)
            P'''_S(g) = mutate P''_S(g)
            P_S(g) = P'''_s(g) + E_S(g)
            Evaluate population P_S(g)
        end for
    end while
end Fuzzy CoCo
```

FIGURE 6. Pseudo-code of Fuzzy CoCo. The line "evaluate population $P_S(g)$" is elaborated in FIGURE 7.

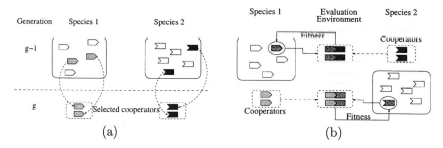

FIGURE 7. Fitness evaluation in Fuzzy CoCo. **(a)** Several individuals from generation $g-1$ of each species are selected to be the representatives, or cooperators, of their species during generation g. **(b)** During the evaluation stage of generation g, each individual is combined with the cooperators of the other species to construct fuzzy systems, which are then evaluated to compute the fitness of the individual.

and real-valued, while rules are discrete and symbolic; (4) these two components are interdependent because the membership functions are indexed by the rules.

Consequently, in Fuzzy CoCo, the fuzzy modeling problem is solved by two coevolving, cooperating species. Individuals of the first species encode values that define the membership functions for all the variables of the system. Individuals of the second species define a set of rules that include the membership functions whose defining parameters are contained in the first species (population). Two evolutionary algorithms control the evolution of the two populations. FIGURE 6 presents the Fuzzy CoCo algorithm in pseudo-code format. The evolutionary algorithms apply fitness-proportionate selection to choose the mating pool and apply an elitist strategy to allow some of the best individuals to survive into the next generation. The elitism strategy extracts individuals—the so-called elite—to be reinserted into the population after evolutionary operators have been applied. Note that the elite is not removed from the population, participating thus in the reproduction process. Standard crossover and mutation operators are applied.

As depicted in FIGURE 7, an individual undergoing fitness evaluation cooperates with one or more representatives of the other species, that is, it is combined with them to construct fuzzy systems. The fitness value assigned to the individual depends on the performance of the fuzzy systems in which it participated (either the average or the maximal value). Representatives, called here *cooperators*, are selected from the previous generation. In Fuzzy CoCo, N_{cf} cooperators are selected according to their fitness, thus favoring the exploitation of known good solutions. Other N_{cr} cooperators are selected randomly from the population to represent the diversity of the species, maintaining in this way exploration of the search space.

Fuzzy CoCo compares favorably with noncoevolutionary approaches, attaining higher performance, while requiring less computation.[3,4]

Introducing Interpretability in Fuzzy CoCo

Fuzzy CoCo allows a high degree of freedom in the type of fuzzy systems it can design, letting the user determine the accuracy-interpretability trade-off. When the interest is to preserve as much as possible the interpretability of the evolved systems, the fuzzy model should satisfy the semantic and syntactic criteria (presented earlier). These strategies—label sharing, orthogonal membership functions, don't-care conditions, and default rule—must guide both the design of the fuzzy inference system and the definition of both species' genomes. Besides, one or more of the linguistic criteria may participate in the fitness function as a way to reinforce the selection pressure towards interpretable systems.

BREAST BIOPSY ANALYSIS: THE WBCD PROBLEM

The WBCD database[15] is the result of the efforts made at the University of Wisconsin Hospital for accurately diagnosing breast masses based solely on a fine needle aspiration (FNA) test.[a] Nine visually assessed characteristics of an FNA sample considered relevant for diagnosis were identified and appraised with an integer value between 1 and 10. The database itself consists of 683 cases, with each entry representing the classification for a certain ensemble of measured values:

Case	v_1	v_2	v_3	...	v_9	Diagnostic
1	5	1	1	...	1	Benign
2	5	4	4	...	1	Benign
...	...	...	...	...	...	...
683	4	8	8	...	1	Malignant

Our own work on the evolution of fuzzy rules for the WBCD problem has shown that it is possible to obtain diagnostic systems exhibiting high performance, coupled with interpretability and a confidence measure.[17]

Thus, the WBCD problem involves classifying a presented case of putative cancer as to whether it is benign or malignant. The solution we propose for this problem is depicted in FIGURE 8. It consists of a fuzzy system and a threshold unit. The fuzzy system computes a continuous appraisal value of the malignancy of a case, based on the input values. The threshold unit then outputs a diagnostic according to the fuzzy system's output. The goal is to evolve a fuzzy model to describe such diagnostic decision, while exhibiting good classification performance and high interpretability.

In order to evolve the fuzzy model, we must make some preliminary decisions about both the fuzzy system and the coevolutionary algorithm.

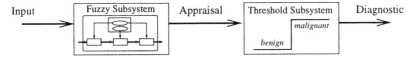

FIGURE 8. WBCD problem: proposed diagnosis system.

[a]FNA is a cost-effective, nontraumatic, and mostly noninvasive outpatient procedure that involves using a small-gauge needle to extract fluid directly from a breast mass.[16]

WBCD Problem: Fuzzy Parameter Setup

Our previous knowledge about the WBCD problem represents valuable information to be used for our choice of fuzzy parameters (TABLE 1). We also take into account the interpretability criteria presented earlier to define constraints on the fuzzy parameters. Referring to TABLE 1, we delineate below the fuzzy-system setup:

- Logical parameters: singleton-type fuzzy systems; min-max fuzzy operators; orthogonal, trapezoidal input membership functions; weighted-average defuzzification.

- Structural parameters: two input membership functions (*low* and *high*); two output singletons (*benign* and *malignant*); a user-configurable number of rules. Relevant variables are evolutionary defined.

- Connective parameters: the antecedents and the consequent of the rules, as well as the consequent of the default rule, are searched by the evolutionary algorithm. All rules have unitary weight.

- Operational parameters: the input membership function values are to be found by the evolutionary algorithm. For the output singletons, we used the values 2 and 4 for *benign* and *malignant*, respectively.

WBCD Problem: Evolutionary Setup

Fuzzy CoCo is thus used to search for four parameters: input membership function values, relevant input variables, and antecedents and consequents of rules. The genomes of the two species are constructed as follows:

- **Species 1:** *Membership functions*. There are nine variables (v_1–v_9), each with two parameters defining the membership function edges.

- **Species 2:** *Rules*. The i-th rule has the form

$$\text{if } (v_1 \text{ is } A_1^i) \text{ and } \dots \text{ and } (v_9 \text{ is } A_9^i) \text{ then } (\textit{output is } C^i).$$

A_1^i can take on the values 1 (*low*), 2 (*high*), or 0 or 3 (*don't care*). C^i bit can take on the values 0 (*benign*) or 1 (*malignant*). Relevant variables are searched for implicitly by letting the algorithm choose *don't-care* labels as valid antecedents. TABLE 2 delineates the parameter encoding for both species' genomes, which together describe an entire fuzzy system.

To evolve the fuzzy inference system, we applied Fuzzy CoCo with the same evolutionary parameters for both species. TABLE 3 delineates the values and ranges of values used for these parameters. The algorithm terminates when the maximum number of generations, G_{max}, is reached (we set $G_{max} = 1000 + 100 \times N_r$, that is, dependent on the number of rules).

The fitness function combines two criteria: (1) F_c, the overall classification performance, is the most important measure, and (2) F_v, the maximum number of variables in the longest rule, which measures the readability. The fitness function is given by $F = F_c - \alpha F_v$, where $\alpha = 0.0015$. The value α was calculated to allow F_v to make a difference only among systems exhibiting similar classification performance. The fitness value of an individual is the maximum fitness obtained by the fuzzy systems it participated in.

TABLE 2. Genome encoding

Parameter	Values	Bits	Qty	Total bits
Species 1: Membership functions				
P	$\{1, 2, ..., 8\}$	3	9	27
d	$\{1, 2, ..., 8\}$	3	9	27
		Total genome length		54
Species 2: Rules				
A	$\{0, 1, 2, 3\}$	2	$9 \times N_r$	$18 \times N_r$
C	$\{1, 2\}$	1	$N_r + 1$	$N_r + 1$
		Total genome length		$19 \times N_r + 1$

NOTE: Genome length for membership functions is 54 bits. Genome length for rules is $19 \times N_r + 1$, where N_r denotes the number of rules.

TABLE 3. Fuzzy CoCo setup for the WBCD problem

Parameter	Values
Population size $\|Ps\|$	[30–90]
Maximum generations G_{max}	$1000 + 100N_r$
Crossover probability P_c	1
Mutation probability P_m	[0.02–0.3]
Elitism rate E_r	[0.1–0.6]
"Fit" cooperators N_{cf}	1
Random cooperators N_{cr}	$\{1, 2, 3, 4\}$

WBCD Problem: Results

A total of 495 evolutionary runs were performed, all of which found systems whose classification performance exceeds 96.7%. In particular, considering the best individual per run, 241 runs led to a fuzzy system whose performance exceeds 98.0% and, of these, 81 runs found systems whose performance exceeds 98.5%. Our top-performance system, which serves to exemplify the solutions found by Fuzzy CoCo, is delineated in FIGURE 9. It consists of 7 rules, with the longest rule including 5 variables, and obtains an overall classification rate (i.e., over the entire database) of 98.98%.

MAMMOGRAPHY INTERPRETATION: THE COBRA TOOL

This section presents the design, based on Fuzzy CoCo, of a tool denominated COBRA: Catalonia on-line breast-cancer risk assessor. It is designed to aid radiologists in the interpretation of mammographies.

The *Catalonia mammography database*, collected at Duran y Reynals Hospital in Barcelona, consists of 15 input attributes and a diagnostic result indicating whether

Database

	v_1	v_2	v_3	v_4	v_5	v_6	v_7	v_8	v_9
P	2	1	1	1	6	1	3	5	2
d	7	8	4	8	1	4	8	4	1

Rule base

Rule 1   **if** $(v_1$ is *Low*) **and** $(v_3$ is *Low*) **then** (*output* is *benign*)

Rule 2   **if** $(v_4$ is *Low*) **and** $(v_6$ is *Low*) **and** $(v_8$ is *Low*) **and** $(v_9$ is *Low*) **then** (*output* is *benign*)

Rule 3   **if** $(v_1$ is *Low*) **and** $(v_3$ is *High*) **and** $(v_5$ is *High*) **and** $(v_8$ is *Low*) **and** $(v_9$ is *Low*) **then** (*output* is *benign*)

Rule 4   **if** $(v_1$ is *Low*) **and** $(v_2$ is *High*) **and** $(v_4$ is *Low*) **and** $(v_5$ is *Low*) **and** $(v_8$ is *High*) **then** (*output* is *benign*)

Rule 5   **if** $(v_2$ is *High*) **and** $(v_4$ is *High*) **then** (*output* is *malignant*)

Rule 6   **if** $(v_1$ is *High*) **and** $(v_3$ is *High*) **and** $(v_6$ is *High*) **and** $(v_7$ is *High*) **then** (*output* is *malignant*)

Rule 7   **if** $(v_2$ is *High*) **and** $(v_3$ is *High*) **and** $(v_4$ is *Low*) **and** $(v_5$ is *Low*) **and** $(v_7$ is *High*) **then** (*output* is *malignant*)

Default   **else** (*output* is *malignant*)

FIGURE 9. The best evolved fuzzy diagnostic system with 7 rules. It exhibits an overall classification rate of 98.98%, and its longest rule includes 5 variables.

or not a carcinoma was detected after a biopsy. The 15 input attributes include 3 clinical characteristics and 2 groups of 6 radiologic features, according to the type of lesion found in the mammography: mass or microcalcifications. A radiologist fills out a reading form for each mammography, assigning values for the clinical characteristics and, usually, for one of the groups of radiologic features. Then, the radiologist interprets the case using a 5-point scale: (1) benign; (2) probably benign; (3) indeterminate; (4) probably malignant; (5) malignant. According to this interpretation, a decision is made on whether to practice a biopsy on the patient or not. The database contains data corresponding to 227 cases, all of them sufficiently suspect to justify a biopsy recommendation. For the purpose of this study, each case was examined by 3 different readers, but only diverging readings were kept. The actual number of readings in the database is 516: 187 positive and 329 negative cases.

Proposed Solution: The COBRA System

The solution proposed, the COBRA system depicted in FIGURE 10, is composed of 4 elements: a user interface, a reading form, a database, and a diagnostic decision unit containing a fuzzy system and a threshold unit.

Based on the 15 input attributes collected with the reading form, the fuzzy system computes a continuous appraisal value of the malignancy of a case. The threshold unit then outputs a biopsy recommendation according to the fuzzy system's output. The threshold value used in this system is 3, which corresponds to an "indeterminate" diagnostic. Fuzzy CoCo is applied to design the fuzzy system in charge of appraising malignancy.[4,18] In the Web-based user interface, the user fills the reading form (see a snapshot in FIG. 11). COBRA provides, in addition to the final biopsy recommendation, information about the appraisal value computed by the fuzzy sub-

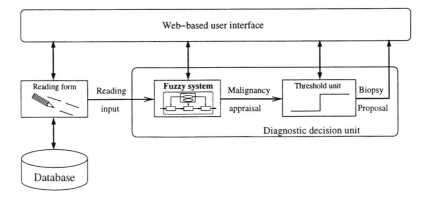

FIGURE 10. The COBRA system comprises a user interface, a reading form, a database of selected cases, and a diagnostic decision unit, in which a fuzzy system estimates malignancy and a threshold unit outputs biopsy recommendations.

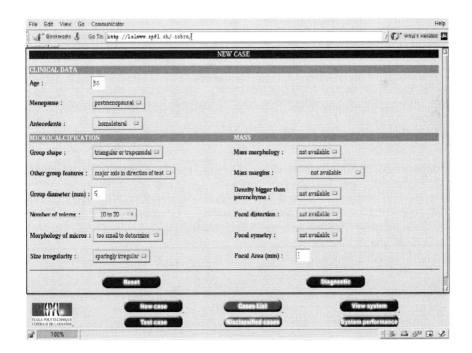

FIGURE 11. User interface: reading form. The snapshot illustrates the reading form through which the COBRA system collects data about a case.

system and about the rules involved in the decision. The tool can be also used to train novel radiologists as the reading form can access previously diagnosed cases contained in the database. The tool is available at http://lslwww.epfl.ch/~cobra/.

COBRA System: Fuzzy Parameter Setup

We used prior knowledge about the Catalonia database to guide our choice of fuzzy parameters. In addition, we took into account the interpretability criteria presented earlier to define constraints on the fuzzy parameters. Referring to TABLE 1, we delineate below the fuzzy system's set-up:

- Logical parameters: singleton-type fuzzy systems; min-max fuzzy operators; orthogonal, trapezoidal input membership functions; weighted-average defuzzification.

- Structural parameters: two input membership functions (*low* and *high*); two output singletons (*benign* and *malignant*); a user-configurable number of rules. The relevant variables are one of Fuzzy CoCo's evolutionary objectives. (Note that *low* and *high* may be further replaced by labels having medical meaning according to the specific context of each variable.)

- Connective parameters: the antecedents and the consequent of the rules are searched by Fuzzy CoCo. The algorithm also searches for the consequent of the default rule. All rules have unitary weight.

- Operational parameters: Fuzzy CoCo searches for the input membership function values. The output singletons are 1 for *benign* and 5 for *malignant*.

COBRA System: Evolutionary Setup

Fuzzy CoCo thus searches for 4 parameters: input membership function values, relevant input variables, and antecedents and consequents of rules. To encode these parameters into both species' genomes, which together describe an entire fuzzy system, it is necessary to take into account the heterogeneity of the input variables as explained below.

Species 1: *Membership functions.* The 15 input variables (v_1–v_{15}) present 3 different types of values: continuous (v_1, v_6, and v_{15}), discrete (v_3–v_5 and v_7–v_{11}), and binary (v_2 and v_{12}–v_{14}). It is not necessary to encode membership functions for binary variables as they can only take on 2 values. The membership function genome encodes the remaining 11 variables—3 continuous and 8 discrete—each with 2 parameters, P_1 and P_2, defining the membership function apices. TABLE 4 delineates the parameters encoding the membership function genome.

Species 2: *Rules.* The i-th rule has the form,

$$\text{if } (v_1 \text{ is } A_1^i) \text{ and } \dots \text{ and } (v_{15} \text{ is } A_{15}^i) \text{ then } (output \text{ is } C^i),$$

where A_j^i can take on the values 1 (*low*), 2 (*high*), or 0 or 3 (*don't care*); C^i can take on the values 1 (*benign*) or 2 (*malignant*). As mentioned before, each database case presents 3 clinical characteristics and 6 radiologic features

TABLE 4. Genome encoding for membership function species

Variable type	Qty	Parameters	Bits	Total bits
Continuous	3	2	7	42
Discrete	8	2	4	64
		Total genome length		106

NOTE: Genome length is 106 bits.

TABLE 5. Genome encoding for rules species

Parameter	Qty	Bits	Total bits
Clinical antecedents	$3 \times N_r$	2	$6 \times N_r$
Radiologic antecedents	$6 \times N_r$	2	$12 \times N_r$
Rule-type selector	N_r	1	N_r
Consequents	$N_r + 1$	1	$N_r + 1$
	Total genome length		$(20 \times N_r) + 1$

NOTE: Genome length is $(20 \times N_r) + 1$ bits, where N_r denotes the number of rules.

according to the type of lesion found: mass or microcalcifications (note that only a few special cases contain data for both groups). To take advantage of this fact, the rule base genome encodes, for each rule, 11 parameters: the 3 antecedents of the clinical data variables, the 6 antecedents of 1 radiological feature group, an extra bit to indicate whether the rule applies for mass or microcalcifications, and the rule consequent. Furthermore, the genome contains an additional parameter corresponding to the consequent of the default rule. Relevant variables are searched for implicitly by allowing the algorithm to choose *don't-care* labels as valid antecedents ($A_j^i = 0$ or $A_j^i = 3$); in such a case, the respective variable is considered irrelevant and removed from the rule. TABLE 5 delineates the parameters encoding the rules genome.

TABLE 6 delineates values and ranges of values of the evolutionary parameters. The algorithm terminates when the maximum number of generations, G_{max}, is reached. (We set $G_{max} = 700 + 200 \times N_r$.)

The fitness definition takes into account medical diagnostic criteria. The most commonly employed measures of the validity of diagnostic procedures are the sensitivity and specificity, the likelihood ratios, the predictive values, and the overall classification (accuracy). TABLE 7 provides expressions for 4 of these measures that are important for evaluating the performance of our systems. Three of them are used in the fitness function; the last one is used in the next subsection to support the analysis of the results. Besides these criteria, the fitness function provides extra selective pressure based on two syntactic criteria: simplicity and readability (see earlier subsection entitled INTERPRETABILITY CONSIDERATIONS)

The fitness function combines the following 5 criteria—(1) F_{sens}: sensitivity, or true-positive ratio, computed as the percentage of positive cases correctly classified;

TABLE 6. Fuzzy CoCo setup for the COBRA system

Parameter	Values
Population size $\|Ps\|$	90
Maximum generations G_{max}	$700 + 200N_r$
Crossover probability P_c	1
Mutation probability P_m	{0.005, 0.01}
Elitism rate E_r	{0.1, 0.2}
"Fit" cooperators N_{cf}	1
Random cooperators N_{cr}	1

TABLE 7. Diagnostic performance measures

Sensitivity	TP/(TP + FN)
Specificity	TN/(TN + FP)
Accuracy	(TP + TN)/(TP + TN + FP + FN)
PPV	TP/(TP + FP)

NOTE: The values used to compute the expressions are as follows—true positive (TP), positive cases detected correctly; true negative (TN), negative cases detected correctly; false positive (FP), negative cases diagnosed as positive; false negative (FN), positive cases diagnosed as negative.

(2) F_{spec}: specificity, or true-negative ratio, computed as the percentage of negative cases correctly classified (note that there is usually an important trade-off between sensitivity and specificity that renders difficult the satisfaction of both criteria); (3) F_{acc}: classification performance, computed as the percentage of cases correctly classified; (4) F_r: rule base size fitness, computed as the percentage of unused rules (i.e., the number of rules that are never fired and can thus be removed altogether from the system); (5) F_v: rule length fitness, computed as the average percentage of *don't-care* antecedents (i.e., unused variables) per rule. This order also represents their relative importance in the final fitness function, from most important (F_{sens}) to least important (F_r and F_v).

The fitness function is computed in 3 steps—basic fitness, accuracy reinforcement, and size reduction—as explained below:

- Basic fitness: Based on sensitivity and specificity, it is given by $F_1 = (F_{sens} + \alpha F_{spec})/(1 + \alpha)$, where $\alpha = 0.3$ reflects the greater importance of sensitivity.

- Accuracy reinforcement: This step reinforces the fitness of high-accuracy systems. It is given by $F_2 = (F_1 + \beta F'_{acc})/(1 + \beta)$, where $\beta = 0.01$. $F'_{acc} = F_{acc}$ when $F_{acc} > 0.7$; $F'_{acc} = 0$ elsewhere.

- Size reduction: Based on the size of the fuzzy system, it is given by $F = (F_2 + \gamma F_{size})/(1 + 2\gamma)$, where $\gamma = 0.01$. $F_{size} = (F_r + F_v)$ if $F_{acc} > 0.7$ and $F_{sens} > 0.98$; $F_{size} = 0$ elsewhere. This step rewards top systems exhibiting a concise rule set, thus directing evolution toward more interpretable systems.

TABLE 8. Diagnostic performance of the average and the top evolved systems

Performance measure	Average	Best system
Fitness	0.8834	0.9166
Sensitivity	98.78% (184.7/187)	100% (187/187)
Specificity	59.69% (196.4/329)	69.30% (228/329)
Accuracy	73.86% (381.1/516)	80.43% (415/516)
PPV	58.32%	64.93% (187/288)

NOTE: In parentheses are the number of cases, leading to each performance measure.

TABLE 9. Rule activation, appraisal, and diagnostic suggestion for the four example cases presented in reference 21

Active rule	Case 1	Case 2	Case 3	Case 4
Rule 1	Benign	–	–	Benign
Rule 2	–	–	–	Benign
Rule 7	Benign	–	–	–
Rule 9	–	–	Benign	–
Rule 13	–	Malignant	–	Malignant
Rule 14	–	Malignant	Malignant	–
Appraisal	1 (benign)	5 (malignant)	3 (indeterminate)	2.33 (prob. benign)
Suggestion	No biopsy	Biopsy	Biopsy	No biopsy

COBRA System: Results

A total of 469 evolutionary runs were performed, all of them searching for systems with up to 20 rules. Considering the best individual per run, all of them found systems whose fitness exceeds 0.83. TABLE 8 shows the diagnostic performance of both the average and the best run of all evolutionary runs. While the usual positive predictive value (PPV) of mammography ranges between 15% and 35%,[19,20] Fuzzy CoCo increases this value to 58.32% for the average system and 64.93% for the best one as shown in TABLE 8.

Even though evolution searched for systems with 20 fuzzy rules, the best system found effectively uses 14 rules. In average, these rules contain 2.71 variables (out of 15), which are, furthermore, Boolean. Note that this latter fact does not contradict the use of a fuzzy approach as Boolean systems are a subset of the more general set of fuzzy systems. In fact, while fuzzy modeling techniques may find Boolean solutions, the contrary does not hold.

To illustrate how COBRA makes a diagnostic decision, we present 4 example cases (more details about these cases are presented in ref. 21). For each case, the system evaluates the activation of each rule and takes into account the values of the proposed diagnostics—that is, 1 for benign and 5 for malignant. The system's malignancy appraisal is computed as the weighted average of these diagnostics. The final biopsy is given to the user together with the rules participating in the decision.

TABLE 9 shows the rules activated for each case, the diagnostic they propose, the appraisal value, and the final biopsy suggestion using 3 (i.e., indeterminate) as threshold.

The system takes into account all active rules to compute a malignancy appraisal, that is, it searches for and considers all possible indicia of benignity and malignancy before making a decision. In particular, cases 3 and 4 illustrate well such behavior.

CONCLUDING REMARKS

We presented Fuzzy CoCo, a fuzzy modeling technique based on cooperative coevolution, along with its application to breast cancer diagnosis. In evolutionary fuzzy modeling, the interpretability-accuracy trade-off is of crucial import, imposing several restrictions on the choice of fuzzy parameters and into criteria included in the fitness function. As Fuzzy CoCo is highly configurable, it facilitates the management of this interpretability-accuracy trade-off.

Applying Fuzzy CoCo to breast cancer diagnosis, we concentrated on increasing the interpretability of solutions applying the proposed strategies, obtaining excellent results. We note, however, that the consistency of the entire rule base and its compatibility with the specific domain knowledge can only be assessed by further interaction with medical experts.

Currently, we are investigating two novel ideas that could improve Fuzzy CoCo (see ref. 4): (1) Island Fuzzy CoCo, where several Fuzzy CoCo instances coexist (each one set to evolve systems with a different number of rules), permitting migration of individuals among them so as to improve both global search capabilities and evolutionary dynamics with respect to simple Fuzzy CoCo; (2) Incremental Fuzzy CoCo, where the number of rules of the sought-after system increases each time that evolution satisfies certain criteria. In this way, the search for more complex systems starts on the basis of some "good" individuals.

Our underlying goal is to provide an approach for automatically producing high-performance, interpretable fuzzy systems for real-world problems.

REFERENCES

1. LINDSKOG, P. 1997. Fuzzy identification from a grey box modeling point of view. *In* Fuzzy Model Identification, pp. 3–50. Springer-Verlag. Heidelberg/Berlin/New York.
2. YAGER, R.R. & L.A. ZADEH. 1994. Fuzzy Sets, Neural Networks, and Soft Computing. Van Nostrand–Reinhold. New York.
3. PEÑA-REYES, C.A. & M. SIPPER. 2001. Fuzzy CoCo: a cooperative-coevolutionary approach to fuzzy modeling. IEEE Trans. Fuzzy Syst. 9(5): 727–737.
4. PEÑA-REYES, C.A. 2002. Coevolutionary Fuzzy Modeling. Ph.D. thesis, École Polytechnique Fédérale de Lausanne–EPFL. [2002 Best Thesis EPFL Prize, Nominee.]
5. KARR, C.L., L.M. FREEMAN & D.L. MEREDITH. 1990. Improved fuzzy process control of spacecraft terminal rendezvous using a genetic algorithm. *In* Proceedings of Intelligent Control and Adaptive Systems Conference. Vol. 1196, pp. 274–288. SPIE.
6. ALANDER, J.T. 1997. An indexed bibliography of genetic algorithms with fuzzy logic. *In* Fuzzy Evolutionary Computation, pp. 299–318. Kluwer. Dordrecht.
7. MICHALEWICZ, Z. 1996. Genetic Algorithms + Data Structures = Evolution Programs. Third edition. Springer-Verlag. Heidelberg/Berlin/New York.

8. HERRERA, F., M. LOZANO & J.L. VERDEGAY. 1995. Generating fuzzy rules from examples using genetic algorithms. *In* Fuzzy Logic and Soft Computing, pp. 11–20. World Scientific. Singapore.

9. VALENTE DE OLIVEIRA, J. 1999. Semantic constraint for membership function optimization. IEEE Trans. Syst. Man Cybernet. **A29**(1): 128–138.

10. GUILLAUME, S. 2001. Designing fuzzy inference systems from data: an interpretability-oriented review. IEEE Trans. Fuzzy Syst. **9**(3): 426–443.

11. ZADEH, L.A. 1975. The concept of a linguistic variable and its applications to approximate reasoning. Inf. Sci. **8**: 199–249 (part I); **8**: 301–357 (part II); **9**: 43–80 (part III).

12. ISHIBUSHI, H., T. NAKASHIMA & T. MURATA. 1999. Performance evaluation of fuzzy classifier systems for multidimensional pattern classification problems. IEEE Trans. Syst. Man Cybernet. **B29**(5): 601–618.

13. PAREDIS, J. 1995. Coevolutionary computation. Artif. Life **2**: 355–375.

14. POTTER, M.A. & K.A. DE JONG. 2000. Cooperative coevolution: an architecture for evolving coadapted subcomponents. Evol. Comput. **8**(1): 1–29.

15. MERZ, C.J. & P.M. MURPHY. 1996. UCI repository of machine learning databases.

16. MANGASARIAN, O.L., W.N. STREET & W.H. WOLBERG. 1994. Breast cancer diagnosis and prognosis via linear programming. Mathematical Programming Technical Report 94-10. University of Wisconsin.

17. PEÑA-REYES, C.A. & M. SIPPER. 1999. A fuzzy-genetic approach to breast cancer diagnosis. Artif. Intell. Med. **17**(2): 131–155.

18. PEÑA-REYES, C.A. & M. SIPPER. 2003. Fuzzy CoCo: balancing accuracy and interpretability of fuzzy models by means of coevolution. *In* Accuracy Improvements in Linguistic Fuzzy Modeling. Vol. 129, pp. 119–146. Physica-Verlag. Würzburg.

19. PORTA, L., R. VILLA, E. ANDIA & E. VALDERRAMA. 1997. Infraclinic breast carcinoma: application of neural networks techniques for the indication of radioguided biopsies. *In* Biological and Artificial Computation: From Neuroscience to Technology. Vol. 1240, pp. 978–985. Springer Pub. New York.

20. OREL, S.G., N. KAY, C. REYNOLDS & D.C. SULLIVAN. 1999. Bi-rads categorization as a predictor of malignancy. Radiology **211**(3): 845–880.

21. PEÑA-REYES, C.A., R. VILLA, L. PRIETO & E. SANCHEZ. 2003. COBRA: an evolved on-line tool for mammography interpretation. *In* Proceedings of the International Work-Conference on Artificial and Natural Neural Networks (IWANN2003). No. 2686, pp. 726–733. Springer Pub. New York.

Bayesian Decomposition

Analyzing Microarray Data within a Biological Context

MICHAEL F. OCHS, THOMAS D. MOLOSHOK, GHISLAIN BIDAUT, AND GARABET TOBY[a]

Bioinformatics, Division of Population Science, Fox Chase Cancer Center, Philadelphia, Pennsylvania 19111, USA

ABSTRACT: The detection and correct identification of cancer, especially at an early stage, are vitally important for patient survival and quality of life. Since signaling pathways play critical roles in cancer development and metastasis, methods that reliably assess the activity of these pathways are critical to understand cancer and the response to therapy. Bayesian Decomposition (BD) identifies signatures of expression that can be linked directly to signaling pathway activity, allowing the changes in mRNA levels to be used as downstream indicators of pathway activity. Here, we demonstrate this ability by identifying the downstream expression signal associated with the mating response in *Saccharomyces cerevisiae* and showing that this signal disappears in deletion mutants of genes critical to the MAPK signaling cascade used to trigger the response. We also show the use of BD in the context of supervised learning, by analyzing the *Mus musculus* tissue-specific data set provided by Project Normal. The algorithm correctly removes routine metabolic processes, allowing tissue-specific signatures of expression to be identified. Gene ontology is used to interpret these signatures. Since a number of modern therapeutics specifically target signaling proteins, it is important to be able to identify changes in signaling pathways in order to use microarray data to interpret cancer response. By removing routine metabolic signatures and linking specific signatures to signaling pathway activity, BD makes it possible to link changes in microarray results to signaling pathways.

KEYWORDS: Bayesian methods; gene expression; microarray; signaling pathways

INTRODUCTION

Despite numerous advances in treatment, cancer remains the second leading cause of death in the United States and throughout the Western world.[1] In order to

Address for correspondence: Michael F. Ochs, Fox Chase Cancer Center, 333 Cottman Avenue, Philadelphia, PA 19111. Voice: 215-728-3660; fax: 215-728-2513.
m_ochs@fccc.edu

[a]Present address: Garabet Toby, Department of Biological Chemistry and Molecular Pharmacology, Harvard Medical School, and Department of Cancer Biology, The Dana Farber Cancer Institute, Boston, MA 02115.

Ann. N.Y. Acad. Sci. 1020: 212–226 (2004). © 2004 New York Academy of Sciences.
doi: 10.1196/annals.1310.018

understand cancer development in individual malignancies, the recovery of the process that led to the specific cellular malfunction present in the cancer cells must be identified. Such development generally involves the cellular signaling networks that control cell growth, differentiation, apoptosis, and motility.[2,3] Because of the extreme underlying biological complexity of these pathways, observed cancers arise from a myriad of different cellular malfunctions.[4,5] It is from this complex background that microarray analysis attempts to glean insight to improve cancer detection and identification.

Cancer detection at early stages remains a critical issue for improving patient survival. Initial uses of microarrays for cancer detection focused on refinement of the identification of the type of cancer using computational and statistical approaches.[6-8] In addition, the discovery of biomarkers in the form of differential levels of production of mRNA has been a focus in a number of studies.[9-11] In general, these methods aim to use microarray technology to detect disease state from tissue samples and thus aim to refine identification of suspect tissues after a biopsy has been performed. Since cancers that presently are typed as similar using current diagnostic and clinical parameters can have drastically different outcomes, refinement of the identification of the subtype of cancer through microarray measurements may aid in therapy and patient survival. Microarrays can also allow the identification of a smaller set of surrogate markers, which can be screened for in a more economical way, increasing the potential for a clinical product.

While the techniques noted above are useful, they have certain limitations as regards more advanced uses in cancer detection. Since cancer is now understood to be primarily a disease involving errors in cellular signaling, newer therapeutics often specifically target proteins involved in signaling pathways.[12-14] These new therapeutics are not always effective, and the reason for failure remains unknown. Possibilities include inherent poor interactions between therapeutic compound and target or complex cellular responses such as activation of other pathways. It therefore becomes critical to understand how the protein target and its associated signaling pathways are affected during treatment in order to identify, for instance, whether the activity of the target has not been affected or whether a different pathway has rescued the cell from apoptosis or senescence. In the first case, a different therapeutic would be needed to target the same pathway; in the second case, additional, simultaneous therapeutics would be needed. Microarray measurements are being used to provide insight into these questions.

Unfortunately, the determination of pathway activity from gene expression requires more complex analysis since signaling protein activity is not typically linked to mRNA expression levels.[15] This makes it difficult to directly infer increased activity of a signaling protein, such as a therapeutic target, and thus of the signaling pathway, from an increase in mRNA expression of the gene encoding the protein. Instead, an analysis must treat changes in mRNA levels as a downstream indicator of activity. The goal in this case is to link observed changes in mRNA levels between two states (e.g., before and after treatment) with specific activity within the signaling pathways of interest.

One method to accomplish this task is to create a model of the signaling network in the cell of interest, including transcription factors and the genes that they transcribe, and test whether the responses seen indicate that the pathway activity has changed. While this can be done in some cases,[16] it is unfortunately of extremely limited use in mammalian studies as the networks are far more complex and too poorly elucidated. In addition, microarray data remain notoriously noisy. Therefore, one faces the reality not only of messy data,[17] but also of muddled models. Both these factors need to be overcome in order to reach the potential promise of microarray data in cancer detection.

BAYESIAN DECOMPOSITION

Within a background of noise, prior knowledge can provide significant enhancement to probabilistic reasoning.[18] The goal of linking expression changes to physiological behavior is especially apt for the inclusion of existing information, since a vast framework of biological knowledge exists, encoded in accessible databases and increasingly using ontologies.[19] This information can be used in multiple ways, including aiding interpretation after computational manipulation or, more importantly, in guiding the computation directly. The advantage of direct incorporation of prior knowledge during the analysis is that links between genes or samples can provide statistical power in the same way that a replicate can, since existing information can be used to encourage genes or samples to share characteristics.

Bayesian Decomposition (BD) is an algorithm developed initially for spectral analysis,[20] which has demonstrated success in microarray analysis.[21–23] The fundamental goal of the algorithm when applied to expression analysis is identification of groups of coexpressed genes even in cases where genes belong to multiple groups. Genes will typically belong to such multiple groups since evolution has led to the reuse of function, allowing many proteins to play roles in different cellular processes (e.g., kinases that function at multiple points in the cell cycle).[24] In addition, the algorithm incorporates prior knowledge in a number of ways, allowing refinement of the algorithm to specific questions posed by noisy microarray data.

The main complication for expression analysis is shown in FIGURE 1. A simplified look at three signaling pathways in yeast is given, together with their links to transcription factors and a few of the genes these factors regulate. As can be seen, even in this less complex organism and with a simplified view, signaling pathways share elements, and genes are regulated by multiple transcription factors, forming overlapping groups of coregulated genes. Processes that force genes into a single group inevitably confuse the link between genes and pathways. The pathway interactions and cooperativity between transcription factors are far more complicated in mammalian systems.

BD addresses this issue by creating a statistical model allowing the behavior of a gene to be explained as arising from multiple fundamental behaviors. In FIGURE 2, the mathematical decomposition performed by BD is demonstrated. The data matrix, D, comprises an $M \times N$ matrix quantifying measurements across M conditions for N genes. BD identifies simultaneously a set of patterns (matrix P) and their distributions or amplitudes (matrix A) that together form a mock matrix, M, which is identical to the data matrix, except for the absence of noise. Essentially, M is the denoised image of the data created from the model (A and P). At this time, the number of patterns (k) must still be specified outside the algorithm. Since the equation described in FIGURE 2 is mathematically degenerate, there cannot be a general analytic solution. Specific analytic solutions can be constructed, such as with principal com-

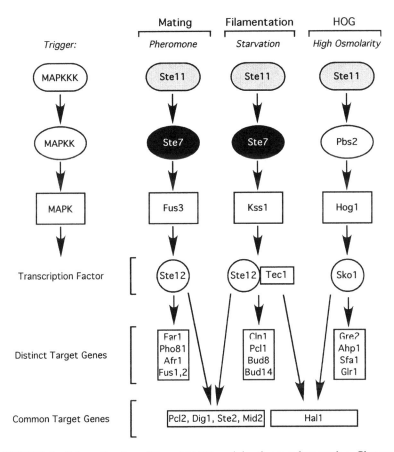

FIGURE 1. Schematic view of three MAPK modules that regulate mating, filamentous growth, and high osmolarity glycerol signaling pathways in the yeast *Saccharomyces cerevisiae.* Activation of these pathways is determined by the state of the cell and exposure to external signals. All three pathways share some signaling components and activate certain genes in common, but they also activate unique sets of genes. This leads to overlapping coregulation groups in gene expression studies.

ponent analysis (PCA). However, for BD, the rows of **P** need not be orthogonal or fulfill other independence criteria, permitting modeling of biological systems that typically have underlying processes that are nonindependent. BD performs a Markov chain Monte Carlo search for probable solutions using a Bayesian statistical framework,[25] which consists of an exploration of a series of likely solutions to the problem under study as described previously.[26]

The Bayesian framework allows introduction of significant prior knowledge in BD through the use of an atomic domain and mappings between it and the model domain (i.e., the **A** and **P** matrices). The atomic domain contains two one-dimensional

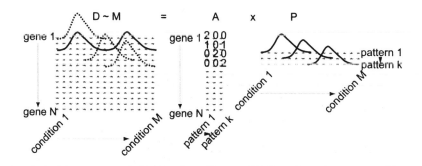

FIGURE 2. The decomposition performed by BD. The algorithm identifies simultaneously a pattern matrix, **P**, and a distribution or amplitude matrix, **A**, which together reconstruct the data within the noise. An example set of patterns is shown in the superimposed curves, with the second data row (*solid line*) showing how two fundamental patterns are combined to recover more complex behavior.

spaces (2^{32} points for computational convenience), one corresponding to the **A** matrix and one to the **P** matrix. Atoms defined solely by position and amplitude are created along these lines according to a prior distribution that is uniform in position and exponential in amplitude. Each atom is mapped to a matrix by a convolution function that describes the allowed relationships between points in the matrices. For example, in a supervised learning case where the conditions represent samples in known groups, some patterns could be step functions representing the known groups, as shown in FIGURE 3. In addition, coregulation of a set of genes can be encoded by having a single atom appear as a set of correlated amplitudes in the columns of the **A** matrix, effectively having all genes within a group change together (note that this does not force them to always track each other in the data as genes can belong to multiple patterns and may appear individually or in other coregulated groups). The prior information is encoded in the atomic domain distributions and in the convolution functions mapping the atoms to the matrices.

The key advantage to this linking of points within the models, whether it is through declaration of samples being related or a priori identification of genes that are coregulated, is that it guides the algorithm into expecting these points to show some coordinated behavior. This is similar (though not identical) to the belief that replicated spots should yield the same value, allowing averaging out of noise as well as estimation of uncertainty. Since there can be large numbers of genes showing coregulation (e.g., genes encoding ribosomal proteins or components of metabolic pathways), the statistical power gained can be significant. Nevertheless, this power is gained without forcing the solutions to behave as expected, since the algorithm is free to ignore this prior knowledge. In practice, the knowledge can significantly impact analysis of messy data where signal-to-noise values are low, but has less impact on high-quality data that are less uncertain. This is desirable as it allows prior knowledge to guide probabilistic reasoning when data quality is poor, but does not force acceptance of a prior bias when data quality is high.

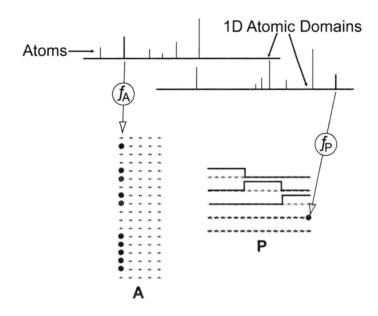

FIGURE 3. The domain structure within BD. The top lines represent the atomic domains that model infinitely divisible one-dimensional lines upon which atoms, defined solely by amplitude and location, are created *ex vacuo*. This space comprises a positive additive distribution that is mapped by convolution functions (shown as *circles* with *f* signs) to the model domain comprising the **A** and **P** matrices. Prior information is encoded in the prior distribution for the atoms (described in the text) and in the convolution functions, which permit linking of points in the model. On the *left*, the convolution function f_A causes an atom to appear in the model as a group of genes (indicated by the *dots*) that vary together (i.e., enforcing coregulation). On the *right*, a different convolution function f_P enforces a classification in 3 of the patterns (*top rows*), while allowing complete independence between samples in 2 additional patterns.

METHODS

We present here the analysis of two separate data sets to demonstrate the potential of BD in microarray analysis. The first set is the yeast deletion mutant data from Rosetta Inpharmatics,[27] which comprises microarray measurements of mRNA levels in yeast cultures with specific genes knocked out. This analysis demonstrates the ability of BD to use minimal prior knowledge and the ability to assign genes to multiple coexpression groups to recover knowledge on pathway activity. The second set is the Project Normal mouse data from the Fred Hutchinson Cancer Research Center,[28] which contains replicated measurements on kidneys, livers, and testes from 6 C57BL6 mice. This analysis demonstrates BD functioning as a supervised learning system and shows its ability to remove metabolic background signals during analysis.

The Rosetta data comprise genome-wide measurements of gene expression across 300 deletion mutants using oligonucleotide microarrays. The data were downloaded from Rosetta Inpharmatics and filtered to remove experiments where less than 2 genes underwent 3-fold changes and to remove genes that did not change by 3-fold across the remaining experiments. The resulting data set comprised 764 genes and 228 experiments. The Rosetta error model[29] provided the estimate of uncertainty for each data point. For this analysis, a direct mapping from the atomic domain to the model domain is used. Since the atomic domain comprises a positive additive distribution, the model (matrices A and P) must be positive, as must the mock data (M) in this case. As such, all data were transformed from log ratios to ratios. In order to determine the number of patterns, BD was applied multiple times positing 3 to 30 patterns. A tree was constructed by comparing the patterns from the positing of $k+1$ patterns to those from positing k patterns. In this way, stable patterns were identified. Analysis of the data in terms of coregulation and pathway activation focused on these stable patterns. For each pattern, the genes that were significantly expressed in each pattern were identified (i.e., the amplitude of their assignment to the pattern was greater than three times the uncertainty in that amplitude). The 50 largest amplitude genes in each pattern were analyzed in terms of cellular role as defined in the Proteome Yeast Database[30,31] in order to assign a function to the pattern. One pattern with a clear function was then validated by analysis of specific deletion mutants from the compendium.

The Project Normal data comprise measurements of the expression of 5406 genes in 3 tissues (kidney, liver, and testis) from 6 genetically identical C57BL6 male mice raised together.[28] The data were downloaded from the Critical Assessment of Microarray Data Analysis (CAMDA) Web site (http://www.camda.duke.edu/CAMDA02/). The raw data consisted of gene expression levels measured in quadruplicate for all samples, and background correction was performed by subtracting the median background intensity from the median foreground intensity. A mean expression ratio and standard deviation of the mean were determined from these corrected values. For data points for which one or fewer ratios were available or for data where the average ratio was negative, the ratio was set to 1.0 and the uncertainty to 100, effectively ensuring that the data point would not influence the model. The third and fourth testis data were removed completely since their average ratios across all genes were 2.74 and 3.11, respectively, as opposed to an average of 1.02 for all other conditions with these data removed. The final data set contained 97,979 points with 4 replicates, 1013 with 3 replicates, and 146 with 2 replicates, with 24 data points eliminated due to lack of replication.

The Project Normal data were analyzed using BD with enforced links between samples as in FIGURE 3 for the P matrix (i.e., enforcing a kidney pattern, a liver pattern, and a testis pattern, respectively), as well as with 1 to 3 additional unconstrained patterns. The final number of patterns to use to describe the data was estimated through use of gene ontology information.[19] Gene ontology (GO) was also used to determine the significance of the unforced patterns as well as to interpret the assignment of genes to the tissue-specific patterns.

RESULTS

The results across many different analyses of the yeast deletion mutant data set using BD were constructed into a tree (figure not shown) and, for each node in the

TABLE 1. Identification of pattern function from the Yeast Proteome Database

Pattern	Genes	Identified	Cellular roles
1	403	36	22: amino acid metabolism 9: other metabolism
2	410	27	7: metabolism 7: DNA/RNA processing 6: transport
4	276	20	No clear pattern
6	297	20	No clear pattern
7	223	23	13: mating response 5: meiosis

NOTE: The results from positing 7 patterns are shown, with pattern 7 representing the early-forming, extremely stable pattern.

tree, genes present in the pattern at the 3σ level were identified. For our analysis, we focused on patterns that were stable across many levels of the tree. The behavior underlying an expression pattern was determined from information on the gene functions, as defined in the Proteome database. The stable patterns are summarized in TABLE 1, showing the number of genes appearing in the pattern at a 3σ level, the number of the strongest 50 genes that have the cellular role identified in the Proteome database, and the cellular roles of these genes. Pattern 7 emerged when there were 4 patterns posited and remained stable through to 30 patterns.

Pattern 7 is of special interest as it is not only stable, but appears strongly linked to the yeast mating response. This is significant since the signaling pathway for the mating response has been worked out in detail,[32] as shown in FIGURES 1 and 4a. The response is triggered by binding of a mating pheromone to the Ste2 or Ste3 membrane receptor. This leads to cleavage of a G protein complex and subsequent triggering of the MAPK cascade involving Ste11, Ste7, and Fus3, which are bound to a scaffolding protein, Ste5. The trigger can be communicated to the MAPK cascade either through the Ste20 protein or directly by the G protein complex. The signal results in activation of the Ste12 transcription factor that initiates transcription of mating response genes. If pattern 7 truly represents this mating response, then deletion mutants that eliminate key elements of the pathway should result in the signal for that pathway disappearing. Essentially, the column of **P** related to that deletion mutant should have no signal for pattern 7, indicating that the mating response is absent. The results for the deletion mutants of interest are shown in FIGURE 4b and are exactly as expected, except for the *Fus3* deletion mutant. However, it is known that Kss1 can substitute for Fus3 in the mating response, and the double mutant eliminating both genes does indeed show loss of the mating response. It is important to note here that none of the genes encoding elements of the signaling pathway for mating response are assigned by BD to this pattern, except *Ste2*, which is known to be regulated by Ste12.[33] This demonstrates that it is not regulation of the pathway genes, but rather the transcriptional response to pathway activation that is being detected. In fact, expression measurements for *Ste20*, *Ste11*, *Ste7*, and *Ste12* are absent from the analyzed data set. A more detailed description of the analysis of this data set has been presented previously.[21]

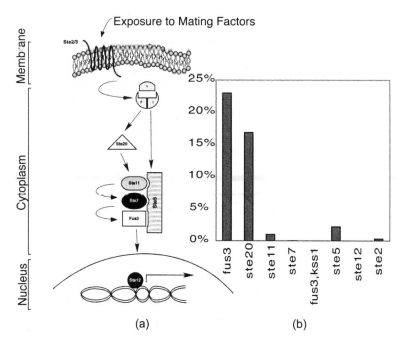

FIGURE 4. The mating response pathway and the results from BD analysis of the Rosetta deletion mutant data. **(a)** The mating response pathway in *S. cerevisiae* is shown. **(b)** The strength of pattern 7, the mating response pattern, for the deletion mutants for genes in the pathway, with the strength of the pattern shown (i.e., how much of the behavior of each deletion mutant is explained by pattern 7). Note that there is no *Ste3* deletion mutant in the data set. See the text for a discussion of these results.

For the Project Normal data set, the BD analysis focused on isolation of patterns related to the individual tissues in the background of ongoing metabolic processes. One issue often overlooked in discussions of supervised learning is the presence throughout all samples of expression linked to routine cellular processes (e.g., metabolic processes, routine synthesis, and transport). The proteins encoded by such genes are likely being made regardless of tissue type or disease state, but they are also likely to vary between individual samples due to biological noise (i.e., differences in states such as point in a metabolic cycle) and stochastic behavior. Even in carefully controlled yeast cultures, some genes are known to vary dramatically in expression with no phenotypic impact.[29] Removing the expression signals of such genes is important to interpretation of results, especially in cases where insight into underlying processes is a goal, as it is when identifying specific cellular malfunctions present in cancerous growth or specific responses to targeted therapies.

Removal of signals that differ significantly between samples, but do not relate to the phenotype of interest, requires that the number of such signals be identified. This is known to be problematic in pattern recognition in gene expression.[34] In order to determine the number of patterns in this set, we analyzed the data positing 4 (i.e.,

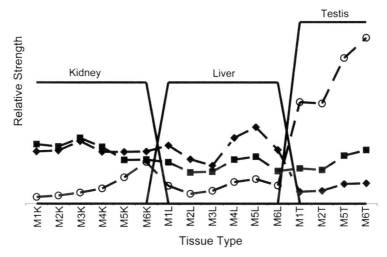

FIGURE 5. The results of BD analysis of the Project Normal data positing 6 patterns. The *solid lines* represent (from left to right) the kidney, liver, and testis tissue-specific patterns encoded in the algorithm. The *dashed line with open circles* shows an unconstrained pattern that is clearly related to differences in the expression in the testis between mice 1–2 and mice 5–6. The *dashed lines with solid squares and solid diamonds* show 2 patterns related to routine cellular processes (see TABLE 2).

1 pattern not related to tissue type) to 6 (i.e., 3 patterns not related to tissue type) patterns. The result with 6 patterns is shown in FIGURE 5. Each nontissue-specific pattern was analyzed by identifying all genes assigned to each pattern at the 3σ level and recovering up-to-date GO information using the ASAP system.[35] The pattern shown with open circles is clearly related to differences in the testis tissue of the first and second versus fifth and sixth mice. The other 2 patterns (closed squares and closed diamonds) correspond to a single pattern from the 5-pattern result.

GO was used to estimate the correct number of patterns by identifying enhancement in GO within each pattern. For all patterns, we determined the number of genes within the pattern assigned to each GO term and compared this to the number of genes assigned to the term within the full data set. In order to avoid false enhancement due to only a few genes being assigned to the GO term, we eliminated all terms represented by less than 5 genes in the data set (leaving 224 terms out of an original 724 terms). We computed the enhancement of the term within the pattern as

$$\text{enhancement} = (N_{patt}{}^{GO}/N_{patt}{}^{TOTAL})/(N_{data}{}^{GO}/N_{data}{}^{TOTAL})$$

where the numerator gives the normalized number of genes with the GO term in the pattern, and the denominator is the normalized number of genes with the GO term in the full data set. The pattern was then analyzed for coordinated enhancement of GO terms relative to related patterns positing more and fewer patterns during BD analysis. The results for 5 and 6 patterns in order of enhancement are shown in TABLE 2. Since the use of 6 patterns appeared to lead to coordinated, logical

TABLE 2. GO enhancement for the patterns related to metabolism and biosynthesis in analyses positing 5 and 6 total patterns

Five patterns: metabolic pattern	Protein secretion, secretory pathway, antiapoptosis, translational initiation, coenzymes and prosthetic group biosynthesis, steroid biosynthesis, N linked glycosylation, lipid biosynthesis, main pathways of carbohydrate metabolism, catabolic carbohydrate metabolism
Six patterns: metabolic pattern 1	Aromatic compound metabolism, main pathways of carbohydrate metabolism, aromatic amino acid family metabolism, catabolic carbohydrate metabolism, energy derivation by oxidation of organic compounds, amino acid catabolism, amine catabolism, coenzymes and prosthetic group metabolism, energy pathways, coenzymes and prosthetic group biosynthesis, microtubule-based process, amino acid derivative metabolism, membrane lipid metabolism, fatty acid metabolism, organic acid metabolism, carboxylic acid metabolism, electron transport, glucose catabolism, carbohydrate catabolism, hexose catabolism, alcohol catabolism, monosaccharide catabolism, protein targeting, protein folding, phospholipid metabolism, regulation of neurotransmitter levels
Six patterns: metabolic pattern 2	Wnt receptor signaling pathway, organic acid biosynthesis, carboxylic acid biosynthesis, oxygen and reactive oxygen species metabolism, polysaccharide metabolism, ectoderm development, epidermal differentiation, histogenesis, secretory pathway, N-linked glycosylation

NOTE: The pattern from the results positing 5 patterns shows 1.3- to 1.4-fold enhancement, while the patterns from results positing 6 patterns show up to 3.4-fold and 2.7-fold enhancement, respectively.

enhancement in mechanisms involving metabolism and biosynthesis, results with 6 patterns were chosen for further analysis.

In TABLE 3, the corresponding enhancement in GO terms is shown for the tissue-specific patterns. The assignment clearly relates to the specific purpose of each tissue, with catabolism and aromatic metabolism occurring in the kidney; amino acid catabolism, cholesterol and sterol metabolism, and hemostasis assigned to the liver; and spermatogenesis and reproduction assigned to the testis. The liver also has over-representation of genes related to embryogenesis and morphogenesis, which may be related to its ability to regenerate tissue. The testis has overrepresentation of cell cycle genes, which is likely related to the ongoing proliferation of sperm cells.

There are numerous further avenues of investigation made possible by the removal of the background metabolic signals and by the ability of BD to identify genes that, through evolution, have come to be involved in multiple processes. For instance, a number of genes involved in spermatogenesis are general-purpose kinases and stress response genes. BD assigns these genes to the testis pattern precisely because they can be assigned to multiple patterns, allowing their testis-specific signal to be recovered once the background metabolic signals are identified. Additional details on this and on identification of genes shared uniquely by two tissue types have been published.[23]

TABLE 3. GO terms enhanced in the tissue-specific patterns

Tissue	Terms enhanced in GO
Kidney	Amino acid catabolism, amine catabolism, aromatic amino acid family metabolism, aromatic compound metabolism, anion transport, chloride transport, inorganic anion transport, oxygen and reactive oxygen species metabolism, amino acid metabolism, main pathways of carbohydrate metabolism, amino acid biosynthesis, endocytosis, catabolic carbohydrate metabolism, amine metabolism, energy derivation by oxidation of organic compounds, electron transport, amino acid and derivative metabolism, amine biosynthesis
Liver	Amino acid catabolism, amine catabolism, aromatic amino acid family metabolism, amino acid metabolism, amino acid biosynthesis, aromatic compound metabolism, amine biosynthesis, amino acid and derivative metabolism, amine metabolism, lipid transport, amino acid derivative metabolism, blood coagulation, hemostasis, electron transport, biogenic amine metabolism, positive regulation of cell proliferation, embryogenesis and morphogenesis, cholesterol metabolism, sterol metabolism, regulation of neurotransmitter levels
Testis	Spermatogenesis, reproduction, gametogenesis, DNA-dependent DNA replication, DNA replication and chromosome cycle, microtubule-based process, S phase of mitotic cell cycle, DNA replication, regulation of cell shape and cell size, nuclear division, cytoskeleton organization and biogenesis, protein kinase cascade, chromatin assembly/disassembly, DNA packaging, nuclear organization and biogenesis, chromosome organization and biogenesis (sensu Eukarya), organelle organization and biogenesis, cell organization and biogenesis, mitochondrion organization and biogenesis, DNA metabolism, cytoplasm organization and biogenesis, M phase of mitotic cell cycle, mitosis, DNA repair, actin filament–based process, sodium transport, translational initiation, calcium ion transport, mitotic cell cycle, regulation of transcription from Pol II promoter, M phase, establishment and/or maintenance of chromatin architecture, pattern specification, phospholipid metabolism, Wnt receptor signaling pathway, di- and trivalent inorganic cation transport

NOTE: The terms are listed in order of enhancement, with all terms shown enhanced at least 2-fold over the level within the full data set.

DISCUSSION

New techniques in molecular and cellular biology coupled to methods under development in bioinformatics offer opportunities to improve cancer detection and identification. Microarray and GeneChip™ technologies can probe the inner workings of cancerous and normal tissues through genome-wide expression measurements. Interpretation of these measurements requires appropriate tools tuned to the goal of the analysis, whether it is identification of patterns related to outcomes or identification of biomarkers. For most studies involving cancer treatment, gene expression is inherently a downstream indicator of signaling pathway activity, so methods that recover pathway activity from gene expression are required for interpretation. BD provides both a method to link observed changes in pathway activity and a way to include prior biological knowledge. Since the data generated by microarrays tend to be extremely noisy, prior knowledge generated over decades of biological investigation can aid in the analysis process. Here, this was demonstrated by the use of gene ontologies to deduce the biological function associated with a pattern and to link a pattern to pathway activity.

New technologies continue to emerge that promise to greatly improve early detection of cancer. Of particular interest is the use of serum proteomics to determine disease state,[36] since such measurements are minimally invasive and do not require prior determination that cancer is probable. These measurements, as well as more detailed measurements of activated and nonactivated protein levels in disease tissue,[37] offer to allow a direct look at the workhorses of the cell in cancerous tissues. Merging these measurements of protein levels and states with microarray measurements of downstream effects of protein activity presents us with the next step forward in understanding cancer and the effects of therapeutics. Integrating these two types of data into a unified framework will be essential to developing a thorough understanding of cancer. Because of its reliance on the inclusion of prior knowledge, BD can provide a method of unifying these data. For instance, changes in the protein states can provide prior knowledge of expected gene expression changes, providing the algorithm with more statistical power to overcome the inherent noise in microarray measurements. The integration of the direct measure of protein activity in the pathways and the indirect measure of transcriptional response will provide a powerful tool to understand individual cancers and their responses to therapy.

ACKNOWLEDGMENTS

We thank the National Institutes of Health/National Cancer Institute (CCCG CA06927 to R. Young), the Pennsylvania Department of Health (grant to M. F. Ochs), and the Pew Foundation for support.

REFERENCES

1. ALISON, M. & C. SARRAF. 1997. Understanding Cancer. Cambridge University Press. Cambridge/London/New York.
2. JACKS, T. & R.A. WEINBERG. 2002. Taking the study of cancer cell survival to a new dimension. Cell 111: 923–925.
3. KOLCH, W. 2000. Meaningful relationships: the regulation of the Ras/Raf/MEK/ERK pathway by protein interactions. Biochem. J. 351(part 2): 289–305.
4. COOPER, G.M. 1992. Elements of Human Cancer. Jones and Bartlett. Boston.
5. MACDONALD, F. & C.H.J. FORD. 1997. Molecular Biology of Cancer. BIOS Sci. Pub. Oxford.
6. ALIZADEH, A.A., M.B. EISEN, R.E. DAVIS et al. 2000. Distinct types of diffuse large B-cell lymphoma identified by gene expression profiling. Nature 403: 503–511.
7. GOLUB, T.R., D.K. SLONIM, P. TAMAYO et al. 1999. Molecular classification of cancer: class discovery and class prediction by gene expression monitoring. Science 286: 531–537.
8. ZHANG, H., C.Y. YU, B. SINGER et al. 2001. Recursive partitioning for tumor classification with gene expression microarray data. Proc. Natl. Acad. Sci. USA 98: 6730–6735.
9. WILLIAMS, N.S., R.B. GAYNOR, S. SCOGGIN et al. 2003. Identification and validation of genes involved in the pathogenesis of colorectal cancer using cDNA microarrays and RNA interference. Clin. Cancer Res. 9: 931–946.

10. KIKUCHI, T., Y. DAIGO, T. KATAGIRI *et al.* 2003. Expression profiles of non-small cell lung cancers on cDNA microarrays: identification of genes for prediction of lymph-node metastasis and sensitivity to anti-cancer drugs. Oncogene **22:** 2192–2205.

11. CARR, K.M., M. BITTNER & J.M. TRENT. 2003. Gene-expression profiling in human cutaneous melanoma. Oncogene **22:** 3076–3080.

12. MAURO, M.J. & B.J. DRUKER. 2001. STI571: targeting BCR-ABL as therapy for CML. Oncologist **6:** 233–238.

13. REPKA, T., E.G. CHIOREAN, J. GAY *et al.* 2003. Trastuzumab and interleukin-2 in HER2-positive metastatic breast cancer: a pilot study. Clin. Cancer Res. **9:** 2440–2446.

14. VON MEHREN, M. 2003. Recent advances in the management of gastrointestinal stromal tumors. Curr. Oncol. Rep. **5:** 288–294.

15. CHEN, G., T.G. GHARIB, C.C. HUANG *et al.* 2002. Discordant protein and mRNA expression in lung adenocarcinomas. Mol. Cell. Proteomics **1:** 304–313.

16. GILMAN, A. & A.P. ARKIN. 2002. Genetic "code": representations and dynamical models of genetic components and networks. Annu. Rev. Genomics Hum. Genet. **3:** 341–369.

17. MILLIKEN, G.A. & D.E. JOHNSON. 1992. Analysis of Messy Data. Van Nostrand–Reinhold. New York.

18. BESAG, J. 1986. On the statistical analysis of dirty pictures. J. R. Stat. Soc. **B48:** 259–302.

19. ASHBURNER, M., C.A. BALL, J.A. BLAKE *et al.* 2000. Gene ontology: tool for the unification of biology—The Gene Ontology Consortium. Nat. Genet. **25:** 25–29.

20. OCHS, M.F., R.S. STOYANOVA, F. ARIAS-MENDOZA *et al.* 1999. A new method for spectral decomposition using a bilinear Bayesian approach. J. Magn. Reson. **137:** 161–176.

21. BIDAUT, G., T.D. MOLOSHOK, J.D. GRANT *et al.* 2002. Bayesian decomposition analysis of gene expression in yeast deletion mutants. *In* Methods of Microarray Data Analysis II, pp. 105–122. Kluwer Academic. Boston.

22. MOLOSHOK, T.D., D. DATTA, A.V. KOSSENKOV *et al.* 2003. Bayesian decomposition classification of the Project Normal data set. *In* Methods of Microarray Data Analysis III. Kluwer Academic. Boston.

23. MOLOSHOK, T.D., R.R. KLEVECZ, J.D. GRANT *et al.* 2002. Application of Bayesian decomposition for analysing microarray data. Bioinformatics **18:** 566–575.

24. WOLFE, K.H. & W.H. LI. 2003. Molecular evolution meets the genomics revolution. Nat. Genet. **33**(suppl.)**:** 255–265.

25. BESAG, J., P. GREEN, D. HIGDON *et al.* 1995. Bayesian computation and stochastic systems. Stat. Sci. **10:** 3–66.

26. OCHS, M.F. 2003. Bayesian Decomposition. *In* The Analysis of Gene Expression Data: Methods and Software. Springer-Verlag. New York/Berlin.

27. HUGHES, T.R., M.J. MARTON, A.R. JONES *et al.* 2000. Functional discovery via a compendium of expression profiles. Cell **102:** 109–126.

28. PRITCHARD, C.C., L. HSU, J. DELROW *et al.* 2001. Project Normal: defining normal variance in mouse gene expression. Proc. Natl. Acad. Sci. USA **98:** 13266–13271.

29. HUGHES, J.D., P.W. ESTEP, S. TAVAZOIE *et al.* 2000. Computational identification of *cis*-regulatory elements associated with groups of functionally related genes in *Saccharomyces cerevisiae*. J. Mol. Biol. **296:** 1205–1214.

30. COSTANZO, M.C., M.E. CRAWFORD, J.E. HIRSCHMAN *et al.* 2001. YPD, PombePD, and WormPD: model organism volumes of the BioKnowledge library, an integrated resource for protein information. Nucleic Acids Res. **29:** 75–79.

31. COSTANZO, M.C., J.D. HOGAN, M.E. CUSICK *et al.* 2000. The yeast proteome database (YPD) and *Caenorhabditis elegans* proteome database (WormPD): comprehensive resources for the organization and comparison of model organism protein information. Nucleic Acids Res. **28:** 73–76.

32. POSAS, F., M. TAKEKAWA & H. SAITO. 1998. Signal transduction by MAP kinase cascades in budding yeast. Curr. Opin. Microbiol. **1:** 175–182.

33. HWANG-SHUM, J.J., D.C. HAGEN, E.E. JARVIS *et al.* 1991. Relative contributions of MCM1 and STE12 to transcriptional activation of a- and alpha-specific genes from *Saccharomyces cerevisiae*. Mol. Gen. Genet. **227:** 197–204.

34. LUKASHIN, A.V. & R. FUCHS. 2001. Analysis of temporal gene expression profiles: clustering by simulated annealing and determining the optimal number of clusters. Bioinformatics **17:** 405–414.

35. KOSSENKOV, A., F.J. MANION, E. KOROTKOV *et al.* 2003. ASAP: automated sequence annotation pipeline for Web-based updating of sequence information with a local dynamic database. Bioinformatics **19:** 675–676.
36. PETRICOIN, E.F., A.M. ARDEKANI, D.A. HITT *et al.* 2002. Use of proteomic patterns in serum to identify ovarian cancer. Lancet **359:** 572–577.
37. SREEKUMAR, A., M.K. NYATI, S. VARAMBALLY *et al.* 2001. Profiling of cancer cells using protein microarrays: discovery of novel radiation-regulated proteins. Cancer Res. **61:** 7585–7593.

InfoEvolve™

Moving from Data to Knowledge Using Information Theory and Genetic Algorithms

GANESH VAIDYANATHAN

Corporate Center for Engineering Research, E. I. DuPont de Nemours & Company, Wilmington, Delaware 19880-0357, USA

ABSTRACT: InfoEvolve™ is a unified suite of data mining and empirical modeling tools capable of discovering low-bias and low-variance solutions to complex processes. The method is based on a common set of principles involving information theory and genetic algorithms. InfoEvolve™ can also discover multiple strategies embedded in complex data sets for achieving a desired target or goal. This latter aspect may prove to be very useful in drug design. The paper analyzes the following: InfoEvolve™ from a theoretical standpoint; a conceptual overview of InfoEvolve™ with a short description of the modeling method; the method using the example of homogeneous identification of DNA from an analysis of its melting curve behavior; and key learnings and additional applications of the technology for both drug design and genome analysis.

KEYWORDS: InfoEvolve™; data; information; theory; genetic algorithm

INTRODUCTION

Data acquisition is rapidly increasing in many different fields. The ability to acquire data has often outstripped the ability to extract useful knowledge from the data, especially when the information is hidden in the midst of significant amounts of noise. Common difficulties include the discovery of the critical inputs to a complex process and the limitations imposed by the bias-variance trade-off. The rule of thumb has always been to sacrifice some accuracy in the learning process (increase bias or training set error) in order to generalize with higher accuracy (decrease variance or test set error). InfoEvolve™ is a unified suite of data mining and empirical modeling tools capable of discovering low-bias and low-variance solutions to complex processes.[a] The method is based on a common set of principles involving information theory and genetic algorithms. Generalized information metrics are used to drive genetic algorithms for finding the most "information-rich" solutions to a wide range of problems. The information metrics are based on the work of Shannon,[1] who used the thermodynamic notion of entropy to measure infor-

Address for correspondence: Ganesh Vaidyanathan, Senior Research Associate, Corporate Center for Engineering Research, E. I. DuPont de Nemours & Co., P. O. Box 80357, Wilmington, DE 19880-0357. Voice: 302-695-3550; fax: 302-695-2747.
  gvaidyanathan@comcast.net
[a]InfoEvolve™ is a trademark of E. I. DuPont de Nemours & Company, Inc.

Ann. N.Y. Acad. Sci. 1020: 227–238 (2004). © 2004 New York Academy of Sciences.
doi: 10.1196/annals.1310.019

mation capacity in communication theory. The use of genetic algorithms also enables the discovery of the critical interactions between inputs that can encode significant amounts of information. Most existing methods measure the importance of inputs in isolation, without including their interactions, or model the interactions using predetermined assumptions. InfoEvolve™ can also discover multiple strategies embedded in complex data sets for achieving a desired target or goal. This latter aspect may prove to be very useful in drug design.

The paper is organized as follows. The first section introduces InfoEvolve™ from a theoretical standpoint. A conceptual overview of InfoEvolve™ is followed by a short description of the modeling method. The next section illustrates the method using the example of homogeneous identification of DNA from an analysis of its melting curve behavior. Finally, key learnings and additional applications of the technology for both drug design and genome analysis are discussed in the last section.

THEORY AND CONCEPTUAL BASIS OF InfoEvolve™

InfoEvolve™ can be classified as a nonparametric and nonregressive modeling methodology. It is based on the assumption that, for most highly dimensional data spaces encountered in real applications, information is localized in many pockets that are distributed throughout the space. In this view, the goal of data modeling is to discover these localized information-rich regions and combine the discovered information in optimal ways to create a successful model. It is not necessary or even desirable to model the structure of the entire data space, which can be computationally expensive due to the exponential growth in the data needed as the dimensionality of the input space increases. This latter problem is commonly known as the "curse of dimensionality". The identification of many locally information-rich regions, of significantly lower dimensionality than the total input space, is consistent with an existence theorem by Kolmogorov and described by Rabitz et al.[2,3] The theorem proves the possibility of decomposing any continuous n-dimensional function into a unique sum of $2n+1$ single-variable functions. InfoEvolve™ uses informational entropy metrics to drive an evolutionary algorithm in order to discover these lower dimensional, information-rich regions.

The InfoEvolve™ family of algorithms includes the following:

- InfoEvolve™ Cluster—data clustering;
- InfoEvolve™ Discovery—identification of the most significant inputs in massive, complex data sets;
- InfoEvolve™ Forecast—forecasting and prediction;
- InfoEvolve™ Strategy—discovering multiple strategies for achieving a desired outcome;
- InfoEvolve™ Publisher—information visualization and knowledge warehousing.

The key elements incorporated into InfoEvolve™ Forecast to discover an optimum model are summarized below:

- Identification of the most information-rich inputs using InfoEvolve™ Discovery;

- Identification of multiple interacting combinations of the most information-rich inputs, where each combination is characterized by a complexity factor;
- Discovery of the optimum sampling resolution of the data space covered by the information-rich input combinations;
- Building a total solution as an optimum combination of multiple, partial solutions spanned by the data subspaces consisting of the information-rich input combinations.

These elements can be viewed through an analogy of taking a good picture in a complex terrain. The required actions are as follows: point the camera in the right overall direction; adjust the f-stop; zoom the camera to more clearly see the scene; reposition the camera slightly in order to center the shot; and trigger the exposure. InfoEvolve™ is unique in the way it optimizes all these steps required to take the best picture.

The key notions of bias and variance are also fundamental to data mining. In most data mining methods, comparing model performance on a training data set and a test data set develops optimal models. The conventional wisdom is that, if the model is overtrained on the training data set (resulting in a low training error bias), it will not perform well on the test data set (resulting in a high test error variance). Most approaches attempt to find the optimum training bias that results in a minimum test variance; this normally results in increasing overall bias in both training and test data sets in order to gain generalizability. This is known as the bias-variance trade-off.[4] In InfoEvolve™, it is possible to discover low-bias/low-variance solutions to complex problems for reasons described below. This can result in lower test error performance in classes of problems where the best solution may lie in the low-bias/low-variance regime.

Discovering the Most Information-Rich Inputs and Input Combinations: "Positioning the Camera" to Overcome the Curse of Dimensionality

Following the camera analogy, we address the important issue of dimensionality reduction. For many complex problems, a key to developing optimum generalizable models is to use only the most information-rich inputs. Otherwise, modeling the noise in the data wastes significant effort. Difficulties that must be overcome include potentially nonlinear relationships between inputs and outputs, as well as inter-actions among inputs. In addition, the relationship between the number of inputs and model performance is not generally monotonic. Too few inputs result in incomplete information, whereas too many inputs results in introduction of unwanted noise. Both these effects degrade model performance.

Existing methods for dimensionality reduction are not well suited to deal with the complications described above. The commonly used principal component analysis (PCA)[5] method is linear and based on input variance, and does not deal explicitly with input-output relationships. Factor analysis[5] is another method of dimensionality reduction based on identifying correlations among inputs, but again does not explicitly take input-output relationships into account. Other nonlinear methods such as the tree-based Branch and Bound Procedure[4] assume a monotonic relationship between number of inputs and model quality. This is not true in general. Decision tree methods generally deal with inputs one at a time and thus miss potentially information-rich input combinations that are diluted across several branches in the tree. It is also difficult in many empirical modeling methods to separate model structure from intrinsic importance of variables as they tend to be intertwined.

In InfoEvolve™, a data preprocessing step based on genetic algorithms for input combination selection has been developed to overcome these difficulties. It is important to note that this step has been separated from the actual model development step so that we can first position the camera properly before taking the picture. A fundamental notion in InfoEvolve™ is that of a pseudogene: a binary bit string that defines a set of input features. The pseudogene in turn can be used to define a feature subspace. Each binary bit in the pseudogene is associated with a corresponding input in the data set. The on/off state of the bit determines whether that input should be included in the feature subspace. In this fashion, a pseudogene can represent any combination of inputs. Each feature subspace can be further segmented into cells (analogous to the segmentation of an image into cells), where a cell is a local region of the subspace. Individual data records from the data set are then projected into the subspace, with each data record ending up in a specific cell. The global information content of the input feature subspace coded for by the pseudogene is then measured using a number-weighted sum of local "cell" entropies. The local cell entropy is a measure of the uniformity of the local output distribution within a cell in the subspace and is calculated using the Nishi informational entropy function[6] based on the definition by Shannon.[1]

The global information content of the feature subspace is used as the fitness function to drive a genetic algorithm[7–9] to evolve a final pseudogene pool typically comprising several thousand pseudogenes and possessing high global information content. A histogram of the frequency of occurrence of each input in this population of information-rich pseudogenes is used to create an *Information Map*. The Information Map is used to select the most important inputs based on the frequency of occurrence in the map. Note that the effects of nonlinear input interactions are included through the discovery of information-rich genes that implicitly contain input interactions.

Identifying Optimum Model Complexity: "Adjusting the f-Stop"

Once dimensionality reduction has been performed, InfoEvolve™ searches to find an optimum model complexity factor if one exists. The complexity factor is defined as the characteristic dimension of the genes that results in the best empirical model. In this context, we should first define a model in InfoEvolve™ as a collection of pseudogenes. This definition is a natural extension of the concept of a gene defined as a collection of inputs. We shall defer the discussion of how an optimum collection of pseudogenes can be discovered, but suggest that such a collection can comprise either a heterogeneous population of pseudogenes of different dimensionalities or a homogeneous population of pseudogenes of the same dimensionality. In the latter instance, this characteristic dimensionality can provide insight into the informational complexity of the data space.

For example, if an optimum model can be developed from a population of 2D pseudogenes, it is simpler in a fundamental sense from a model developed from a group of 5D pseudogenes due to the smaller number of input interactions. In decision tree methods, the notion of a common number of nodes for every branch of the tree is hard to implement since the tree is grown a single input at a time and the notion of a pseudogene is missing. In neural networks, the network architectures combine all the inputs at each node, making the identification of a characteristic interaction complexity difficult, if not impossible.

Identifying Optimum Sampling Resolution: "Adjusting the Lens Zoom"

After an optimum model complexity has been discovered, InfoEvolve™ proceeds to discover the best quantization conditions for cell definition within each input feature subspace coded by a pseudogene. In our camera analogy, this relates to adjusting the camera zoom. If the lens is zoomed in too much, it will miss the full data object that we are trying to capture in an image. Conversely, if the lens is zoomed out too far, the data object will be an indistinguishable blur. Optimum sampling resolution relates directly to the bias-variance trade-off for best model generalizability. Too fine a resolution is analogous to overfitting the training data set, resulting in poor generalizability.

In InfoEvolve™, often the best models result from extremely high sampling resolutions, where cell population statistics resemble a Poisson distribution with most cells containing either a single or no data record. In other modeling methods, this type of overfitting results in poor generalizability. The root of the apparent paradox lies in the observation that, in these other methods, there is only one prediction for the output in an individual model unit. This results in the need to have sufficient data support associated with the single prediction and, thus, the bias-variance trade-off emerges quite naturally. In InfoEvolve™, each model unit is defined as a collec-

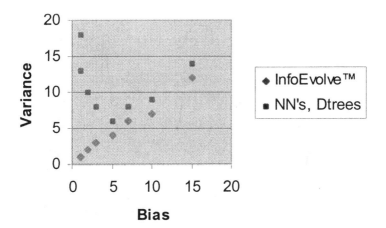

FIGURE 1. Qualitative positioning of different modeling methods in bias-variance space. The *squares* indicate how existing technologies generally behave in different portions of the solution space. For these methods, the variance tends to decrease initially as the bias decreases. However, below a certain minimum bias, the variance starts to increase rapidly. InfoEvolve™, indicated by the *diamonds*, can find solutions in the lower left portion of the bias-variance space, resulting in the best models for complex problems. If a low-bias/low-variance solution does not exist, higher bias, but still lower variance solutions are found. Note that the bias and variance are qualitatively represented in arbitrary units.

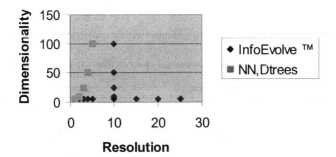

FIGURE 2. Qualitative plot of regions of dimensionality/resolution space sampled by different modeling methods. InfoEvolve™ first performs a sharp dimensionality reduction indicated by the vertical drop at resolution 10. It then scans all of the resolution space to find the optimum solution. This is indicated by the horizontal line at a low dimensionality value. Other methods, such as decision trees and neural networks, try to simultaneously find the optimal dimensionality and resolution, but only search a small portion of the dimensionality-resolution space, as indicated by the parabolic-like curve in the left portion of the graph.

tion of genes, where each gene makes a partial prediction of the output. Since there are many genes comprising a model, each gene can afford to be sampled at a high resolution due to the multiplicity of predictions. This has profound consequences for final model performance as it enables the development of low-bias/low-variance models that are beyond the scope of most other methods (see FIGS. 1 and 2).

Finally, the idea of a model as being represented by an optimum collection of relatively low complexity pseudogenes implies that some of the information in a complex process is encoded in the pseudogene-pseudogene interactions. This is analogous to our earlier observation that information may also be encoded in input-input interactions. The notion of information being encoded in a hierarchy of inter-actions between evolutionary objects provides a foundational basis for the process of distributed hierarchical evolution described by InfoEvolve™.

Evolving the Final Model: "Repositioning the Camera and Clicking the Picture"

Once a gene pool of the most information-rich input feature combinations has been evolved against the training data set, the final empirical model can be evolved in a second evolutionary stage. In model evolution, a subset of the information-rich genes in the gene pool is evolved that best explains the test data set. An error score is calculated based on the actual versus predicted test output states. An inverse measure of this error score is used to drive the model evolution phase to select an optimal subset of the genes in the information-rich gene pool, which minimizes the predicted error in the test set. This final (sub)collection of genes defines a model.

The notion of a model being defined as an optimal group of interacting genes, with each gene in turn being defined as an optimal group of interacting inputs, has several important advantages. First and foremost, the notion of *redundancy and multiplicity* is built within a single model unit. This allows each subspace coded for by a gene to be superresolved beyond the limits imposed by the conventional bias-variance trade-off.

Inverse Modeling: Discovery of Multiple Microstrategies

In addition to predicting an output from a given set of inputs, information-rich clusters that map to a specific output *state* can also be discovered to reveal unique *input patterns* associated with specific outcomes. This type of microstrategy discovery is widely used in the financial industry for the analysis of financial signals in time to make real-time buying and selling decisions. In a pharmaceutical context, microstrategies can be used to discover pattern combinations of chemical descriptors and the associated ranges of their values that map strongly to a desired activity or biochemical function.

The key idea in microstrategy discovery is based on gene dissection. Once a family of information-rich genes has been evolved using the methods described earlier, the resulting genes can be either aggregated to define a model or dissected to reveal underlying strategies. Dissecting a gene involves examination of each of the hyper-cells comprising the subspace coded for by the gene and measuring its information content and underlying data support. Information content is again measured by entropy measures. A list of the most information-rich cells with the highest data support can be constructed during the gene dissection process, with each cell encoding a specific combination of input features and their associated ranges. In effect, each cell encodes a microstrategy for achieving a specific output *state* with a very high probability. The discovery of multiple cells reinforces the general conclusion that complex problems can be analyzed or viewed in many ways and that many information-rich solutions are possible.

Data Clustering: Discovery of Macrostrategies

We now discuss InfoEvolve™ Cluster, a data clustering algorithm based on the same underlying principles of entropy and genetic algorithms that characterize the empirical modeling algorithms described earlier. Data clustering is a very important function within the overall scope of empirical modeling that deals with segregating a data set into smaller data subsets based on the similarity of their inputs. Clustering is often used in biomedical applications for identifying characteristics of normal and abnormal populations.[6] It can also be used to group genes, proteins, and other molecules based on the similarity of their biochemical descriptors.

Many data clustering algorithms such as the well-known K-means algorithm require the user to specify the number of desired clusters in advance. This may pose problems in situations where it is difficult or impossible to make such an estimate. Other agglomerative algorithms work in a tree-like hierarchical fashion where extremely small, highly uniform clusters are found first and gradually merge to create larger, less uniform clusters. In these algorithms, there is usually a trade-off: the larger the clusters, the less uniform they tend to be, and this is generally a monotonic relationship. Subjective methods are then to decide which clusters to retain. InfoEvolve™ Cluster does not require the user to specify the number of clusters in advance and it tends to find the most uniform clusters beyond a predetermined minimum size as the earliest clusters during its searching process. The algorithm is guided by minimum and maximum cluster size parameters and will first find the most uniform clusters and then leave a remainder suboptimal cluster that is iteratively searched for further clusters until no more clusters can be found.

The initial stages of the cluster discovery process are guided by finding extremely uniform or tight data clusters. In this stage, clusters are grown by maximal differential improvement in cluster uniformity when a new data member is added. In this way, the best clusters are evolved first as they absorb the most information-rich members (uniformity is again based on entropy). A residual remainder cluster (or sometimes clusters) usually emerges as part of this process and is iteratively searched for further clusters. Once clusters satisfying the size constraints can no longer be found in the residual remainder cluster, the algorithm searches this cluster using a different criterion for cluster growth. In this final stage, clusters are grown by maximal total cluster uniformity of each cluster, resulting in the breakup of the residual remainder cluster into more uniform subclusters. The two-pronged strategy of the clustering algorithm results in a final population of optimal clusters with many superb clusters and no final suboptimal cluster.

The method for calculating cluster uniformity using entropy-based metrics within InfoEvolve™ works equally well for both categorical and continuous input variables. This has proven to be a difficulty with many other clustering paradigms and is an important strength of InfoEvolve™.

Another critical issue in clustering deals with the assignment of weights to each of the input features to drive cluster development. For example, if certain inputs are more important to specific problems, they should be weighted more heavily than other, less important features. These weights are often assigned subjectively or by using other feature selection methods that may be suboptimal. Here, InfoEvolve™ Discovery is used to first create Information Maps from which weights to individual input features can be assigned based on their frequency of occurrence in the map. This provides a natural, elegant solution to a major problem in cluster analysis and illustrates the way in which the different InfoEvolve™ tools can work effectively together.

IDENTIFICATION OF TARGET DNA

Description of Problem

Analytical tools used to detect specific genes are in common use today for the diagnosis of disease as well as many research and even industrial applications. Traditional methods for DNA-based analysis have involved gel electrophoresis that can be time-consuming and error-prone. Newer methods for DNA identification include the analysis of the temperature dependence of fluorescence emerging from fluorescent labels intercalated between the double strands of the DNA helix. Empirical modeling of this temperature spectrum is the key to identifying the presence or absence of the targeted gene. This application illustrates the use of InfoEvolve™ Forecast in DNA identification.

Data Characteristics

The data set consists of the fluorescence-temperature spectrum for 2088 samples that may (state 1) or may not (state 0) have the desired DNA target. The raw spectrum has been preprocessed to reduce some of the noise. There are 250 temperature inputs in the spectrum, and the data set is divided into a training set consisting of

1566 samples and a validation set consisting of 522 samples. Although the input feature set is information-rich, it is an interesting problem in that the desired accuracy needs to be extremely high (~99%).

Population Statistics

See TABLE 1 for the population statistics.

TABLE 1. Population statistics

	Output state	Population
Training data	0	586
	1	980
Validation data	0	196
	1	326

Identification of Important Features

Following the methodology described above, a pseudogene pool consisting of the most information-rich input feature combinations was evolved from the training set using a genetic algorithm. A histogram of the frequency of occurrence of each input feature in the final pseudogene pool is shown in FIGURE 3. This histogram is also known as an Information Map and indicates the importance of each input through its interactions with other inputs. These interactions can be potentially very nonlinear. The Information Map for this example is highly structured, and significant dimensionality reduction is possible. Thirteen temperature inputs, corresponding to the peak locations, were selected from this map to perform the modeling using InfoEvolve™. Models are developed on the training data set that has been parsed with these 13 inputs and subsequently validated on the validation data set.

Prediction Accuracy on the Validation Data Set

InfoEvolve™ misclassified 6 out of the 522 validation cases for an error of 1.1%. The confusion matrix is shown in TABLE 2.

TABLE 2. The confusion matrix

Actual/Predicted	0	1
0	192	4
1	2	324

The high accuracy of InfoEvolve™ in this example illustrates its capability of successfully searching a large input data space, identifying the most important inputs, and subsequently developing a low-bias/low-variance model. The dimen-

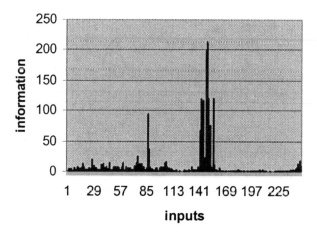

FIGURE 3. Information Map for temperature inputs in the fluorescence-temperature example given in the text. The sharp structure in the map shows that only certain temperature regions are important for revealing the presence of a target.

sionality reduction of the original 250-point temperature spectrum down to 13 selected inputs in this example demonstrates an important advantage of InfoEvolve™ in being able to identify the most information-rich inputs *through their interactions* in a multidimensional input space. The fundamental notion of a gene as a group of interacting inputs implicitly encodes input interactions in a natural fashion without any predetermined assumptions. The subsequent evolution of a subset of information-rich genes in the reduced dimensional data space defines a model where there are partial output predictions emerging from *each* gene in the subset. The multiplicity of predictions built within a single model unit enables the discovery of low-bias/low-variance models: Each gene comprising the model can be superresolved, leading to a low bias in the training set. The combination of the predictions from all the genes can lead to low variance in the test set.

DISCUSSION AND POSSIBLE EXTENSIONS

In this paper, we have introduced InfoEvolve™, a new empirical modeling frame-work based on the marriage of information theory and genetic algorithms. We have framed our discussion around the key notions of bias and variance and have shown how it is possible within this new paradigm to identify solutions to complex data modeling problems in the low-bias/low-variance region of the solution space that may be precluded using other modeling methods. We have illustrated the capabilities of InfoEvolve™ on the DNA Identification problem where the validation set error was ~99%, comparable to the best results obtainable from gel electrophoresis.

The DNA Identification problem described above illustrates the capabilities of the InfoEvolve™ Discovery and Forecast tools. The Strategy and Cluster tools can also be used in pharmaceutical applications for both drug discovery as well as genomics. In drug discovery, an important need is to determine the information-rich inputs such as biochemical and structural descriptors that are associated with a desired target function. The Cluster tool can be used to first segregate a compound-assay database into groups of compounds that are similar at a macrolevel based on assay response. Each group of compounds can then be expressed in terms of bio-chemical and structural descriptors at a microlevel. A specific assay (or group of assays) may be targeted as an output response domain, and the Strategy tool can then be used within each compound group to discover descriptor combinations that map optimally to a desired target response (or set of responses). The layering of the discovery process into macrostrategy (Cluster) and microstrategy (Strategy) stages can significantly reduce computational complexity and also can enhance process understanding.

In genomics, areas well matched to the strengths of InfoEvolve™ include the empirical modeling of gene expression profiles from microarray data for predicting phenotypes. This is a data-rich domain with complex gene-gene interactions responsible for function. The discovery of the key interactions can occur naturally within the genetic framework offered by InfoEvolve™ through the evolution of the information-rich pseudogene pool from which the Information Map is constructed. Each pseudogene elaborates a specific information-rich interaction among the input features whose corresponding bits are turned on in the pseudogene.

The unification by InfoEvolve™ of key aspects of knowledge discovery and data mining into a single conceptual framework provides a natural and elegant integration over the entire empirical modeling spectrum. The multiplicity of partial predictions built into a single model can be used to circumvent the limitations of the bias variance trade-off. Finally, the powerful dimensionality reduction capabilities built into InfoEvolve™ can be used to search a very highly dimensional input space and discover the key, relatively low order interactions that, working together, ultimately influence function.

ACKNOWLEDGMENTS

I am indebted to Dennis J. Underwood of the DuPont Pharmaceutical Corporation for suggesting this topic for presentation at the conference and to members of the DuPont Pattern Discovery Group and many other colleagues throughout DuPont for valuable discussions and access to real data that have aided the development of this methodology.

REFERENCES

1. SHANNON, C.E. 1948. A mathematical theory of communication. Bell Syst. Tech. J. **27:** 379–423; 623–656.
2. RABITZ, H., O.F. ALIS, J. SHORTER & K. SHIM. 1999. Efficient input-output model representations. Comput. Phys. Commun. **117:** 11–20.
3. RABITZ, H. & O.F. ALIS. 1999. General foundations of high-dimensional model representations. J. Math. Chem. **25:** 197–233.
4. BISHOP, C.M. 1995. Neural Networks for Pattern Recognition. Oxford University Press (Clarendon). London/New York.

5. DUDA, R.O. & P.E. HART. 1973. Pattern Classification and Scene Analysis. Wiley. New York.
6. HAYASHI, T. & T. NISHI. 1991. Morphology and physical properties of polymer alloys. *In* Proceedings of the International Conference on Mechanical Behaviour of Materials VI, Kyoto, p. 325.
7. HOLLAND, J.H. 1975. Adaptation in Natural and Artificial Systems. University of Michigan Press. Ann Arbor.
8. GOLDBERG, D.E. 1989. Genetic Algorithms in Search, Optimization, and Machine Learning. Addison–Wesley. Reading, MA.
9. MITCHELL, M. 1997. An Introduction to Genetic Algorithms. MIT Press. Cambridge, MA.

Applications of Machine Learning and High-Dimensional Visualization in Cancer Detection, Diagnosis, and Management

JOHN F. McCARTHY, KENNETH A. MARX, PATRICK E. HOFFMAN, ALEXANDER G. GEE, PHILIP O'NEIL, M. L. UJWAL, AND JOHN HOTCHKISS

AnVil, Incorporated, Burlington, Massachusetts 01803, USA

ABSTRACT: Recent technical advances in combinatorial chemistry, genomics, and proteomics have made available large databases of biological and chemical information that have the potential to dramatically improve our understanding of cancer biology at the molecular level. Such an understanding of cancer biology could have a substantial impact on how we detect, diagnose, and manage cancer cases in the clinical setting. One of the biggest challenges facing clinical oncologists is how to extract clinically useful knowledge from the overwhelming amount of raw molecular data that are currently available. In this paper, we discuss how the exploratory data analysis techniques of machine learning and high-dimensional visualization can be applied to extract clinically useful knowledge from a heterogeneous assortment of molecular data. After an introductory overview of machine learning and visualization techniques, we describe two proprietary algorithms (PURS and RadViz™) that we have found to be useful in the exploratory analysis of large biological data sets. We next illustrate, by way of three examples, the applicability of these techniques to cancer detection, diagnosis, and management using three very different types of molecular data. We first discuss the use of our exploratory analysis techniques on proteomic mass spectroscopy data for the detection of ovarian cancer. Next, we discuss the diagnostic use of these techniques on gene expression data to differentiate between squamous and adenocarcinoma of the lung. Finally, we illustrate the use of such techniques in selecting from a database of chemical compounds those most effective in managing patients with melanoma versus leukemia.

KEYWORDS: data mining; exploratory data analysis; machine learning; visualization; bioinformatics; biomedical informatics; cheminformatics; genomics; proteomics; molecular medicine; cancer

INTRODUCTION

Cancer has emerged as one of the most significant public health problems of the twenty-first century. This has arisen in part due to a substantial increase in the average life expectancy of the population and the strong positive correlation

Address for correspondence: John F. McCarthy, 2 Devonshire Drive, Canton, MA 02021. Voice: 781-828-4230.
jmccarthy@verizon.net

Ann. N.Y. Acad. Sci. 1020: 239–262 (2004). © 2004 New York Academy of Sciences.
doi: 10.1196/annals.1310.020

between cancer and age. Globally, approximately 10 million new cancer patients are diagnosed each year, with a doubling of this number expected by the year 2020.[1] As a consequence, radical new approaches to cancer detection, diagnosis, and management are necessary if we are to successfully alleviate both the social and economic burden of this devastating disease.

The development of cancer results from the accumulation of DNA changes in some of the approximately 40,000 chromosomal genes that may potentially lead to functional alterations in several of the 100,000 to 10 million proteins coded for by these genes.[2] Recent advances in molecular technology have resulted in the availability of large sets of genomic, proteomic, and chemical data. Clearly, there is a pressing need for new analytical approaches to help in exploring this immense hypothesis space and to provide clinically useful results.[3]

In this paper, we explore the use of machine learning and high-dimensional visualization as exploratory data analysis tools within this domain. These techniques are first described, followed by three successful clinical applications of their use in cancer detection, diagnosis, and management, respectively. In order to further demonstrate the breadth and scope of these techniques for molecular medicine, three distinctly different types of data sets are considered.

DATA ANALYSIS BY MACHINE LEARNING

Overview of Machine Learning and Visualization

Machine learning is the application of statistical techniques to derive general knowledge from specific data sets by searching through possible hypotheses exemplified in the data. The goal is typically to build predictive or descriptive models from characteristic features of a data set and then use those features to draw conclusions from other similar data sets.[4] In cancer detection, diagnosis, and management, machine learning helps identify significant factors in high-dimensional data sets of genomic, proteomic, chemical, or clinical data that can be used to understand or predict underlying disease, in addition to providing possible insights into effective disease management strategies. Machine learning techniques serve as tools for finding the "needle in the haystack" of possible hypotheses formulated by studying the correlation of protein or genomic expression with the presence or absence of disease. These same techniques can also be used to search chemical structure databases for correlations of chemical structure with biological activity.

In the process of analyzing the accuracy of the general concepts extracted from a specific data set, high-dimensional visualizations give the researcher timesaving tools for analyzing the significance, biases, and strength of possible hypotheses. In dealing with a potentially discontinuous high-dimensional concept space, the researcher's intuition benefits greatly from a visual validation of the statistical correctness of a result. The visualizations can also reveal sensitivity to variance, nonobvious correlations, and unusual higher-order effects that are scientifically important, but would require time-consuming mathematical analyses to discover.

Effective cancer detection, diagnosis, and management involve a group of techniques in machine learning called classification techniques. Classification is supervised learning. The classes of objects are already known and are used to train the system to learn the attributes that most effectively discriminate among members of different classes. For example, given a set of gene expression data for samples with known classes of disease, a supervised learning algorithm might learn to classify disease states based on patterns of gene expression. In unsupervised learning, either there are no predetermined classes or the class assignments are ignored, and data objects are grouped together by cluster analysis based on a wide variety of similarity measures. In both supervised and unsupervised learning, an explicit or implicit model is created from the data to help to predict future data instances or understand the physical processes responsible for generating the data. Creating these models can be a very computationally intensive task, given the large size and dimensionality of typical biological data sets. As a consequence of the large number of descriptors and low number of samples, many such models are prone to the flaw of "overfitting", which may reduce the external validity of the model when applied to other data sets of similar type. Feature selection and reduction techniques help with both computation time and overfitting problems by reducing the number of data attributes used in creating a data model to those most important for characterizing the hypothesis.

In the three cancer examples to be presented, combinations of both supervised and unsupervised learning, as well as feature reduction, are used and will be described. In addition, we will discuss the use of high-dimensional visualization in conjunction with these analytical techniques. One particular visualization, RadViz™, incorporates machine learning techniques with an intuitive and interactive visual display. Two other high-dimensional visualizations, parallel coordinates and PatchGrid™ (similar to heatmap) are also used to analyze and display results.

Below, we summarize the classification, feature reduction, validation, and visualization techniques we use in the examples that follow. Particular emphasis is placed on explaining the techniques of RadViz™ and Principal Uncorrelated Record Selection (PURS), which have been developed by the authors.

Machine Learning Techniques

Classification techniques vary from simple testing of sample features for statistical significance to sophisticated probabilistic modeling techniques. The supervised learning techniques used in the following examples include Naïve Bayes, support vector machines, instance-based learning (K-nearest neighbor), logistic regression, and neural networks. Much of the work presented in the following examples utilizes the supervised learning method. However, some instances of unsupervised hierarchical clustering using Pearson correlations are also shown. There are many excellent texts giving detailed descriptions of the implementations and use of these techniques.[4]

Feature Reduction Techniques

In machine learning, a data set is usually represented as a flat file or table consisting of m rows and n columns. A row is also called a record, a case, or an n-dimensional data point. The n columns are the "dimensions", "features", "attributes", or "variables" of the data points. One of the dimensions is typically the "class" label used in supervised learning. Machine learning classifiers do best when the number of dimensions is small (less than 100) and the number of data points is large (greater than 1000). Unfortunately, in many biochemical data sets, the number of dimensions is large (e.g., 30,000 genes) and the number of data points is small (e.g., 50 patient samples). The first task is to reduce the dimensions or features of the data set so that machine learning techniques can be used effectively. There are a number of statistical approaches to feature reductions that are quite useful. These include the application of pairwise t and F statistics to select the features that best discriminate among classes.

A more sophisticated approach is one we call Principal Uncorrelated Record Selection (PURS). PURS is a technique that limits the amount of correlation among selected features. It can be used to reduce the complete set of features to a subset that incorporates the major differences in the feature space, or it can be used to reduce a preselected set of "significant" features to a subset that incorporates representatives of all the classes and important subclasses. PURS is initialized with a correlation parameter, a subset (possibly all) of the features, and one or more seed features in the selection set. At each step, features that correlate highly with any feature in the current selection set (i.e., with correlation higher than the correlation parameter) are deleted. One of the remaining features is then chosen for addition to the selection set. This new feature may be chosen randomly from those that remain, or based on an initial statistical, biological, or chemically relevant rank ordering of features. The process is repeated until there are no features remaining to be considered for possible addition to the selection set. The value of the correlation parameter will determine the size of the final selection set of features. The desired result is a small set of features, capturing the most relevant variability in the data and limiting redundancy.

Validation Techniques

Perhaps the most significant challenge in the application of machine learning to biological data is the problem of validation, or the task of determining the expected error rate from a classifier when applied to a new data set. The data used to create a model cannot be used to predict the performance of that model on other data sets. In order to evaluate the external validity of a given model, the features selected as important for classification must be tested against a different data set, one that was not used in the creation of the original classifier. An easy solution to this problem is to divide the data into a training set and a test set. However, since biological data are usually expensive to acquire, large data sets, sufficient to allow this subdivision and still have the statistical power to generalize knowledge from the training set, are hard to find. In order to overcome this problem, a common machine learning technique called 10-fold cross-validation is sometimes used. This approach divides the data into 10 groups, creates the model using 9 of the groups, and then tests it on the remaining group. This procedure is repeated in an iterative fashion until each of the 10 groups has served as a test group. The 10 error estimates are then averaged to give an overall sense of the predictive power of the classification technique on that data set.

Another technique used to help predict performance in limited data sets is an extension of the 10-fold validation idea called "leave-one-out" validation. In this technique, one data point is left out of each of the iterations of model creation and is subsequently used to test the model. This is repeated until every data point in the data set has been used once as test data. This approach is unbiased by the class distribution within the data as compared to 10-fold cross-validation, which requires the careful random stratification of the 10 groups. In contrast to the 10-fold approach, however, it does not give as useful a characterization of the accuracy of the model for some distributions of classes within the data sets.

High-Dimensional Visualization

Although there are a number of conventional visualizations that can help in understanding the correlation of a small number of dimensions to an attribute, high-dimensional visualizations have been difficult to understand and use because of the potential loss of information that occurs in projecting high-dimensional data down to a two- or three-dimensional representation.

There are numerous visualizations and a good number of valuable taxonomies of visual techniques.[5] The authors frequently make use of many different visualization techniques in the analysis of biological data, especially matrices of scatterplots,[6] heatmaps,[6] parallel coordinates,[7] RadViz™,[8] and principal component analysis (PCA).[9] Only RadViz™, however, is uniquely capable of dealing with ultrahigh-dimensional (>10,000 dimensions) data sets, and very useful when used interactively in conjunction with specific machine learning and statistical techniques to explore the dimensions critical for accurate classification.

RadViz™ is a visualization, classification, and clustering tool that uses a spring analogy for placement of data points, while incorporating machine learning and feature reduction techniques as selectable algorithms. The "force" that any dimension exerts on a sample point is determined by Hooke's law: $f = kd$. The spring constant, k, ranging from 0.0 to 1.0, is the value of the scaled dimension for that sample, and d is the distance between the sample point and the perimeter point on the RadViz™ circle assigned to that feature. The placement point of a sample is the point where the total vector force, determined from all features, is zero.

In the RadViz™ layout illustrated in FIGURE 1, there are 15 variables or dimensions associated with the one data point plotted; an addition dimension is used to color and/or shape the data points. Fifteen imaginary springs are anchored to the points on the circumference and attached to this one data point. In this example, the spring constants (or dimensional values) are higher for the darker springs and lower for the lighter springs. Normally, many data points are plotted without showing the spring lines. The values of the dimensions are normalized to be between 0 and 1 so that all dimensions have "equal" weights. This spring paradigm layout has some interesting features:

- it is intuitive—higher-dimension values "pull" the data points closer to that dimension on the circumference;
- points with approximately equal dimension values will lie close to the center;
- points with a balanced pattern of high and low values around the circle will also lie near the center;
- points that have one- or two-dimension values greater than the others lie closer to those dimensions in the display;
- the relative locations of the dimension anchor points can drastically affect the layout;
- a line in *n*-dimensional space is mapped to a line (or single point) in RadViz™;
- convex sets in *n*-space map into convex sets in RadViz™.

The RadViz™ display combines the *n* data dimensions into a single point for the purpose of clustering. It should be noted that many points in *n*-space will map to the

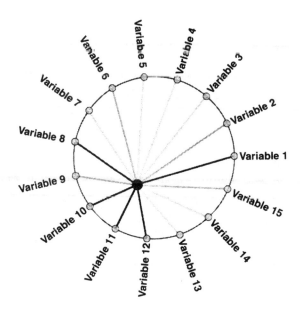

FIGURE 1. One point with 15 dimensions in RadViz™. Spring lines (not usually shown) are colored by value (k) for that variable (dark is higher, light is lower). The point is plotted where the sum of the forces is zero. Since variables 10, 11, and 12 have higher values (scaled to between 0 and 1), the point is pulled closer to those variables around the circumference of the circle.

same position on the RadViz™ display. This represents a nonlinear transformation of the data that preserves certain symmetries and produces an intuitive display. In addition, RadViz™ also integrates analytic embedded algorithms in order to intelligently select and radially arrange the dimensional axes. This arrangement is performed through a set of algorithmic procedures based upon a dimension's statistical significance, which optimizes clustering by maximizing the distance separating clusters of points. The default arrangement is to have all dimensions equally spaced around the perimeter of the circle. However, the feature reduction and class discrimination algorithms subsequently optimize the arrangement of features in order to increase the separation of different classes of sample points. The feature reduction technique used in the present work is based on the t statistic with Bonferroni correction for multiple tests. The RadViz™ circle is divided into n equal sectors or "pie slices", one for each class. Features assigned to a class are spaced evenly within a sector in a counterclockwise order with respect to statistical significance. For a 3-class problem, features are assigned to class 1 based on the sample's t statistic that compares class 1 samples with class 2 and 3 samples combined. Class 2 features are assigned based on the t statistic comparing class 2 values with class 1 and 3 values combined, and class 3 features are assigned based on the t statistic comparing class 3 values with class 1 and class 2 combined. Occasionally, when large portions of the perimeter of the circle have no features assigned to them, the data points would all cluster on the opposite side of the circle, pulled by the unbalanced force of the features present in the other sectors. In this case, a variation of the spring force calculation is used where the features present are effectively divided into qualitatively different forces comprising high and low k value classes. This is done by requiring k to range from -1.0 to 1.0. The net effect is to make some of the features "pull" (high or $+k$ values) and others "push" (low or $-k$ values) the points within the RadViz™ display space, while still maintaining their relative point separations.

The t statistic significance test is a standard method for feature reduction in machine learning approaches. RadViz™ has this machine learning feature embedded in it and is responsible for the selections carried out here. The advantage of RadViz™ is that one immediately sees a "visual" clustering of the results of the t statistic selection. Generally, the amount of visual class separation correlates to the accuracy of any classifier built from a reduced feature set. The additional advantage of this visualization technique is that subclusters, outliers, and misclassified points can quickly and easily be seen in this unique graphical display. One of the standard techniques to visualize clusters or class labels is to perform a PCA and show the points in a two- or three-dimensional scatterplot using the first few principal components as axes. Often, this display shows clear class separation, but the most important features contributing to the PCA are not easily determined as the PCA axes represent a linear combination of the original feature set. RadViz™ is a "visual" classifier that can help one understand important features and how these features are related within the original feature space, thus preserving the domain-dependent context of significantly correlated features and maximizing the scientific insight to be derived from the analysis.

APPLICATIONS

A Classifier for Detection of Ovarian Cancer Using Proteomic Data

Introduction to the Proteomics Problem

It is less than a decade since the term proteomics was suggested to describe genome-wide protein expression. Traditionally, much of the differential proteome expression (disease versus normal state) has been analyzed by two-dimensional polyacrylamide gel electrophoresis (2D-PAGE) on immobilized pH gradients and visualized by staining. The differentially expressed proteins were identified using mass spectrometry. Despite its utility, there are several disadvantages. In recent times, in the quest for rapid identification of biomarkers for early-stage disease detection, mass spectrometry has been adopted as a method of choice for its higher sensitivity and high-throughput capabilities.[10] The two most widely used ionization techniques in mass spectrometry in the area of biological application are electron spray ionization and matrix-assisted laser desorption/ionization (MALDI), permitting almost any high-molecular-weight, nonvolatile, and thermally labile compound to be converted into a gas-phase ion. SELDI-TOF is a type of mass spectrometry that combines on-chip fractionation of a biological fluid sample, or cell lysates, with MALDI. Subsequent time-of-flight (TOF) separation then yields distinct proteomic patterns.

The segregation of these unique signature patterns between disease versus normal samples can be very instructive in the identification of biomarkers for disease.

Machine learning and high-dimensional visualization techniques have been shown to be extremely valuable in deciphering these complex spectral patterns. In the original studies, on the use of proteomic patterns in serum to identify ovarian cancers, combinations of genetic algorithms (GA) and Kohonen self-organizing maps (SOM) were used.[11] Similarly, a predictive model on the diagnostic potential from such spectral signatures for prostate cancer has been derived using a decision tree algorithm.[12,13] A neural net implementation of proteomic pattern data on SELDI chips for human tumors was reported by Ball.[14] Unified Maximum Separability Analysis (UMSA) algorithm successfully extracted the unique serum biomarker pattern for breast cancer using affinity-based SELDI.[15]

The specific goal of this project was to classify patients with ovarian cancer on the basis of their SELDI-TOF mass spectroscopy signature derived from patients' whole sera after processing on the Ciphergen (Fremont, CA) WCX2 protein array. The methods for data collection and the general approach as described by Petricoin is the first documented attempt at applying machine learning techniques to the analysis of clinical proteomic data.[11] The data set used here is not the same as in the original paper, but a similar one labeled 8-07-02, provided by the authors.[16] The authors indicate that this data set is less variable than the original data as a result of using an improved protein chip coupled with totally automated processing by a robotic instrument.

The data consist of over 15,000 mass-charge ratio (m/z) intensity measures, below the 20,000 m/z range, on 253 patient samples: 162 of these samples were from patients with ovarian cancer and 91 were from controls. The major objective was to select a set of m/z values that best distinguish cancer cases from controls. Since the number of features is much larger than the number of samples, it is important to do this in a principled manner to avoid classifying on the basis of noise.

Two aspects of this data set pose interesting technical challenges in its analysis. The first is the low signal-to-noise ratio (S/N) associated with many of the features, and the second is the high degree of correlation between different features. There are at least two sources of correlation. One, illustrated in FIGURE 2 for m/z ratios near 417, is the high correlation between neighboring features in the vicinity of a peak. Such correlation may be due to the inherent resolution limitations of the instrumentation in resolving two adjacent peaks when separated by less than some minimum spectral difference. The other, illustrated in FIGURE 3, is correlation between data at peaks where one m/z ratio is almost exactly half the other m/z ratio. The graph at the right of FIGURE 3 shows the spectrum in the m/z range from 5300 to 10,600, while the left graph shows the range from 2650 to 5300, exactly half the range of the right graph. All of the peaks of the left graph are repeated in the right graph, consistent with molecules with the same mass and twice the charge, suggesting production of doubly ionized forms of the original protein fragments. These figures illustrate the power of visualization for data exploration. Clearly there is a high degree of noise and redundancy in the data. Such data attributes can be problematic for feature reduction and thus reduce the accuracy of the predictive model under development.

Specific Methods Used

Initially, each sample was randomly assigned (with 50% probability) to either a "train" group or a "test" group. This resulted in a training group of 88 ovarian cancer

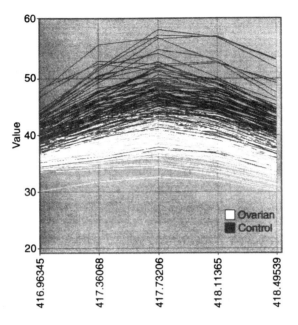

FIGURE 2. This is a parallel coordinate's display of a peak at 417.732 and its closest neighbors. The intensities at nearby *m/z* values are very similar. The correlation between this peak and its two nearest neighbors is about 0.97, and the correlation with the next two neighbors is about 0.91, illustrating one source of redundancy in the data.

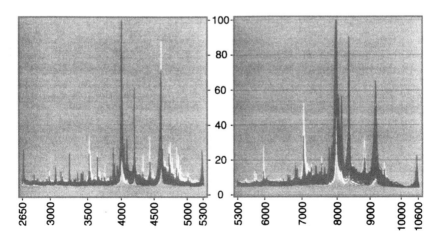

FIGURE 3. The *left graph* shows the portion of the spectrum from *m/z* of 2650 to 5300, while the *right graph* shows the portion from 5300 to 10,600. Thus, the range at the left is exactly half the range at the right. Notice that all peaks in the right graph are repeated in the left graph. This is consistent with molecules with the same mass and twice the charge, suggesting production of doubly ionized forms of the original protein fragments. This is a second source of redundancy in the data.

samples and 49 controls, and a test group of 74 ovarian cancer samples and 42 controls. In order to avoid any influence of test group data on the classification results, all feature reduction and modeling were done on the basis of training group data only.

The first step in feature reduction was to improve the S/N by eliminating all m/z ratios less than 350, as well as those for which the maximum intensity value (in the train group) was less than 17.5. This was done in order to minimize the possibility of choosing a feature based on noise alone and resulted in a reduction from over 15,000 to less than 4000 features. The next step was to perform a t test on the remaining features to determine which features showed a significant difference between cancer patients and controls. We kept features with significance of $P < .001$ after Bonferroni correction for multiple tests. This left over 400 features, many of which were redundant in the sense discussed above.

Simply choosing the most significant 5 or 10 features could incorporate this redundancy into the classifier and could lead to poor performance. In order to address this problem, we applied the PURS feature reduction technique with a correlation parameter of 0.90 and initialized with two features, the most significant feature for each of the two classes. The result was a set of 12 features. We trained two neural network models using SPSS Clementine. One used all 12 features; the other used the top 6 features.

Results and Discussion

Both neural network models classified cancer patients and controls perfectly in both the training and test groups. FIGURE 4 shows a RadViz™ display of the test data, using the 6-feature model, which visually confirms the high degree of discrimination that can be obtained between patients. On the NCI Clinical Proteomics Program Web site, Petricoin *et al.* present a set of 7 m/z values that also result in perfect classification.[16] These were chosen by means of a GA. Our past experience with GA and microarray data has shown us that GA are susceptible to classification by noise. Microarray data are similar to the proteomic data in that the number of features (genes) is far greater than the number of samples. With this level of imbalance, it is possible to find perfect classifiers in randomly generated data. Although having an independent test set helps to weed out the really noisy models, when you consider the number of ways of choosing 7 features out of 15,000 ($>10^{25}$), you begin to see that the chance of finding a set of 7 "good" features is extremely small. At a minimum, features should show a statistically significant difference between the 2 classes. Of the 7 features given on the Web site, 2 are not even marginally significant before correcting for multiple tests. These contribute mostly noise to the classifier. Two or 3 more features would fail our strict $P < .001$ standard after a Bonferroni correction. This is an arbitrary standard; however, since it still leaves more than 400 "good" features, there is no good reason to relax it.

FIGURE 5 shows parallel coordinate displays of the 2 feature sets. On the left are the data for the 7 features given on the Web site. On the right are the data for the 6 features that we selected. Five of the 7 features on the left in FIGURE 5 have very low intensities. We eliminated these in the first step of feature reduction because they failed to reach the 17.5 threshold.

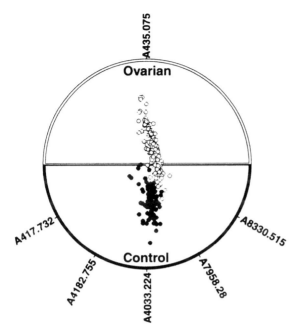

FIGURE 4. This is a RadViz™ class discrimination display of the samples using the 6 selected features. Ovarian cancer samples are shown in *white*. Controls are shown in *black*. The 2 classes are reasonably well separated by these features, indicating that the features can be used for classification. A neural network model based on these 6 features classified both the training set and the test set perfectly.

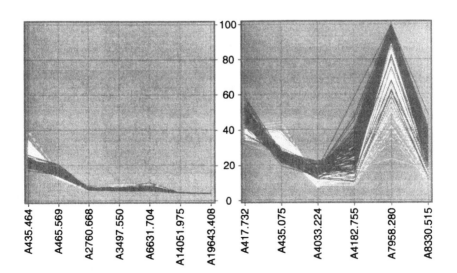

FIGURE 5. On the *left* are the 7 *m/z* ratios selected by Petricoin *et al.* On the *right* are the 6 features selected by the present authors. Data from ovarian cancer patients are displayed in *white*. Data from controls are displayed in *black*. Several of the features on the left have very low intensities. Some, but not all, of the features on the left show visible differences between the 2 groups of samples. There is a significant difference between the 2 groups for all of the features on the right.

Conclusions

It is clear that there are significant differences in proteins in serum between ovarian cancer patients and controls, and that mass spectroscopy is potentially a very useful ovarian cancer detection tool. Because of differences in machines and instrumentation, the applicability of our model to a new data set is an open question. However, by applying intelligent feature reduction to mass spectroscopy data using high-dimensional visualization prior to classification, the development of clinically accurate and useful models for cancer screening and detection using proteomic data should be possible.

A Classifier for the Diagnosis of Lung Cancer Using Gene Expression

Introduction to the High-Throughput Gene Expression Problem

Completion of the Human Genome Project has made possible the study of the gene expression levels of over 30,000 genes.[17,18] Major technological advances have made possible the use of DNA microarrays to speed up this analysis. Even though the first microarray experiment was only published in 1995, by October 2002 a PubMed query of microarray literature yielded more than 2300 hits, indicating explosive growth in the use of this powerful technique.[19] DNA microarrays take advantage of the convergence of a number of technologies and developments, including robotics and miniaturization of features to the micron scale (currently 20–200 μm surface feature sizes for spotting/printing and immobilizing sequences for hybridization experiments), DNA amplification by PCR, automated and efficient oligonucleotide synthesis and labeling chemistries, and sophisticated bioinformatics approaches.

An important application of microarray technology is the identification and differentiation of tissue types using differential gene expressions, either between normal and cancerous cells or among tumor subclasses. The specific aim of this project was to explore the potential for using machine learning and high-dimensional visualization in building a diagnostic classifier that could differentiate normal lung tissue from the various subclasses of non–small cell lung cancer (non-SCLC) using microarray-based differential expression patterns. We have recently reported on using such techniques to successfully construct classifiers that can solve the more general 2-class detection problem of differentiating non-SCLC from normal tissue with accuracy greater than 95%.[20] However, the analysis of the 3-class diagnostic problem of distinguishing normal lung tissue from the 2 subclasses of non-SCL carcinoma (adenocarcinoma and squamous cell carcinoma) was not fully addressed. Our ultimate aim was the creation of gene sets with small number of genes that might serve as the basis for developing a clinically useful diagnostic tool.

In collaboration with the NCI, we examined 2 data sets of patients with and without various lung cancers. The first data set was kindly provided by Dr. Jin Jen of the Laboratory of Population Genetics at the NCI Center for Cancer Research and included 75 patient samples. This set contained 17 normal samples, 30 adeno-carcinomas (6 doubles), and 28 squamous cell carcinomas (2 doubles). Doubles represent replicate samples prepared at different times, using different equipment, but derived from the same tissue sample. A second patient set of 157 samples was obtained from a publically available data repository.[21] This set included 17 normal samples, 139 adenocarcinomas (127 of these with supporting information), and 21 squamous cell carcinomas. Both data sets included gene expression data from tissue samples using Affymetrix's Human Genome U95 Set;[22] only the first of 5 oligonucleotide-based GeneChip® arrays (Chip A) was used in this experiment. Chip A of the HG U95 array set contains roughly 12,000 full-length genes and a number of controls. Because we were dealing with 2 data sets, both from different sources and microarray measurements taken at multiple times, we needed to consider a normalization procedure. For this particular analysis, we kept with a simple mean of 200 for each sample. This resulted in a set of 9918 expressed genes, of which approximately 2000 were found to be statistically significant ($P < .05$) in differentiating normal lung tissue from non-SCLC. This differentially expressed set of genes was then used as the starting point for further analysis as described below.

Specific Methods Used

Because the combinatorial scale of trying all possible gene sets requires a significant amount of time and computational power, we undertook an approach using sample gene sets defined by 3 different gene selection methods. First, we defined and analyzed the results from 10 independent random gene sets drawn from the set of approximately 2000 differentially expressed genes as previously described. These random selections provided a lower predictive bound for each gene set size. Second, we selected only genes that demonstrated high statistical significance by a standard *F* test. Finally, we applied the previously described proprietary RadViz™ technique to identify sets of genes that best distinguish differences among the subclasses of samples. Applying these 3 approaches to the available expression data, we were able to generate gene sets that ranged in size from 1 to 100 genes. The construction of gene sets was accomplished using a collection of custom scripts written in Python.

To evaluate the resulting sets of genes, we applied a collection of predictive algorithms to each gene set using a 10-fold cross-validation testing methodology since an initial comparison of both 10-fold and hold-one-out cross-validation showed that they result in essentially the same predictive accuracy. The predictive algorithms used in this analysis included (but were not limited to) variations on neural networks, support vector machines, Naïve Bayes, and K-nearest neighbors, all implemented using the publically available Weka application program.[23] Throughout our process of evaluating the various gene sets we kept the 2 data sets separate in order to perform and evaluate 2 distinct testing scenarios. First, we used the NCI data set for cross-validation as described above; second, we used the Meyerson data set as an independent validation set.

As a final validation of the biological significance of the genes in our 3-way classifier, we mined the scientific literature for references that associated the selected genes with specific keywords found in association with lung cancer. To aid our analysis, we have used a combination of tools available both in the public domain and directly licensed from academic sources, such as OntoExpress.[24] Briefly Onto-Express assigns GO (gene ontology) terms to gene accession numbers and examines the role of functionally related genes based on hypergeometric distribution of preselected and precalibrated categories of functionally related genes. Typically, a list of differentially expressed genes from a gene expression profiling experiment, or one derived from a predictive model, is mapped to the terminal nodes on the GO hierachy via the Unigene and LocusLink databases. The exploratory environment of DAVID (Database for Annotation, Visualization, and Integrated Discovery) provides some very useful tools for such functional annotation and was extensively used in this analysis.[25] The co-occurrence relationships in the corpus of 11 million MEDLINE literature articles for a given disease term, associated with a specific gene, were determined using InPharmix text mining tools.[26] InPharmix maps the relationships between a human disease and genes associated with that disease, as well as cross-mapping all disease terms associated with genes by generating a co-citation matrix. The rank order of the genes to a given disease term is scored on the basis of nonparametric tests like the chi-square statistic and Fisher's exact test ($\alpha < 0.05$, 1 df).

Results and Discussion

Distinguishing normal and two tumor types. Our analysis of the general 2 class problem for distinguishing between normal lung tissue and non-SCLC samples has been reported elsewhere.[20] Unlike the 2-class problem, however, the 3-class problem is more challenging. This problem involves distinguishing normal lung tissue from 2 subclasses of non-SCLC: adenocarcinoma and squamous cell carcinoma. Our best gene sets performed with an average accuracy of around 88% for the NCI data set and 96% for the Meyerson data set, both resulting in between 8 to 10 misclassifications. As shown in FIGURE 6, sets constructed from genes that are highly significant for the 3-class problem using the F statistic performed better overall than gene sets constructed from randomly selected genes. Also shown in this figure is the fact that the RadViz™ selection method generally outperforms randomly selected genes and genes selected on the basis of high statistical significance using the F test. The

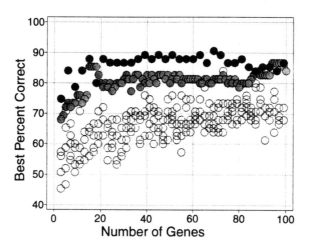

FIGURE 6. Classification results for the NCI data set showing the size of the gene sets compared to their associated best percent correct. Notice how the RadViz™ algorithm selected genes (*black*) generally perform better than either the top F statistic genes (*gray*) or the randomly selected genes (*white*). As the gene set sizes increased from 1 to about 20 genes, there was a shared increase in classification accuracy. In addition, as more random genes are selected, their associated performance increases.

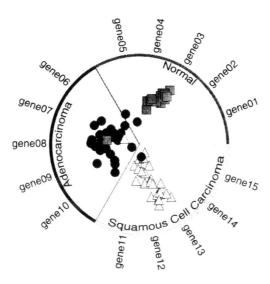

FIGURE 7. A RadViz™ display showing an example of a selected set of 15 genes from the Meyerson data set defined by a balanced layout for the 3 classes: normal (*gray squares*), adenocarcinoma (*black circles*), and squamous cell carcinoma (*white triangles*). Ideally, the patient samples displayed by their associated representative glyph should fall within their respective regions; however, some samples clearly fall into other regions, thus being visually misclassified. This particular gene set performs very well with about 6 misclassifications visually. After applying our collection of classification algorithms, this gene set performed with 8 misclassifications.

RadViz™ display for the 3-class problem as shown in FIGURE 7 clearly demonstrates near perfect discrimination between normal lung tissue and the 2 non-SCLC subclasses using as few as 15 genes.

Identification of problematic samples. Besides examining the classification results for each gene set independently, we looked at the consistency of classification of samples across gene sets using different machine learning algorithms as previously described. Surprisingly, we identified a few samples in both data sets that were consistently misclassified. FIGURE 8 shows an example visualization of the results of the various classification algorithms (displayed horizontally) for each sample (displayed vertically) within the NCI data set. The 2 continuous vertical lines, which are readily visible, represent 2 samples that have been consistently misclassified by all the classification algorithms. Although it appears likely that these samples were improperly labeled, we had no supporting information for these patients and thus could not clinically validate these findings. In contrast, upon analysis of the Meyerson data set, we were able to identify 6 misclassified patients. After reviewing these patients' supporting information, we found that 2 of these samples consisted of mixed tissue types and that the classification algorithms caught this clinical anomaly.

Validation using biological relevance. Biological validation of any set of predictor genes, resulting from the analysis of gene expression data, is paramount in developing

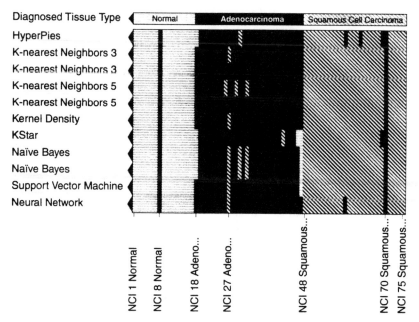

FIGURE 8. Example classification results for a selected set of genes aimed at distinguishing NCI patient samples, displayed here using the PatchGrid visualization technique. The top row identifies the diagnosed tissue types for the NCI samples, which are presented vertically and sorted by the 3 types: normal (*horizontal strips*), adenocarcinoma (*solid*), and squamous cell carcinoma (*diagonal strips*). Sample misclassifications for 1 of the 11 classification algorithms, listed vertically on the left, are represented as short vertical bars that are displayed using the appropriately misclassified tissue type. Notice how we can clearly see 2 continuous vertical bars: one under normal and the other under squamous cell carcinoma; these represent 2 samples that have been misclassified by all the classification algorithms and indicate samples that either contain mixed tissue types or have been misdiagnosed.

reliable and reproducible disease markers if these predictive gene sets are to be adapted for routine clinical diagnostics. One useful approach to validation is through establishing the biological relevance of selected gene sets through text mining the vast corpus of biomedical literature that has been electronically captured in vast public databases like MEDLINE. The last few years have witnessed a great deal of interest in mining literature to extract protein-protein interaction[27] or extract relationships between genes, proteins, drugs, and other molecular entities.[28] InPharmix maps the relationships between a human disease and genes associated with that disease. Our analysis in the 15-gene model has yielded that adenocarcinoma was significantly ($P < .05$) associated with von Willebrand's factor (VWF), followed by fibroblast activation protein, alpha (FAP1), and collagen type XI/alpha 1 (COLL11A1) in decreasing order of statistical significance. Surprisingly, squamous cell carcinoma was also associated with VWF, albeit with a significantly lower P value ($<.0001$) than that previously discussed for its association with adenocarcinoma. Melanoma antigen, family D,1 (MAGED1) was found to be only slightly less significant for squamous cell carcinoma when ranked in a similar fashion. It must be cautioned that text mining has its own pitfalls when the context in which these terms are evaluated is not stringently set.

While a substantial amount of biomedical knowledge is recorded in the free-text form, there is a strong need for developing controlled vocabularies for gene annotation. GO consortium has been involved in these efforts. GO is a hierarchical set of codes organized across three broad categories: molecular function, cellular location, and biological process. Gene sets in several of our predictive models have been mapped to GO terms in an attempt to extract relationships of gene sets to defined molecular function and biological processes. The 15-gene model in our 3-class classification mapped to some of the processes that have been shown to be directly involved in the progression of lung cancer, namely, oncogenesis and induction of apoptosis ($P < 5.00E-3$), and thus lend a degree of significant biological validation to our model. The DAVID tools permit semantic mappings to be obtained at different depths within the GO hierachy. Interestingly, when physiological processes are chosen as the top level node within GO, 60% of the probes map to disruption of the cellular hemostasis and <26% map to developmental processes. Furthermore, the genes in "binding" function outscored other molecular functions, even when thresholds were set fairly high. Although general and indirect, this functional evidence is consistent with alterations in the physiological processes know to be associated with neoplastic transformation.

Conclusions

This microarray high-throughput gene expression example demonstrates the usefulness of the machine learning and high-dimensional visualization approach to the identification of genes that may play a significant role in the pathogenesis of non-SCLC. We have shown that the RadViz™ technique is extremely useful in identifying genes with significant differential gene expression that can be used as the basis for a clinically useful and accurate diagnostic model incorporating measurements from as few as 15 genes. Our validation of the various gene sets we constructed and tested included the use of domain knowledge in an attempt to support the biological relevance of the selected gene set on the basis of literature references that associated the selected genes with lung cancer. Finally, we have provided the basis for a comprehensive pipeline-based microarray analysis system incorporating the selection, evaluation, and relevance of genes for multiclass problems in cancer diagnosis.

Mining the NCI Cancer Cell Line GI$_{50}$ Database for Chemical Knowledge

Introduction to the Cheminformatics Problem

Important objectives in the overall process of molecular design for drug discovery are (1) the ability to represent and identify important structural features of any small molecule and (2) to select useful molecular structures for further study, usually using linear quantitative structure activity relationship (QSAR) models and based upon simple partitioning of the structures in n-dimensional space. To date, partitioning using nonlinear QSAR models has not been widespread, but the complexity and high-dimensionality of the typical data set require them. The machine learning and visualization techniques that we describe and utilize here represent an ideal set of methodologies with which to approach representing structural features of small molecules, followed by selecting molecules via constructing and applying nonlinear QSAR models. QSAR models might typically use calculated chemical descriptors of compounds along with computed or experimentally determined compound physical properties and interaction parameters (ΔG, Ka, kf, kr, LD_{50}, GI_{50}, etc.) with other large molecules or whole cells. Thermodynamic and kinetic parameters are usually generated *in silico* (ΔG) or via high-throughput screening of compound libraries against appropriate receptors or important signaling pathway macro-molecules (Ka, kf, kr), whereas the LD_{50} or GI_{50} values are typically generated using whole cells that are suitable for the disease model being investigated. When the data have been generated, then the application of machine learning can take place. We provide a sample illustration of this process below that has potential relevance to the selection of optimal chemotherapy for the clinical management of cancer patients.

The NCI's Developmental Therapeutics Program maintains a compound data set (~500,000 compounds) that is currently being systematically tested for cytotoxicity in generating 50% growth inhibition (GI_{50}) against a panel of 60 cancer cell lines representing 9 clinically defined tissue types. Therefore, this data set contains a wealth of valuable information concerning potential cancer drug pharmacophores. In a data mining study of the 8 largest public domain chemical structure databases, it was observed that the NCI compound data set contained by far the largest number of unique compounds of all the databases.[29] The application of sophisticated machine learning techniques to this unique NCI compound data set represents an important open problem that motivated the investigation we present in this report. Previously, this data set has been mined by supervised learning techniques such as cluster correlation, PCA, and various neural networks, as well as statistical techniques.[30,31] These approaches have identified distinct subsets within a variety of different classes of chemical compounds.[32–35] More recently, gene expression analysis has been added to the data mining activity of the NCI compound data set[36] to predict chemosensitivity, using the GI_{50} test data for each compound, for a few hundred compound subset of the NCI data set.[37] After we completed our initial data mining analysis using the GI_{50} values,[38] gene expression data on the 60 cancer cell lines were combined with NCI compound GI_{50} data and also with a 27,000 chemical feature database computed for the NCI compounds.[39]

In this study, we use microarray-based gene expression data to first establish a number of "functional" classes of the 60 cancer cell lines via a hierarchical clustering technique. These functional classes are then used as class labels in supervising a 3-class learning problem, using a small, but complete subset of 1400 of the NCI compounds' GI_{50} values as the input to a clustering algorithm using the RadViz™ technique. We then identify 2 unique subsets of derivatized quinone compounds: one effective against melanoma, the other against leukemia cell lines.

Specific Methods Used

For the ~4% missing values found in the 1400 compound data set, we tried and compared two approaches to missing value replacement: (1) record average replace-ment; (2) multiple imputation using Schafer's NORM software.[40] Since applying either missing value replacement method to our data had little impact on the final results of our analysis, we chose the record average replacement method for all subsequent analysis.

Clustering of cell lines was done with R-Project software using the hierarchical clustering algorithm with "average" linkage method specified and a dissimilarity matrix computed from (1 – the Pearson correlations) of the gene expression data. The RadViz™ technique was used for feature reduction and initial classification of the cell lines based on the compound GI_{50} data. The selected features were validated using several classifiers as implemented in the Weka software application program.[23] The classifiers used were IB1 (first nearest neighbor), IB3 (three nearest neighbors), logistic regression, Naïve Bayes Classifier, support vector machines, and neural network with back-propagation. Both ChemOffice 2000 (CambridgeSoft Corp.) and the NCI Web site were used to identify compound structures via their NSC numbers. Substructure searching to identify quinone compounds in the larger data set was carried out using ChemFinder ultra 7.0 (CambridgeSoft Corp.).

Results and Discussion

Identifying functional cancer cell line classes using gene expression data. Based on gene expression data, we identified cancer cell line classes that we could use in a subsequent supervised learning approach. In FIGURE 9, we present a hierarchical clustering dendrogram using the (1 – Pearson) distances calculated from the 1376 gene expression values determined for the 60 NCI cancer cell lines.[41] There are 5 well-defined clusters observed in this figure. Clusters 2–5 respectively represent pure renal, leukemia, ovarian, and colon rectal cancer cell lines. Only in cluster 1, the melanoma class instance, does the class contain 2 members of another clinical tumor type—the 2 breast cancer cell lines, MDA-MB-435 and MDA-N. The 2 breast

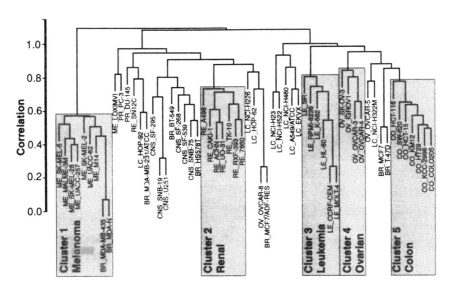

FIGURE 9. Cancer cell line functional class definition using a hierarchical clustering (1 – Pearson coefficient) dendrogram for 60 cancer cell lines based upon gene expression data. Five well-defined clusters are shown highlighted. We treat the highlighted cell line clusters as the truth for the purpose of carrying out studies to identify which chemical compounds are highly significant in their classifying ability.

cancer cell lines behave functionally as melanoma cells and seem to be related to melanoma cell lines via a shared neuroendocrine origin.[41] The remaining cell lines in this dendrogram, those not found in any of the 5 functional classes, are defined as being in a sixth class: the non–melanoma, leukemia, renal, ovarian, colorectal class. In the supervised learning analyses that follow, we treat these 6 computationally derived functional clusters as ground truth.

3-Class cancer cell line classifications and validation of selected compounds. High class number classification problems are difficult to implement in cases where the data are not clearly separable into distinct classes. Thus, we could not successfully carry out a 6-class classification of cancer cell lines based upon the starting GI_{50} compound data. Alternatively, we implemented a 3-class supervised learning classification using RadViz™.[8,42,43] Starting with the small 1400 compounds' GI_{50} data set that contained no missing values for all 60 cell lines, we selected those compounds that were effective in carrying out a 3-way class discrimination at the $P < .01$ (Bonferroni corrected t statistic) significance level. A RadViz™ visual classifier for

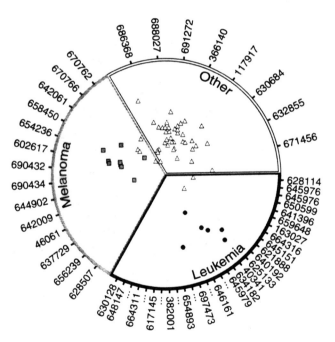

FIGURE 10. RadViz™ result for the 3-class problem of classification of melanoma (*gray squares*), leukemia (*black circles*), and other [nonmelanoma/nonleukemia] (*white triangles*) cancer cell types at the $P < .01$ criterion. Cell lines are symbol coded as previously described and appear inside the circle. Compounds are numerically coded and appear around the circumference of the circle. A total of 14 compounds (*left side of layout*) were most effective against melanoma and are displayed on the melanoma sector (counterclockwise from most to least effective). For leukemia (*bottom of layout*), 30 compounds were identified as most effective and are displayed in that sector. Some 8 compounds (*top of layout*) were found to be most effective against other [nonmelanoma/nonleukemia] cell lines and are displayed in that sector.

the melanoma, leukemia, and other (nonmelanoma/nonleukemia) classes is shown in FIGURE 10. A clear and accurate class separation of the 60 cancer cell lines can be seen. There were 14 compounds selected as being most effective against melanoma cells and 30 compounds selected as being most effective against leukemia cells. Similar classification results were obtained for the 2 separate 2-class problems: melanoma vs. nonmelanoma and leukemia vs. nonleukemia. For all other possible 2-class problems, we found that few to no compounds could be selected at the significance level we had previously set.

In order to validate our list of computationally selected compounds, we applied 6 additional analytical classification techniques, as previously described, to the original GI_{50} data set using the same set of chemical predictors and a hold-one-out cross-validation strategy. Using these selected compounds resulted in a greater than 6-fold lowered level of error compared to using the equivalent numbers of randomly selected compounds, thus validating our selection methodology.

Quinone compound subtypes. Upon examining the chemical identity of the compounds selected as most effective against melanoma and leukemia, an interesting observation was made. For the 14 compounds selected as most effective against melanoma, 11 were *p*-quinones and all have an internal ring quinone structure as shown in FIGURE 11A. Alternatively, there were 30 compounds selected as most effective against leukemia, of which 8 contain *p*-quinones. In contrast to the internal ring quinones in the melanoma class, however, 6 out of the 8 leukemia *p*-quinones were external ring quinones as shown in FIGURE 11B. In order to ascertain the uniqueness of the 2 quinone subsets, we first determined the extent of occurrence of *p*-quinones of all types in our starting data set via substructure searching using the ChemFinder 7.0 ultra software. The internal and external quinone subtypes represent a significant fraction: 25% (10/41) of all the internal quinones and 40% (6/15) of all the external quinones in the entire data set.[38]

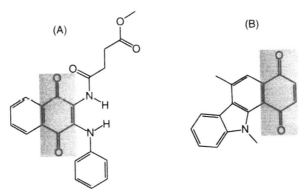

FIGURE 11. (A) Quinones effective against melanoma cell lines are of the "internal" type, where the quinone ring (*highlighted*) is flanked by either adjacent fused ring structures or ortho- and/or meta-substituents in the molecule. The example shown, NSC 670762, is the most potent compound in this class. **(B)** Quinones effective against leukemia cell lines are of the "external" type, where the quinone ring is terminally positioned in the molecule. The most potent member of this class, NSC 648147, is shown.

Conclusions

With this cheminformatics example, we have demonstrated that the machine learning approach described above utilizing RadViz™ has produced 2 novel discoveries. First, a small group of chemical compounds, enriched in quinones, were found to effectively discriminate among melanoma, leukemia, and other (nonmelanoma/nonleukemia) cell lines on the basis of experimentally measured GI_{50} values. Second, 2 quinone subtypes were identified that possess clearly different and specific toxicity to the leukemia and melanoma cancer cell types. We believe that this example illustrates the potential of sophisticated machine learning approaches to uncovering new and valuable relationships in complex high-dimensional chemical compound data sets that may have relevance for the clinical management of cancer patients on chemotherapy.

CONCLUDING REMARKS

In this paper, we have discussed and shown by way of 3 heterogeneous examples the applicability of machine learning and high-dimensional visualization in providing clinically useful knowledge concerning the underlying molecular etiology of cancer. Using proteomic, genomic, and chemical data, respectively, we derive classifiers that can be used in cancer detection, diagnosis, and management.

In the first example, proteomic data from patient sera were analyzed to derive a unique mass spectrometry signature that could differentiate patients with ovarian cancer from normal healthy individuals. Unlike known biomarkers, commonly used in cancer detection, the identity of the proteins comprising this unique signature is currently unknown. Still, the 2-class model previously described provides a clinically useful screening tool for ovarian cancer detection using just 6 features.

In the second example, we show how exploratory data analysis techniques can be used to construct a 3-class predictive model for lung cancer which can differentiate between normal lung tissue and 2 subclasses of non–small cell carcinoma. Although such a model can also be used to detect the presence of lung cancer, independent of subclass, its real value is as a diagnostic tool in distinguishing squamous cell carcinoma from adenocarcinoma. The ability to firmly establish a cancer diagnosis, at the subclass level, may have important prognostic as well as therapeutic implications. Unlike the previous example, the sequences of the 15 predictor genes used to construct this model are known. In many cases, as our biological validation has shown, the functions of these genes are also known, providing valuable knowledge about the underlying molecular mechanisms involved in neoplastic development.

Finally, our last example using the NCI 60 cancer cell line GI_{50} compound database illustrates how cell-specific cytotoxicity relates to compound structure. We have shown how our exploratory approach to data analysis resulted in the discovery of new knowledge regarding the substructural elements responsible for the differential cytotoxicity exhibited between melanoma and leukemia in response to various chemical compounds. Such knowledge can provide useful insight into the clinical management of cancer patients undergoing chemotherapy.

Although this paper has dealt exclusively with the application of data mining and high-dimensional visualization to cancer biology at a molecular level, recent advances in biomedical informatics and clinical data management will soon make possible the inclusion of clinical and epidemiological data as additional model dimensions. Applying the exploratory approaches discussed in this paper to such high-dimensional data sets should bring us one step closer to understanding and successfully dealing with cancer as a major public health issue.

ACKNOWLEDGMENTS

AnVil, Inc., and the authors gratefully acknowledge support from two SBIR Phase I grants (R43 CA94429-01 and R43 CA096179-01) from the National Cancer Institute. We also wish to thank Dr. Jin Jen and Dr. Tatiana Dracheva, from the NCI Laboratory of Population Genetics, for allowing us to use their microarray data on lung cancer in this study.

REFERENCES

1. SIKORA, K. 1999. Developing a global strategy for cancer. Eur. J. Cancer **35:** 1870–1877.
2. BAAK, J.P. *et al.* 2003. Genomics and proteomics in cancer. Eur. J. Cancer **39:** 1199–1215.
3. HAQUE, S. *et al.* 2002. Advances in biomedical informatics for the management of cancer. Ann. N.Y. Acad. Sci. **980:** 287–297.
4. WITTEN, I.H. & E. FRANK. 2000. Data Mining: Practical Machine Learning Tools and Techniques with Java Implementations. Morgan Kaufmann. San Francisco.
5. SHNEIDERMAN, B. 1996. The eyes have it: a task by data type taxonomy of information visualization. Presented at the IEEE Symposium on Visual Languages '96, Boulder, CO.
6. TUKEY, J.W. 1977. Exploratory Data Analysis. Addison–Wesley. Reading, MA.
7. INSELBERG, A. 1985. The plane with parallel coordinates. Special Issue on Computational Geometry: The Visual Computer **1:** 69–91.
8. HOFFMAN, P. & G. GRINSTEIN. 1999. Dimensional anchors: a graphic primitive for multidimensional multivariate information visualizations. Presented at the Workshop on New Paradigms in Information Visualization and Manipulation (NPIV '99).
9. HOTELLING, H. 1933. Analysis of a complex of statistical variables into principal components. J. Educ. Psychol. **24:** 417–441, 498–520.
10. WULFKUHLE, J.D., L.A. LIOTTA & E.F. PETRICOIN. 2003. Proteomic applications for the early detection of cancer. Nat. Rev. Cancer **3:** 267–275.
11. PETRICOIN, E.F. *et al.* 2002. Use of proteomic patterns in serum to identify ovarian cancer. Lancet **359:** 572–577.
12. BANEZ, L.L. *et al.* 2003. Diagnostic potential of serum proteomic patterns in prostate cancer. J. Urol. **170:** 442–446.
13. ADAM, B.L. *et al.* 2002. Serum protein fingerprinting coupled with a pattern-matching algorithm distinguishes prostate cancer from benign prostate hyperplasia and healthy men. Cancer Res. **62:** 3609–3614.
14. BALL, G. *et al.* 2002. An integrated approach utilizing artificial neural networks and SELDI mass spectrometry for the classification of human tumors and rapid identification of potential biomarkers. Bioinformatics **18:** 395–404.
15. LI, J. *et al.* 2002. Proteomics and bioinformatics approaches for identification of serum biomarkers to detect breast cancer. Clin. Chem. **48:** 1296–1304.
16. NCI. 2003. NCI Clinical Proteomics Web Site [http://clinicalproteomics.steem.com/download-ovar.php/].
17. VENTER, J.C. *et al.* 2001. The sequence of the human genome. Science **291:** 1303–1351.
18. LANDER, E.S. *et al.* 2001. Initial sequencing and analysis of the human genome. Nature **409:** 860–921.
19. STOECKERT, C.J. *et al.* 2002. Microarray databases: standards and ontologies. Nat. Genet. **32:** 469–473.

20. JEN, J. *et al.* 2004. Distinguishing lung tumors based on small number of genes using flow-through-chips. In preparation.
21. MATTHEW MEYERSON LAB, DANA-FARBER CANCER INSTITUTE. 2003. http://research.dfci.harvard.edu/meyersonlab/lungca/data.html/.
22. AFFYMETRIX, INC. (SANTA CLARA, CA). 2003. http://www.affymetrix.com/.
23. WEKA (WAIKATO ENVIRONMENT FOR KNOWLEDGE ANALYSIS), UNIVERSITY OF WAIKATO. 2003. http://www.cs.waikato.ac.nz/~ml/.
24. KHATRI, P. *et al.* 2003. Profiling gene expression using OntoExpress. Genomics **79**: 1–5.
25. DENNIS, G., JR. *et al.* 2003. Database for annotation, visualization, and integrated discovery. Genome Biol. **4**: 3–14.
26. INPHARMIX DATABASE. 2003. http://www.inpharmix.com/.
27. JENSSEN, T. *et al.* 2001. A literature network of human genes for high-throughput analysis of gene expression. Nat. Genet. **28**: 21–28.
28. RINDFLESCH, T.C. *et al.* 2000. EDGAR: extraction of drugs, genes, and relations from biomedical literature. Pac. Symp. Biocomput. **5**: 517–528.
29. VOIGT, K. & R. BRUGGEMAN. 1995. Toxicology databases in the metadatabank on online databases. Toxicology **100**: 225–240.
30. WEINSTEIN, J.N. *et al.* 1997. An information-intensive approach to the molecular pharmacology of cancer. Science **275**: 343–349.
31. SHI, L.M. *et al.* 2000. Mining and visualizing large anticancer drug discovery databases. J. Chem. Inf. Comput. Sci. **40**: 367–379.
32. BAI, R.L. *et al.* 1991. Halichondrin B and homohalichondrin B, marine natural products binding in the vinca domain of tubulin: discovery of tubulin-based mechanism of action by analysis of differential cytotoxicity data. J. Biol. Chem. **266**: 15882–15889.
33. CLEVELAND, E.S. *et al.* 1995. Site of action of two novel ramidine biosynthesis inhibitors accurately predicted by COMPARE program. Biochem. Pharmacol. **49**: 947–954.
34. GUPTA, M. *et al.* 1995. Eukaryotic DNA topoisomerases mediated DNA cleavage induced by new inhibitor: NSC 665517. Mol. Pharmacol. **48**: 658–665.
35. SHI, L.M. *et al.* 1998. Mining the National Cancer Institute Anticancer Drug Discovery Database: cluster analysis of ellipticine analogs with p53-inverse and central nervous system–selective patterns of activity. Mol. Pharmacol. **53**: 241–251.
36. ROSS, D.T. *et al.* 2000. Systematic variation of gene expression patterns in human cancer cell lines. Nat. Genet. **24**: 227–235.
37. STAUNTON, J.E. *et al.* 2001. Chemosensitivity prediction by transcriptional profiling. Proc. Natl. Acad. Sci. USA **98**: 10787–10792.
38. MARX, K.A. *et al.* 2003. Data mining the NCI cancer cell line compound GI_{50} values: identifying quinone subtypes effective against melanoma and leukemia cell classes. J. Chem. Inf. Comput. Sci. **43**: 1652–1667.
39. BLOWER, P.E. *et al.* 2002. Pharmacogenomic analysis: correlating molecular substructure classes with microarray gene expression data. Pharmacogenomics J. **2**: 259–271.
40. SCHAFER, J.L. 1997. Analysis of Incomplete Multivariate Data. No. 72 of Monographs on Statistics and Applied Probability. Chapman & Hall/CRC. London.
41. SCHERF, W. *et al.* 2000. A gene expression database for the molecular pharmacology of cancer. Nature **24**: 236–247.
42. HOFFMAN, P. 1997. DNA visual and analytical data mining. *In* The Proceedings of the IEEE Visualization '97 (Phoenix, AZ), pp. 437–441.
43. HOFFMAN, P. & G. GRINSTEIN. 2000. Multidimensional information visualization for data mining with application for machine learning classifiers. *In* Information Visualization in Data Mining and Knowledge Discovery. Morgan Kaufmann. San Francisco.

Applications of Bioinformatics in Cancer Detection: A Lexicon of Bioinformatics Terms

ASAD UMAR

Division of Cancer Prevention, National Cancer Institute, Bethesda, Maryland, USA

ABSTRACT: This paper compiles a list of numerous bioinformatics terms for the Applications of Bioinformatics in Cancer Detection conference. It should be helpful as a lexicon for the volume as a whole.

KEYWORDS: bioinformatics; cancer; detection; prevention; technique

ALGORITHM

Algorithm is a procedure consisting of a sequence of algebraic formulas and/or logical steps to calculate or determine a given task. Alternatively, a computable set of steps to get a desired result or rules or a process, particularly in computer science, is considered algorithm. In medicine, it is a step-by-step process for reaching a diagnosis or ruling out specific diseases. Algorithm may be expressed as a flowchart in either sense. The word comes from the Persian author, Abu Ja'far Mohammed ibn Mûsâ al-Khowârizmî, who wrote a book with arithmetic rules dating from about 825 A.D. Greater efficiencies in algorithms, as well as improvements in computer hardware, have led to advances in computational biology.[1,2]

Algorithm development for bioinformatics applications combines mathematics, statistics, computer science, as well as software engineering to address the pressing issues of today's biotechnology and build a sound foundation for tomorrow's advances. Algorithms are required for dealing with the large amounts of data produced in sequencing projects, genomics, or proteomics. Moreover, they are crucial ingredients in making new experimental approaches feasible.

Genetic and Evolutionary Algorithms

Evolutionary algorithm incorporates aspects of natural selection or survival of the fittest and utilizes theory- and data-driven approaches.[3] With the advent of a large number of high-throughput multiplex techniques and their consistent and productive use in the field of cancer detection and cancer prevention, biomedical researchers need, first of all, the expertise to marry information technology to biology in a productive way.

Address for correspondence: Asad Umar, D.V.M., Ph.D., Division of Cancer Prevention, National Cancer Institute, 6130 Executive Boulevard, Bethesda, MD 20892-7317. Voice: 301-594-2684; fax: 301-435-6344.
asad.umar@nih.gov

Ann. N.Y. Acad. Sci. 1020: 263–276 (2004). © 2004 New York Academy of Sciences.
doi: 10.1196/annals.1310.021

It is clear from current publications in the arena of early detection of cancers and characterization of risk and response that new hardware and software will be needed, together with support and collaboration from experts in multiple allied fields. Inevitably, those needs will grow as biology moves increasingly from a bench-based to a computer-based science and as bioinformatics models replace increasingly more and more experiments and at the same time complement many others. This era brings us a new opportunity in the field of cancer prevention and early detection, where it seems that single researchers are increasingly being supplemented by inter-disciplinary teams that include biomedical researchers as well as statisticians and computer informatics experts to form complete bioinformatics teams. This calls for an urgent need for the fusion of biomedicine and informatics in a coherent fashion to fully utilize the promise of multiplexed data acquisition and analysis.

Genetic algorithm similarly refers to a computer simulation of Darwinian evolu-tion, where the outcome is "survival" of the fittest in terms of the data in a sample. For example, the genetic algorithm for proteomic patterns may start by randomly selecting many proteomic patterns within the training data for analysis. Each chosen pattern is eventually tested to see how well it can discriminate affected from unaffected in the training set, by cluster analysis. In the end, successful proteomic patterns are kept and recombined (also referred to as being "mated"), whereas futile patterns are discarded. Ultimately, a best pattern emerges after several successive iterations by the algorithm. This finely evolved proteomic pattern, which best segregates the training sets, is used to classify diagnostically unknown samples.

ARTIFICIAL NEURAL NETWORKS (ANNs)

ANN, also known as "neural network" or "neural net", is a network of many simple processors ("units" or "neurons"), each possibly having a (small amount of) local memory.[3] The units are connected by unidirectional communication channels ("connections"), which carry numeric (as opposed to symbolic) data. The units operate only on their local data and on the inputs they receive via the connections.

A neural network is a processing device, either an algorithm or actual hardware, whose design was inspired by the design and functioning of brains and components thereof. Most neural networks have some sort of "training" rule whereby the weights of connections are adjusted on the basis of presented patterns. In other words, neural networks "learn" from examples, just like as young kids learn to recognize the type of a dog from previous encounters with different dogs, and exhibit some structural capability for generalization.

The term "neural net" should logically—but in common usage never does—also include biological neural networks, whose elementary structures are far more complicated than the mathematical models used for ANNs.

BAYESIAN DECOMPOSITION

Bayesian algorithms are a variation of the maximum likelihood classifiers, based on the Bayes law of probability. The Bayesian classifier allows the application of a priori weighting factors, representing the probabilities that a given event will be assigned to each class. Originally developed for spectroscopic analysis, Bayesian decomposition includes two features that make it useful for microarray data analysis: the ability to assign genes to multiple coexpression groups and the ability to encode biological knowledge into the system.[4]

BIOINFORMATICS

Bioinformatics is a broad term that encompasses the application of computer technology to investigate biological processes from high-dimensional data generated from multiple sources. Bioinformatics research takes place in large part *in silico* and includes the development and testing of the software tools necessary to analyze the data as it is usually the creation of new knowledge from existing data.[5,6] The practice of bioinformatics can be considered as interplay between knowledge of empirically derived data, bioinformatics tools, and human decision making. Exactly which information and tools are to be accessed is dependent on the nature of the question of interest.

Bioinformatics is a conceptualizing biology in terms of molecules (in the sense of physical chemistry) and applying "informatics technique" (derived from disciplines such as applied computer science and statistics) to understand and organize the information associated with these molecules, on a large scale. In short, bioinformatics is a management information system for molecular biology and has many practical applications.

BIOPAX

A more recent effort to develop a standard exchange format for pathway data is BioPAX.[7] BioPAX is a community-based effort created to enable sharing of pathway information, such as signal transduction, metabolic, and gene regulatory pathways, using a standard data exchange format.

BIOPERL

Bioperl is a tool kit of perl modules useful in building bioinformatics solutions in perl. It is built in an object-oriented manner so that many modules depend on each other to achieve a task.[8] The collection of modules in the bioperl-live repository consists of the core of the functionality of bioperl.

BLACK-BOX MODELING

Black-box model is constructed entirely from data using little additional a priori knowledge. A nonlinear black-box structure for a dynamical system is a model structure that is prepared to describe virtually any nonlinear dynamics. Neural network black-box modeling is usually performed using nonlinear input-output models. During the past few years, the use of neural networks for the black-box modeling of nonlinear dynamical systems has been suggested. There has been considerable recent interest in this area with structures based on ANNs, as well as wavelet transform-based methods and models based on fuzzy sets and fuzzy rules.[9,10] The problem of designing a mathematical model of a process using only observed data has attracted much attention.

Gray-box modeling, on the other hand, takes into account certain prior knowledge of the modeled system to provide the black-box models with human-interpretable meaning. This is especially valuable whenever a knowledge-based model exists, but is not fully satisfactory and cannot be improved by further analysis. The gray-box modeling combines knowledge-based modeling, whereby mathematical equations are derived in order to describe a process, based on a physical (or chemical, biological, etc.) analysis, and black-box modeling, whereby a parameterized model is designed, whose parameters are estimated solely from measurements made on the process. Similarly, *white-box modeling* (fuzzy logic) approaches assume that everything about the system is known a priori, expressed either mathematically or verbally.

COMPUTER-AIDED DETECTION (CAD) AND COMPUTER-AIDED DIAGNOSIS (CADX)

The development of modern computerized schemes for detection and characterization of lesions in mostly (but not limited to) radiologic images that are based on computers and sophisticated algorithms defines a new era in the future medical practice.[11,12] Computer-aided detection and diagnosis (CAD/CADX) may be defined as a diagnosis made by a physician who takes into account the computer output as a second opinion. The purpose of CAD is to improve the diagnostic accuracy and the consistency of the radiologist's image interpretation.

CAD methods may provide research physicians with tools to obtain more accurate diagnoses for a number of cancers. Future knowledge-based CAD systems will provide detailed analysis of the related conditions of different organs, and diagnostic analysis of preoplastic and neoplastic lesions. These systems need to be improved by knowledge-based engineering, which is difficult to implement and requires model refinement and optimization based on a large database of cases. Research is needed to develop these methods rather than comparing prototype systems with current practices.

COMPUTER-AIDED MOLECULAR DESIGN (CAMD)

This involves all computer-assisted techniques used to discover, design, and optimize compounds with desired structure and properties, also known as molecular modeling or computational chemistry, and uses computers to analyze and model the physicochemical properties of a molecule. CAMD programs allow integrated molecular design to take drug discovery to a new level by using a more cross-functional team approach to drug research and development. Furthermore, they can also improve efficiency and conserve human and experimental resources by allowing researchers to consider and test fewer options.

COMPUTER-ASSISTED DRUG DESIGN (CADD)

This involves all computer-assisted techniques used to discover, design, and optimize biologically active compounds with a putative use as drugs. Software is being developed for lead optimization by considering both receptor binding and pharmacologically important properties. The GenMol program, for example, performs an extensive conformational search in a protein's binding site to find the optimal positioning of ligands. Large trial sets of ligands are automatically generated from a virtual library of more than 1000 compounds and each ligand is screened for desired druglike properties with the integrated software program. A scoring function is used to rate the binding affinity or activity for each trial ligand.

CANCER GENOME ANATOMY PROJECT (CGAP)

In 1996, the National Cancer Institute implemented the Cancer Genome Anatomy Project (CGAP) to accelerate the advances in cancer genomics.[13,14] The idea of the CGAP was built on the concept that molecular signatures are unique for cancer type and that each signature is the manifestation of the changes that occurred in the cellular genome. It is expected that new research strategies and approaches would initiate new technologies that would empower early detection, diagnosis, prevention, and treatment of cancer.

CATALONIA ON-LINE BREAST CANCER RISK ASSESSOR (COBRA)

COBRA is designed to aid radiologists in the interpretation of mammography to decide whether to perform a biopsy on a patient or not, while providing a human-friendly explanation of the underlying reasoning.[15] From a diagnostic point of view, the tool exhibits high performance measures (i.e., sensitivity, specificity, and positive predictive value). The on-line breast-cancer risk assessor provides rule-based explanations (based on fuzzy logic), allowing the radiologists to understand the suggested diagnostic whether they agree or not with it. Moreover, as it possesses an integrated base of real cases, this tool could be used together with the corresponding mammograms as a tutor to train radiology residents in diagnosing mammograms exhibiting breast diseases.

CLUSTER ANALYSIS

Cluster analysis (*hierarchical clustering* or *pattern clustering*) is a method of grouping or clustering gene expression or protein patterns that are similar or differ from each other. It may be unsupervised (with no a priori knowledge) or supervised, where a set of known "training" samples are used to segregate the data into two groups (or clusters): those containing samples from affected and unaffected individuals. The pattern of an unknown sample is diagnostically classified by its similarity to the diseased or unaffected clusters found in the training set.

DATA MINING

Data mining refers to the analysis and extraction of data from a database and may involve the use of tools that look for trends or anomalies without knowledge of the meaning. The new computational algorithms emerging in the data mining literature, in particular, the self-organizing map (SOM) and principal component analysis (PCA), offer health science and cancer researchers tools for analyzing large amounts of data.

DIAGRAMMATIC CELL LANGUAGE

Diagrammatic cell language (DAC) is a complete diagrammatic language for large-scale network visualization and simulation.[16] Using VisualCell, which is a tool for large-scale cellular network definition, visualization, and modeling in the proprietary Gene Network Sciences, DAC can describe biological computation rather precisely. This is usually achieved by using DAC's modular, scalable, and graphical language, and biologists can often describe biological computation in a mathematically precise way.

EARLY CANCER DETECTION

Early cancer detection represents a multidisciplinary approach to recognizing symptoms, performing self-exams, getting regular checkups/screenings, surveillance, and detection of surrogate markers in the blood (e.g., PSA, CA-125, etc.). With the advancement of technology in data mining and bioinformatics approaches, early detection of cancer and precancer is in a promising arena and this volume describes applications of bioinformatics in cancer detection.

FUZZY LOGIC

Fuzzy logic methodology refers to the simultaneous evolution of two or more species of logic with coupled fitness. Such coupled evolution favors the discovery of complex solutions whenever complex solutions are required. Whereas conventional logic is concerned with complete truth, fuzzy logic is extended to handle gray areas that include the concept of partial truth—truth values between "completely true" and "completely false".

When analyzing gene expression patterns or proteomic profiles, the answer is more than just simply present or not, but rather an infinite number of possibilities in between. For the purpose of early detection and cancer prevention, consider if a biomarker is present or absent in the cancer, or if one can use that as a surrogate (intermediate) biomarker of chemopreventive response that can be handled by conventional (Boolean) logic.

Fuzzy logic was introduced in the 1960s as a mean to model the uncertainty associated with language.[17,18] This involves that fuzzy logic should not be considered as a single theory, but rather the process of "fuzzification" should be considered as a continuous form rather than a specific theory. This concept has been extended to introduce fuzzy calculus, fuzzy mathematics, fuzzy differential equations, etc.

To date, fuzzy expert systems are the most common use of fuzzy logic. Fuzzy sets and logic must be viewed as a formal mathematical theory for the representation of uncertainty. Uncertainty is crucial for the management of real systems. They are used in biological and other wide-ranging fields, including the following:

- linear and nonlinear control,
- pattern recognition,
- operation research,
- data analysis.

GENE ONTOLOGY (GO)

The GO project is a collaborative effort to address the need for consistent descriptions of gene products in different databases.[19] Three structured, controlled vocabularies (ontologies) are being developed that describe gene products in terms of their associated biological processes, cellular components, and molecular functions in a species-independent manner.[19]

GENECARDS

GeneCards™ is a database of human genes, their products, and their involvement in diseases.[20] It offers concise information about the functions of all human genes that have an approved symbol, as well as selected others. As related terms, *GeneLoc* presents an integrated map for each human chromosome, based on data integrated by the GeneLoc algorithm, and GeneNotes™ describes expression profiles in healthy tissues.

GENOMICS

Genomics may be defined as the study of any (molecular) biology experiment taken to the whole genome scale ideally in a single experiment. Not including splice variants, it is estimated that human genome has between 30,000 and 40,000 genes, potentially encoding 40,000 different proteins. Examples of genomic experiments include genome sequencing or DNA microarray analysis of gene expression.

JAVA

Java technology is both a programming language and a selection of specialized platforms; hence, it is ideal as a cross-platform Internet tool. As such, it standardizes the development and deployment of the kind of secure, portable, reliable, and scalable applications required by the networked economy. The *Java programming language* lets one write powerful programs that run in the browser, from the desktop, on a server, or on a consumer device. Java programs are run on (interpreted by) another program called the *Java Virtual Machine* (Java VM). Rather than running directly on the native operating system, the program is interpreted by the Java VM for the native operating system. This means that any computer system with the Java VM installed can run a Java program regardless of the computer system on which the application was originally developed.

K-MEANS CLUSTERING

This non-hierarchical method initially takes the number of components of the population equal to the final required number of clusters. In this step itself, the final required number of clusters is chosen such that the points are mutually farthest apart. Next, it examines each component in the population and assigns it to one of the clusters depending on the minimum distance. The centroid's position is recalculated every time a component is added to the cluster and this continues until all the components are grouped into the final required number of clusters. K-means clustering minimizes the variability within each cluster. It partitions *n* genes into *k* clusters, where *k* has to be predetermined.

KOHONEN SELF-ORGANIZING MAPS (SOMs)

In some ways, this is similar to K-means in that a set number of cells are defined at the outset. SOM is a neural network approach to clustering using a one- or two-dimensional map. However, Kohonen SOM clustering not only groups data into clusters, but uses a two-dimensional representational map of the clusters to order them. It does this in such a way as to place adjacent to each other clusters that are most nearly alike. This can have advantages when associating results with classifications.

LASER-CAPTURED MICRODISSECTION (LCM)

LCM technology provides researchers with a means of isolating a specific population of cells from heterogeneous tissue specimens. Developed by Michael Emmert-Buck and colleagues at NCI/NIH, LCM is basically an inverted microscope fitted with a low-power near-infrared laser that provides enough energy to transiently melt thermoplastic film in a precise location, binding it to the targeted cells. After the cells have been selected, the film and adherent cells are removed, and protein or RNA is extracted.

LOCUSLINK

LocusLink provides a single query interface to curated sequence and descriptive information about genetic loci. It presents information on official nomenclature, aliases, sequence accessions, phenotypes, EC numbers, MIM numbers, UniGene clusters, homology, map locations, and related Web sites. Pathway databases provide a view of biology that is distinct from that offered by sequence, expression, or structure databases, or collections of encyclopedic gene/protein pages such as LocusLink.[21]

MACHINE LEARNING

The study of computer algorithms that improve automatically through experience is machine learning. Applications of machine learning range from data mining software that discovers general rules in large data sets to information filtering systems that automatically learn users' interests.

MICROARRAY DATA MANAGER (MADAM)

MADAM is a Java-based application designed to load and retrieve microarray data to and from a database that is also supplied with the software.[22] MADAM provides data entry forms, data report forms, and additional applications necessary to maintain microarray data for further analysis. MADAM often loads and retrieves microarray data to and from a database.

META-ANALYSIS

A meta-analysis is a statistical procedure for combining the results of a number of studies. Although meta-analysis is widely used in medicine today, a meta-analysis of a medical treatment was not published until 1955. In the 1970s, more sophisticated analytical techniques were introduced in educational research.[23–25] Because the results from different studies investigating different dependent variables are measured on different scales, the dependent variable in a meta-analysis is some standard measure of effect size, such as a standard score equivalent to a difference between means or an odds ratio.

A weakness of the method is that sources of bias are not controlled by the method. A good meta-analysis of badly designed studies will still result in bad statistics.

MULTIDIMENSIONAL SCALING (MDS)

MDS is a statistical technique often used in data visualization. It is a procedure for reducing the dimensionality of the data to produce lower-dimensional data suitable for graphing or 3D visualization from a high-dimensional data set, while preserving some of the most prominent "distance" relationships of the data set.

MULTIEXPERIMENT VIEWER (MEV)

This is a Java application designed to allow the analysis of microarray data to identify patterns of gene expression and differentially expressed genes. It provides a large number of different data mining tools.

MULTIVARIATE ANALYSIS

Multivariate analysis is concerned with the analysis of multiple measurements, made on one or several samples of individuals: for example, to measure length, width, and weight of a product.

NEURO-FUZZY LOGIC

The neuro-fuzzy algorithm is a supervised learning algorithm that develops fuzzy rules that can be modified by experts. As combinations of fuzzy rules give continuous output functions, these methods are best applied to modeling as opposed to classification problems.

ONCOMINE DATABASE

The Oncomine project developed by the Chinnaiyan Lab (University of Michigan, Ann Arbor, MI) is focused on using high-throughput genomic and proteomic technologies to analyze human disease[26] to curate publicly available cancer microarray studies and provide data mining tools to efficiently query genes and data sets of interest, as well as meta-analyze groups of studies. Oncomine is a bioinformatics infrastructure for the cancer biologist and incorporates links to several bioinformatics resources, including Unigene, Swissprot, Biocarta, HPRD, and KEGG, among others.

ORTHOLOGOUS PATHWAYS

This is a linked list of interconnected nodes and is represented usually in a two-dimensional format. While homologous pathways are defined as the pathway genes or proteins with good alignment, the orthologous pathways will represent genes and proteins performing the same function in different species.

PRINCIPAL COMPONENT ANALYSIS (PCA)

Here, the goal is the identification of key variables (principal components) that best explain the differences between observations. It is a method of reducing the dimensionality of data, by selecting the principal components that contain the majority of the variance.

PROTEIN LYSATE ARRAYS AND ANTIBODY ARRAYS

Protein lysate arrays are whole cell lysates that are placed in a low-density format to allow for the multiplex analysis of protein expression in multiple samples. Conversely, antibody arrays are made by depositing multiple antibodies onto a substrate, allowing the monitoring of expression levels for multiple proteins in a single sample.

PROTEOMIC FINGERPRINTING

A set of proteins gives a fingerprint that describes a discriminating pattern formed by a small key subset of proteins or peptides buried among the entire repertoire of thousands of proteins represented in the sample spectrum. This pattern of proteins can be from a traditional proteomic pattern such as a 2D gel pattern or from mass spectrometric patterns. The proteomic pattern of mass spectrometry like SELDI/MALDI-TOF is defined by peak amplitude values only at key mass/charge (m/z) positions along the spectrum horizontal axis.

PROTEOMICS

Alternative RNA splicing and posttranslational modification may lead to an increase from a genome size of 30,000–40,000 genes to approximately 2 million proteins or protein fragments. It is expected that the proteome is far more complex than the genome.

Proteomics can be considered a scientific discipline that evaluates proteins that are associated with a disease by means of their altered levels of expression between control and disease states. Proteome research permits the discovery of new protein markers for diagnostic purposes and of novel molecular targets for drug discovery.

SURFACE-ENHANCED LASER DESORPTION/IONIZATION (SELDI) AND MATRIX-ATTACHED LASER DESORPTION/IONIZATION TIME OF FLIGHT (MALDI-TOF)

Surface-enhanced laser desorption/ionization (SELDI) time of flight (TOF) and matrix-assisted laser desorption/ionization (MALDI) are mass spectrometric methods for profiling a population of proteins in a sample according to the size or mass (m) and electrical charge (z) of the individual proteins.[27,28] The results of such analysis from a protein-based sample are a spectrum of peaks. The position of an individual protein in the spectrum corresponds to its "time of flight" because the small proteins fly faster and the large proteins fly more slowly. The main difference between SELDI and MALDI is in the method of sample introduction into the mass spectrometer; however, SELDI can be considered a refinement of MALDI as the proteins are pre-selected from the sample by allowing them to bind to the treated surface of a metal bar, which is coated with a specific chemical that binds a subset of the proteins within the serum sample.

SINGLE NUCLEOTIDE POLYMORPHISMS (SNPs)

A single nucleotide polymorphism (SNP) is a small genetic change, or variation, that can occur within DNA sequence. The genetic code is specified by the four nucleotide "letters": A (adenine), C (cytosine), T (thymine), and G (guanine). SNP variation occurs when a single nucleotide, such as an A, replaces one of the other three nucleotide letters—C, G, or T. It is estimated that, on average, SNPs occur in the human population more than 1% of the time. SNPs may or may not lead to a change in the code of DNA that translates into proteins.

SUPPORT VECTOR MACHINES (SVMs)

SVMs are classification tools where previous knowledge of gene function can be used to identify functions of unknown genes. The concept of SVMs is based on strong mathematical functions like the statistical learning theory that results in simple, yet very powerful algorithms. SVMs are a new generation of learning systems that deliver the state-of-the-art performance in biological applications such as image classification, biosequence classification, analysis of DNA microarray data, sequence data, phylogenetic information, and promoter region information.

SUPERVISED CLUSTERING

Supervised classification, also known as *discriminant analysis* in statistics, requires the knowledge of the classes and seeks to find the rule that will best separate the groups based on the measured variables. The classes are predefined and the task is to understand the basis for the classification from a set of labeled objects. This information is then used to classify future observations. Unsupervised classification (see below), on the other hand, also known as *cluster analysis*, involves detecting previously unknown clusters in the data.

Hence, supervised clustering can be defined as grouping of variables (usually genes), controlled by information about the variables, that is, for example, the tumor types of the tissues. The objective here is to find differences in the measured variables among the classes. Differences here might be actual separations between classes on a variable or linear combination of variables. In order to perform this supervised clustering, first numerous candidate groups are generated by unsupervised hierarchical clustering. Then, the average expression profile of each cluster is considered as a potential input variable for a response model, and the few gene groups that contain the most useful information for tissue discrimination are identified. The second step makes the clustering supervised as the selection process relies on external information about the tissue types. The algorithm iteratively extracts the most discriminative cluster within the genes. The discriminative capability of a cluster specifies how much a cluster discriminates between sample classes, that is, how differently the genes in that cluster are expressed across sample classes.

SYSTEMS BIOLOGY MARKUP LANGUAGE (SBML)
AND CELL MARKUP LANGUAGE (CellML)

A machine-readable format for representing computational models is systems biology computational models. This format is intended for software tools, not for humans.[29] Although it is text-based and therefore readable, it is intended to be a tool-neutral exchange language for software applications in systems biology.

Systems Biology Markup Language (SBML) is an XML-based language for describing simulations in systems biology. The language is oriented towards representing biochemical networks common in research on a number of topics, including cell signaling pathways, metabolic pathways, biochemical reactions, gene regulation, and many others. Similarly, the *Cell Markup Language* (CellML) is an open standard based on the XML markup language. CellML is being developed to store and exchange computer-based biological models. CellML allows scientists to share models even if they are using different model-building software. It also enables them to reuse components from one model in another, thus accelerating model building.

UNSUPERVISED CLUSTERING

Unsupervised clustering aims at determining the optimum number of clusters without previous knowledge. Many classical clustering algorithms presume that the number of clusters is known. However, in practice, the number of clusters may not be known. This problem is called *unsupervised clustering*. A recent example of such an approach is based on *competitive agglomeration*, which starts by partitioning the data set into an overspecified number of clusters. Then, as the clustering progresses, adjacent clusters compete against each other for data points, and clusters that lose in the competition gradually become depleted and vanish.

REFERENCES

1. NIST. 2004. Dictionary of algorithms and data structures. http://www.nist.gov/dads/.
2. HYPERDICTIONARY. 2004. Algorithm: dictionary entry and meaning. http://www.hyper-dictionary.com/dictionary/algorithm/.
3. FOLDOC. 2004. Artifical neural network. http://foldoc.doc.ic.ac.uk/foldoc/foldoc.cgi?query=artificial+neural&network=search/.
4. BROOKS, S.P. 2003. Bayesian computation: a statistical revolution. Philos. Trans. Ser. A Math. Phys. Eng. Sci. **361**: 2681–2697.
5. YU, U. *et al.* 2004. Bioinformatics in the post-genome era. J. Biochem. Mol. Biol. **37**: 75–82.
6. BLUEGGEL, M., D. CHAMRAD & H.E. MEYER. 2004. Bioinformatics in proteomics. Curr. Pharm. Biotechnol. **5**: 79–88.
7. BIOPAX. 2004. BioPAX: biological pathways exchange. http://www.biopax.org/.
8. BIOPERL. 2004. Bioperl. http://bioperl.org/.
9. TU, J.V. 1996. Advantages and disadvantages of using artificial neural networks versus logistic regression for predicting medical outcomes. J. Clin. Epidemiol. **49**: 1225–1231.
10. GEERAERD, A.H. *et al.* 1998. Application of artificial neural networks as a non-linear modular modeling technique to describe bacterial growth in chilled food products. Int. J. Food Microbiol. **44**: 49–68.
11. MALICH, A. *et al.* 2001. Tumour detection rate of a new commercially available computer-aided detection system. Eur. Radiol. **11**: 2454–2459.
12. MICHENER, C.M. *et al.* 2002. Genomics and proteomics: application of novel technology to early detection and prevention of cancer. Cancer Detect. Prev. **26**: 249–255.
13. NIH. 2004. Cancer Genome Anatomy Project (CGAP). http://cgap.nci.nih.gov/.
14. BORNSTEIN, S.R., H.S. WILLENBERG & W.A. SCHERBAUM. 1998. Progress in molecular medicine: "laser capture microdissection". Med. Klin. (Munich) **93**: 739–743.
15. COBRA. 2004. Catalonia online breast cancer risk assessor (COBRA). http://lslwww.epfl.ch/~penha/catalonia.html/.
16. GNS. 2004. Diagrammatic cell language. http://www.gnsbiotech.com/.

17. ZADEH, L.A. 1965. Fuzzy sets. Information Control **8**: 338–353.
18. ZADEH, L.A. 1982. A note on prototype theory and fuzzy sets. Cognition **12**: 291–297.
19. GO. 2004. Gene ontology (GO) project. http://www.geneontology.org/.
20. GENECARDS. 2004. GeneCards. http://bioinfo.weizmann.ac.il/cards/.
21. NCBI. 2004. LocusLink. http://www.ncbi.nih.gov/LocusLink/.
22. TIGR. 2004. Microarray data manager. http://www.tigr.org/software/tm4/madam.html/.
23. SMITH, M.L. & G.V. GLASS. 1977. Meta-analysis of psychotherapy outcome studies. Am. Psychol. **32**: 752–760.
24. SPARLING, P.B. 1980. A meta-analysis of studies comparing maximal oxygen uptake in men and women. Res. Q. Exercise Sport **51**: 542–552.
25. POSAVAC, E.J. 1980. Evaluations of patient education programs: a meta-analysis. Eval. Health Prof. **3**: 47–62.
26. CHINNAIYAN, A. 2004. Oncomine project. http://www.oncomine.org/.
27. LENNON, J.J. & K.A. WALSH. 1999. Locating and identifying posttranslational modifications by in-source decay during MALDI-TOF mass spectrometry. Protein Sci. **8**: 2487–2493.
28. CAPUTO, E., R. MOHARRAM & B.M. MARTIN. 2003. Methods for on-chip protein analysis. Anal. Biochem. **321**: 116–124.
29. SBML. 2004. Systems biology markup language (SBML). http://www.sbml.org/.

Index of Contributors